HEALTH THROUGH OCCUPATION

Theory and Practice
in
Occupational Therapy

HEALTH THROUGH OCCUPATION

Theory and Practice in Occupational Therapy

GARY KIELHOFNER, M.A., DR. P.H., O.T.R.
DIRECTOR OF GRADUATE STUDIES AND ASSISTANT PROFESSOR
DEPARTMENT OF OCCUPATIONAL THERAPY
VIRGINIA COMMONWEALTH UNIVERSITY
RICHMOND, VIRGINIA

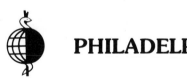

F. A. DAVIS COMPANY   PHILADELPHIA

Library of Congress Cataloging in Publication Data
Main entry under title:

Health through occupation.

    Includes bibliographical references and index.
    1. Occupational therapy. I. Kielhofner, Gary, 1949-
    [DNLM: 1. Occupational therapy. WB 555 H434]
RM735.H39 1983   615.8'515   82-18255
ISBN 0-8036-5317-4

For Harold and Luella, my parents,
for having taught me life's most
important lessons: to love deeply,
to work hard, and to play joyfully.

PREFACE

The reader will likely find this to be a different type of occupational therapy text than those to which he or she is accustomed. As an applied field, occupational therapy's literature focuses on the knowledge and techniques for therapy in a most practical way. For the most part, therapists encounter books that describe why and how to deliver occupational therapy services.

While this volume does not divorce itself from this central focus, it attempts to approach the issue from a more detached and global view. It is a contemplation of occupational therapy which seeks to discover in a fundamental sense what occupational therapy is all about, who it serves, why the service works, and what its place in society is. The reader is challenged to step back from the immediacy of teaching, learning about, or practicing occupational therapy, to reflect and to envision where the field originated and where it is headed.

It is my profound hope as editor and as a contributor that the issues, arguments, proposals, and challenges of this book will help to infuse occupational therapy with a growing sense of pride and purpose, that it will support efforts toward the refinement and betterment of the field's service, and perhaps more importantly, that it will help readers achieve a better sense of their identity as occupational therapists.

Despite the variety of contributors—a sociologist, physicians, and occupational therapists from different areas of clinical practice and education—the volume coheres around several themes. In order to orient readers to these themes, I would like to briefly comment on them.

The first theme is the recognition that occupational therapy has a mission and that it is neither so obscure nor so unimportant as we have sometimes believed. By exploring the history of the field, its place in current medicine, and its potentials in clinical practice, we assert that the maintenance and restoration of human meaning and function by means of occupation is the singular purpose of occupational therapy, and we conclude that it is a necessary and noble mission whose importance will grow in coming decades. We believe strongly that occupational therapy works and that it is a necessary service for patients; our discussions of its knowledge, its relevance to health, and its clinical properties reflect this conviction.

A second theme concerns what occupational therapists should know. Together we assert that occupational therapy must embrace science without sacrificing scholarship, humanism, and holistic perspective, and we call for an organization of occupational therapy knowledge around the central concern for occupation in human life. Its understanding of the occupational nature of humans and of occupational dysfunction, in concert with its expert ability to use occupation as a health-giving measure, is proposed as the essence of the field's knowledge. It is further noted that this constitutes a large and challenging body of information which must be developed and refined through *both* scholarly activity and conventional science. The latter refers to the methods of empirical inquiry that brought first the physical sciences and, more recently, the biological, psychological and social sciences to maturity. Science is recognized as an indispensable method for refining occupational therapy knowledge. At the same time, we argue that science, as we know it today, is only part of a larger enterprise that has advanced human values, knowledge, and technology. The broader intellectual activity is scholarship. It is the contemplative, rational, intuitive, and systematic manipulation of ideas, experiences, and facts. In this book we employ a number of scholarly modes in our examination of occupational therapy. We seek to penetrate and illuminate occupational therapy in new ways. Our scholarly presentation is intended to augment a process of extending the breadth and depth of the field while maintaining its coherence. Since our purpose is large, we have not achieved all we would like to, but the volume should help to point the way for further efforts.

A third theme recognizes that occupational therapy exists in a rapidly changing world. The transformation of society, of science and scholarship, and of the health care system in the coming years, places a complex set of demands on the field; we have attempted to identify what they are and how they might be met. It is argued that occupational therapy exists in and is influenced by a rapidly changing cultural and intellectual climate. The mechanistic mental models that have dominated both science and popular thought for several hundred years are now slowly making way for a new science and a new world view that recognizes wholeness, that acknowledges the importance of ends over means, of values over efficiency, and that provides new tools for thinking that will revolutionize human knowledge and technology. This volume reflects an attempt to keep occupational therapy abreast of these sweeping changes. Further, several discussions give the reader an opportunity to gaze into the future and to visualize both a changed world and a changed occupational therapy playing a vital role in the world.

A fourth theme is our proposal that the efforts of occupational therapy have value only in terms of what they do for clients and patients. This volume argues on behalf of the patients and clients and their unique *experiences and perspectives* as the beginning and end of therapy. Contributors pursue the theme that the patient or client's experience as he or she behaves in therapy and in daily life is the ultimate criteria, the ultimate goal of therapy. Several chapters bring greater appreciation of this aspect of occupational therapy as the summit of the field's knowledge for practice, exploring it in some detail. It is articulated in several ways. First, there is discussion of what "meaningful activity" is about. This is occupational therapy's most important, yet least explored element. Second, the themes of competence, independence, and control are examined. Occupational therapy processes and their relation to these goals for patients and clients are explored. It is proposed that the field, along with most of health care, has fallen short of fully addressing them. Thus, new directions, orientations, and principles are offered.

The fifth theme is that of unity. There is a call for greater coherence in occupational therapy. As noted above, it is proposed that the field rally its efforts around the study of occupation and its health-giving potential, and that it identify its service with the use of occupation as therapy. Some will see this argument as confining and as setting arbitrary boundaries on occupational therapy, while others may wonder about the room for necessary diversity and individual creativity. To such persons we offer the argument that the practitioner with a clear and confident sense of his or her professional identity, mission, and skills is best suited to branch out and create a diverse practice. Without the original unifying and supporting perspective, the individual is sentenced to search haphazardly, if not frantically, for both a professional sense of self and an individual expression of personal effort. My experience confirms for me that the possession of a strong and unified ideological foundation is the best and most comfortable foundation from which to express diversity in one's personal professional practice. And this conviction resounds through the volume.

A final, recurring theme is occupational therapy's relationship to medicine. The book chronicles occupational therapy's emergence from both ancient and more recent medical institutions. And it ponders future relationships with the ideas and work of medicine. There is a clear message that occupational therapy must emancipate itself from an intellectual and operational symbiosis with mainstream medicine and relate itself to the larger issue of health and health care. At the same time there is a recognition that important ties will continue to exist between occupational therapy and medicine. The reader will find that the book offers many perspectives on this issue, which should begin to pave the way for occupational therapy's consideration of how it will exist autonomously, rather than as a part of the retinue of traditional medicine.

The first part of *Health Through Occupation* is devoted to identifying issues, content, and processes relevant to organizing knowledge for the broad commitment of the field to human occupation as a health concern. A number of important themes, including the history of the field, its diversion from original aims and purposes, the interdisciplinary process, and general systems theory are discussed in depth. This section is an overview of the current strengths, weaknesses, needs, and goals for knowledge in occupational therapy.

The second part of the book examines occupational therapy's relationship to the larger health care system, to society, and to the rapid changes occurring in both. The relevance of themes identified in the first section to the real world which confronts occupational therapy are explored. The underlying theme is that occupational therapy can successfully survive the turbulent times of the present and future if it is sufficiently centered on a unifying theory that defines, explains, and directs practice, and that orients the field to a specific human need for occupation and its changing manifestations and disruptions.

The final section of the book is devoted to illustrating the process of operationalizing theoretical knowledge in clinical practice. These chapters introduce some new orientations for clinical service, offer ways of organizing practice to reflect theory, and present a broader grasp of what it means to have a humanistic service.

I do not anticipate that the reader will find this an easy volume. In some cases there will be a need to struggle with an usual vocabulary, different modes of conceptualizing, and novel ideas. As editor I hoped to achieve a balance between easy readability and each chapter's faithful and accurate rendition of theories, concepts, and arguments. I have tough-minded faith in the ability and willingness of therapists and students to struggle with important ideas that require substantial cerebral effort. Further, I believe such willingness is necessary if we are to survive as a profession. In a world of rapidly expanding knowledge that grows in volume and sophistication, we must as a group of educators, students, practitioners, and researchers become literate in the ways of the world's best thinkers. This volume strives toward this end. Thus, it is my ardent hope that readers will find the contents as exciting and uplifting as they are exacting. Writing this book was for all of us both a struggle and a growing process. If the reader shares some small part of our experience, our efforts will have served their purpose.

Gary Kielhofner

FOREWORD

At last! A textbook on occupational therapy that is conceptually whole and that shows the interrelatedness of the components of this practice-minded profession. This book offers a vote of confidence both for the current knowledge in the field and for the rapidly developing potential of occupational therapy. The knowledge base required for practice and research in occupational therapy is still in an early stage of development. It will continue to be developed through practice and research, while educational processes will continue to refine knowledge and transmit it through new modes which further stimulate practitioners and researchers. This volume provides a vital link in the continuum of practice, education, and research.

Historically, occupational therapists have been service-oriented, dedicated to providing help in areas fundamental to humans' self-esteem, sense of personal worth, and roles as achievers and doers. This dedication reflected an identification on the part of the therapist with the same basic needs, and thus the profession grew from an intuitive recognition of principles now encompassed in the occupational behavior model. Early writers recognized these principles, but they were never organized into a conceptual whole.

Slowly but surely during the past few decades occupational therapists have been solving problems, identifying unknowns, trying out new ideas, and refining their practice while adding to the accumulated wisdom. As a result, the field now has a respectable body of knowledge around which to cohere and from which carefully documented rationales for therapeutic intervention may be developed. The special contribution of this book is the coherent framework it provides for integrating knowledge as well as looking at the history of occupational therapy, its accomplishments, its beliefs, and its potential. From such a compilation, movement towards true professionalism may proceed.

In the same sense that occupational therapy is holistically concerned with the disabled person, this book is devoted to an examination of the full range of knowledge that has accrued through practice and research relative to the field of occupational therapy.

Health Through Occupation will be of value to the clinician in several important ways. The history of occupation therapy suggests neglected technology, media that have exciting potential in today's world. It also explains *why* occupation works—an explanation too often unavailable in therapists' minds as they struggle to justify the use of a seemingly mundane task, craft, or game.

This book provides a consistent frame of reference from which to examine the logic of one's own clinical practice, thus permitting the development of a justifiable sequence of professional actions, including evaluation, treatment goals, selection of methods, and predictable outcomes.

To the vast majority of occupational therapists, the clinic or similar therapeutic environments are everyday facts of life. Concerns about how to help persons who are temporarily or permanently dysfunctional dominate most of one's professional thinking. Solutions to these problems are sought in imaginative ways. The clinician will find Part III of this book helpful in the development of such solutions. Each chapter discusses, from a different perspective, how knowledge about human occupation can be used to develop creative solutions to dysfunctional states presented by patients. If one's primary role is one of consultant or program supervisor, the issues presented in Part II will be of considerable interest. This section deals with the significance of the context of treatment, the value systems of society which impinge upon the practice of helping profession.

Persons with academic commitments bear a heavy share of responsibility for the continuous development of a practice profession. They are charged with the protection of the future, as they provide both the knowledge base for practice and an enlightening professional socialization process. In addition, educators must bear the responsibility for integrating that which is newly discovered in the field with already established concepts and methods. This is made infinitely easier by a coherent frame of reference, so that all the pieces of the whole may be matched and resynthesized into a workable body of knowledge. Such is the contribution of this book to the educators in occupational therapy.

Health Through Occupation provides a framework for teaching the whole—a congruent, integrated body of knowledge which may provide both the questions and some of the answers for practice and research in occupational therapy. It will serve as a guide for the planning and development of curricula by identifying those interdisciplinary studies that should *precede* and those that must *be integrated with* the study of occupational therapy per se.

In the finest educational tradition, Chapter 3 identifies the necessary relationship between acquiring professional knowledge and skills and those processes of critical thinking and scholarly inquiry that lead to development of reasoned clinical judgement. Educators may find it useful to work back and forth between Chapter 3 and other chapters in Part I; this will permit an examination of current curricula, while identifying components, sequences, and teaching strategies that may be combined to offer the most challenging style of professional education. Chapter 4 is particularly useful in this regard, as it presents the rules for interdisciplinary scholarship, demonstrating the process by borrowing concepts from other fields and using them to develop a definition of occupational therapy. Through challenge comes critical thinking; through critical thinking are developed the tenets of a profession. In thinking through the issues presented in Chapter 5, educators may find reassurance that both the humanistic and the technologic aspects of the field can be taught through careful scholarship and reasoned critique.

The whole of Part II is well suited to serve as the basis for courses about the health care delivery system, for examining the relationships between occupational therapy and society, medicine, and the consumer movement.

Health Through Occupation has rich offerings for the student. It provides a perspective on the profession by making meaningful the historical development of occupational therapy. In the process of identifying the foundational beliefs of the field, it leads one towards a stronger identification with the values of occupational therapy. Incorporation of values strengthens one's professional identity and leads to further seeking of knowledge and skill.

Part I helps to identify the relevance of occupational therapy to concepts borrowed from other disciplines; it suggests ways in which these concepts may enhance the study of human occupation. It may also suggest some important areas of study for graduate work or for a significant research contribution to the study of human occupation.

To complement more technical readings, Part III examines clinical problems in a different way. It provides an excellent basis for re-examination of the concepts and processes used in activity analysis.

An important function of the book is to heighten one's awareness of the critical relationship between theory and practice and to provide guidance in the pursuit of practical knowledge which has been solidly grounded conceptually. Closely related are the ways in which a professional thinks: How are the links made between theory and practice? Through problem identification, followed by the pursuit of observation, documentation, and analysis of problematic situations until understanding has been achieved. Then, the posing of alternate solutions, each supported from the theory base: intervention, based on reasoned principles, may then follow, together with a new cycle of observation. Thus, practice, education, and research unite to contribute new units of knowledge for the profession.

Critical thinking and problem solving are the basis for both creative practice and research; these skills must be developed as an integral part of the learning process. In any profession, at any given time, there are concepts and facts that have been verified through scholarly study; there are also established "truths" developed through tradition and practice. These truths must be tested in the context of theory and integrated or discarded according to their relevance for the whole. Conceptual gaps must be identified through the practice of the field, and new principles established to provide rational explanation for practice. Both the methods of science and those of the more classic studies in the humanities—often referred to as "scholarship"—will be required to develop and test the knowledge base of occupational therapy.

Health Through Occupation provides a framework through which the profession of occupational therapy may examine its practice, its ideals, and its principles. As you read, rise to the challenges set forth herein; you and your profession will be rewarded and enhanced.

Nedra P. Gillette, M. Ed., O.T.R., F.A.O.T.A.

FOREWORD

The dual themes of this book are sounded clearly and early on. First, occupational therapy has lost the credibility of its earliest premises and promise, and must reorganize professional knowledge for practice around a unified and renewed commitment to the founders' belief in occupation as a central determinant of health. Second, a scientific revolution in both principles and practice is required to resolve the crisis state of occupational therapy at this crossroads of development.

Changes in the health care system, particularly the technologic drive in medicine that characterized science at mid-century, are identified as external forces responsible for the profession's loss of credibility. Internal responses by occupational therapy include such developments as the growth of specialization and the urge toward a more scientific explanation of the discipline. Both gain attribution as causes leading to fragmentation and a loss of identification with unifying principles of the profession.

Analaysis of these diverting developments in the evolution of occupational therapy knowledge and practice has led the editor and principal author to postulate a scientific revolution as essential to reorganizing knowledge for practice. Such reorganization is required to provide coherence in the range of information and technology that characterizes current practice, and to redirect a straight-line future development anchored in the field's basic traditions and principles. The method proposed for accomplishing reorganization is the paradigm which, he argues, is an increasingly used means of defining and expressing the knowledge related status and activities of a field.

Health Through Occupation starts with a probing of history for the core and rationale of occupational therapy. The depth of historical research behind it is evident in the many quotations from our professional pioneers. The analytic skills employed take this section beyond a chronologic history to an examination of repeated themes, distilling from them the values in which our past is cloaked. Directions of change in both principles and practices of occupational therapy are identified at this beginning stage. Commentary on the influence these changes have exerted on development of the profession over its 65-year life to date is also offered.

This chapter makes good reading for occupational therapists who appreciate the impact of history and value its spirit as well as its substance. It will be exciting to the believer in the field's basic professional tenets and to the reader-convert to the case it provides for renewed commitment to them. For professionals who "have lost confidence and enthusiasm for occupational therapy," it may provide reassurance in the validity of their convictions that the noble philosophies conceived by the pioneers of their profession have enduring values. To the agnostic who sees further strengthening of the profession, if not survival itself, requiring exclusive use of reductionist scientific methods of investigation, it should be provocative.

Inferences drawn from this ringing recall to the beliefs of the founders provide the backdrop for the second chapter. In his "Paradigm for Practice," Kielhofner responds to the challenge laid down in the opening chapter. Newcomers to the concept of paradigm in the framework of systems theory may find the chapter technical and demanding. However, understanding is facilitated by its clear logic, precise sequencing, and articulate expression.

Remaining space will therefore be used for comments on implications of this book for the profession. To do so, I shall address both issues raised by authors and questions the reader may wish to probe beyond the scope of this volume. Those selected will be discussed in the approximate order in which they are presented in the book; a fortuitous coincidence is that their order accords with their importance in this commentator's view.

The rationale and applicability of the Kuhnian concept of paradigm to accomplish resolution of the crisis-defined state in occupational therapy is introduced in the first few pages and examined in detail in subsequent chapters. With lucid and persuasive citations, support is developed for acceptance of the author's proposals as feasible routes to the resolution of conflicting viewpoints within the field and to achieve unity under a single paradigm. The period between first publication of several papers on occupational behavior and general systems theories and this expanded and integrated revisit to those concepts is approximately five years and has produced a response in support of parts of the paradigm process, while proposing alternative approaches to solving others.* The contribution of this second view is its explication of a contrasting methodology and application to the field for comparison with the model proposed in *Health Through Occupation*.

A second issue is found in arguments supporting return to the holistic or occupational paradigm over the reductionist paradigm of inner mechanisms. These are forceful in beginning chapters, reflecting the authors' belief in their verity and their strong commitment to winning the field's acceptance of this view. They are presented as competing propositions, with censure of the reductionist scientific method shown as leading to fragmentation and disunity in occupational therapy. Alternately, however, the new paradigm is designed to accommodate opposing views rather than to ignore or replace them. Reassurance to professionals who may feel that exact science in occupational therapy is

---

*The Occupational Journal of Research, 1:115, 1981.

not valued is found at the outset in the stated imperative to add the technology of the mechanistic paradigm, as well as knowledge not available earlier, to the new paradigm. Reinforcing these initial pledges are the beliefs of other authors that the scientific investigation and scholarly study of occupation are as essential as they are compatible and perhaps are best viewed as "two terrains in the geography of one profession."

The third issue revolves around problems in the reorganization of knowledge for practice, including those identified by the authors and related questions that may be inferred by readers. In the former category is the negotiation that will be required between specialty areas of practice and also in integrating differentiated functions in the curative, restorative, preventive, and health promotion sectors to which occupational therapists provide service. Although a detailed development of how occupational therapy knowledge might be organized to support a unified paradigm for practice is presented, it is qualified "as a first attempt to illuminate the range and nature of what will be required." The impact of this statement is more fully realized when the relatively small amount of knowledge already available for reorganization is compared with the far greater amount yet to be ordered and organized from our own and other disciplines. Thus, some readers may wish for more detailed answers and a more definitive statement of what is needed. Others will see the need for identification of a sufficient number of professionals who are committed to developing knowledge that has not previously been attempted and for which the field has limited resources. Readers may also wonder how occupational therapy educators will be involved in the process so that they may be more effective implementers of curriculum reorganization. Chapter 3 responds to this question.

The fourth and final issue to be discussed here concerns the use of varying terms to encompass intervention strategies of practice. This book firmly proposes *occupation* as the most suitable, descriptive, and unifying substitute for such formerly used terms as activity, purposeful activity, and functional activity. The authors identify a focus on *purposeful activity* as a force leading to the reductionist era and consequent loss of initial commitment to the more generic concepts of occupation. They also note that when the term *functional activity* replaced purposeful activity, human performance was made mechanistic. In "Occupation as the Common Core of Occupational Therapy"* it was resolved "that there be universal acceptance and implementation of the common core of occupational therapy as the active participation of the patient/client in occupation for purposes of improving performance. . . ." Congruence of the rationale for standard terminology as explored in this book with official policy of the national professional organization supports the broader term, occupation, for both internal unity and extra-professional delineation of core concepts and the nature of practice.

These and other issues and questions merit serious study. That they will stimulate a great deal of dialogue as clinicians, educators, theorists, and students continue to debate them seems certain. They must also find resolution through the involvement of professional historians, philosophers, and scholars to replace our earlier dependence on organization-authored white papers and position statements. Effective as these have been in the developmental phases of the profession, it is books of the character and quality of *Health Through Occupation* that develop principles which subsequently provide the basis for

---

*Resolution 532-79, *American Journal of Occupational Therapy,* 12:785, 1979.

policies formulated by the national professional organization for its support and promotion. Such a progression will lead the way toward greater self reliance of the individual professional, as well as increased maturity of the association of professionals.

The grand scheme of this book will seem unrealistically ambitious and wide ranging to some, but others may feel as I do, that it achieves a considerable degree of success. It is a tribute to Mary Reilly's influence on the development of occupational therapy. With this ideological updating of history and proposed plan for strengthening therapy around the theme of occupation, the authors have effectively restated and added credence to Reilly's 1962 challenge that "Occupational Therapy Can Be One of the Great Ideas of Twentieth Century Medicine." In Kielhofner's and Burke's words at the conclusion of Chapter 1, "We know it could. Furthermore, we think it will."

My faith in the future of occupational therapy strongly supports the goals and ideals of these statements and, in my opinion, *Health Through Occupation* makes a scholarly and significant contribution toward their realization. There is a splendid reach in this book to a timely and compelling invocation for our concerted attention to professional self-direction. The work is therefore highly recommended for critical study and response by all occupational therapists who will be active participants in the future promise of their profession.

Wilma L. West, M.A., O.T.R.

ACKNOWLEDGEMENTS

As editor of this volume I feel especially privileged. To work on a project which attempts to make important statements about one's field with colleagues whom I respect and admire, has been the high point of my professional career.

Anyone who puts together a book is indebted to a large number of individuals. While it is not possible to acknowledge everyone who gave input, I will mention here those whose support and efforts were most important to this project. My wife, Nancy, had never-ending faith in me and tolerated my frantic periods and long hours of writing and editing; she shared deeply in all that went into the emotional side of this volume. Mary Reilly has given me a set of ideas to believe in and sound concepts to write about. I can do very little in occupational therapy which is not profoundly influenced by her writing, teaching, and personal advice and guidance. I am especially indebted to the contributors whose hard work and substantial expertise have made this volume possible. They can tell stories about how onerous I made the task of writing for this book as I sought to maintain the highest standards. Additionally, many contributors had important roles in the development of this volume. Patti Maurer, my department chairperson, supports and encourages the kind of scholarly effort which makes writing a work like this possible. Roann Barris, Charles Christiansen, Nedra Gillette, Janet Watts, and Wilma West read and made extensive and invaluable comments that assisted substantially in the development of the book. My students, Jill Leffler, Larry Maddy, Janet Magruder, Karen Mock and Mary Oley made helpful comments and assisted in phases of manuscript development. Marian Kavanagh, student and colleague, volunteered untold hours and much expertise to reviewing, criticizing, and correcting the manuscript and galleys. June Brown often worked above and beyond the call of a secretary's duty to prepare portions of the manuscript. I am indebted to Bob Martone, Dick Heffron, and Wendy Bahnsen at F.A. Davis for their faith in this project and their efforts toward making this a quality volume. The American Journal of Occupational Therapy which held copyright on portions of chapters graciously granted permission to reprint material.

Gary Kielhofner
Richmond, Virginia
August, 1982

CONTRIBUTORS

ROANN BARRIS, M.S., ED.D., O.T.R.
Assistant Professor
Department of Occupational Therapy
Virginia Commonwealth University
Richmond, Virginia

JANICE POSATERY BURKE, M.A., O.T.R.
Director of Training in Occupational Therapy
University Affiliated Program, Children's Hospital
Los Angeles, California

CYNTHIA COOPER, M.F.A., M.A., O.T.R.
Director
Hand Rehabilitation Center of Lakewood
Lakewood, California

H. TRISTRAM ENGELHARDT, JR., PH.D., M.D.
Rosemary Kennedy Professor of the Philosophy of Medicine
Center for Bioethics, Kennedy Institute of Ethics
Georgetown University
Washington, D.C.

GAIL S. FIDLER, O.T.R.
Rehabilitation Consultant
New Jersey State Division of Mental Health Hospitals
Consultant, Department of Occupational Therapy
New York University
New York

JAY W. FIDLER, M.D.
Private Practice in Psychiatry

NEDRA P. GILLETTE, M.ED., O.T.R., F.A.O.T.A.
Director of Research
American Occupational Therapy Foundation
Rockville, Maryland

DAVID A. GOODE, PH.D.
Assistant Professor
Department of Sociology and Anthropology
Wilkes College
Wilkes Barre, Pennsylvania

GARY KIELHOFNER, M.A., DR. P.H., O.T.R.
Director of Graduate Studies and Assistant Professor
Department of Occupational Therapy
Virginia Commonwealth University
Richmond, Virginia

JERRY A. JOHNSON, M.B.A., ED.D., O.T.R.
Professor and Elias Michael Director
Program in Occupational Therapy
Washington University
St. Louis, Missouri

WENDY MACK, M.A. (CAND.), O.T.R.
Occupational Therapist
Speech and Language Development Center
Buena Park, California

ZOE MAILLOUX, M.A., O.T.R.
Instructor
Department of Occupational Therapy
University of Southern California
Los Angeles, California

SHAWN MIYAKE, M.A., O.T.R.
Senior Occupational Therapist
Ventura County Mental Health
Oxnard, California

JOAN C. ROGERS, M.A., PH.D., O.T.R.
Associate Professor
Department of Occupational Therapy
University of North Carolina, Chapel Hill
Chapel Hill, North Carolina

GERALD W. SHAROTT, M.A., O.T.R.
Instructor
Department of Occupational Therapy
University of Southern California
Los Angeles, California

WILMA L. WEST, M.A., O.T.R.
President Emeritus
American Occupational Therapy Foundation
Rockville, Maryland

ELIZABETH J. YERXA, ED.D., O.T.R.
Chairperson and Professor
Department of Occupational Therapy
University of Southern California
Los Angeles, California

CONTENTS

PART 1

WHAT THE PRACTITIONER MUST KNOW: THE KNOWLEDGE BASE OF OCCUPATIONAL THERAPY

CHAPTER 1

THE EVOLUTION OF KNOWLEDGE AND PRACTICE IN OCCUPATIONAL THERAPY: PAST, PRESENT AND FUTURE*

Gary Kielhofner
Janice Posatery Burke

EDITOR'S INTRODUCTION

Many writers today agree that mental health requires a good sense of personal history. It is not far fetched to extrapolate that the "mental health" of the professional is abetted by an appreciation of the history of the profession. Occupational therapy's history is a singularly exciting one, full of interesting personalities and dramatic changes. This chapter aims to inform the occupational therapist and the occupational therapy student about the rich heritage of the field. The chapter attempts to preserve this element of the field's history while also providing a scholarly approach to understanding change in the field. The reader may find the concern with the concept of paradigm challenging, but it is important for several reasons to become familiar with this theme. An understanding of paradigm enriches appreciation of what is really taking place as a field develops and changes, making its history more meaningful to those who comprehend the theoretical framework used for historical analysis. The theme of paradigm is an especially fertile one which the reader is likely to encounter with growing frequency in the literature of many fields. For readers not already familiar with the concept of paradigm, this chapter will serve as an introduction to the idea. In addition, the concept of paradigm appears throughout this volume as both a latent and explicit theme. Getting a good sense of it at the outset will facilitate reading subsequent sections.

While the chapter provides detailed articulation of the concept, the reader might find it helpful to think of the paradigm as the world view which characterizes a group. Just as we acquire ways of thinking and attitudes from our immediate experiences, scientists acquire

---

*An abbreviated version of this paper originally appeared in the *American Journal of Occupational Therapy*, 31: 675, 1977.

perspectives for doing their work from the socializing experiences of education and practical training. For the occupational therapist the paradigm comprises the commonsense and know-how accumulated through education, fieldwork, and early work experiences. As noted above, the chapter attempts to preserve many of the qualitative features of the field's history, and for this reason it is lengthy and often detailed in its descriptions of concepts, viewpoints, and practice techniques. To retain a picture of the historical process, the reader may find it helpful to refer to the diagrams that summarize sections and portray changes as they occur at a macro level. The summary and conclusion will also give a sense of how the description will proceed and the story it will tell.

The thrust of the chapter is thus to identify dramatic and consequential shifts which took place in the underlying paradigm of the field. The reader may be surprised to find that the story is not entirely one of progress or advancement of ideas and techniques. Part of the work of this history is to reveal fertile ideas which were not fully developed and which have grown dormant over the years. Many of these concepts will reappear in later chapters where they are updated for current practice.

Because Chapter 1 unearths some important but forgotten concepts and techniques, it should also be a valuable stimulus to the clinician. One cannot read the early literature of the field without noting that many of today's most burning clinical issues were addressed with great acumen and seeing that the resultant solutions were lost along the way. Thus, the history should be suggestive for practice.

The reader may also find that the chapter provides a means of understanding where practice techniques and bodies of knowledge have come from. It sheds new light on mysteries such as the jack-of-all trades nature of occupational therapy, the importance of purposeful activity as a central force of the field's heritage, and the ubiquitous lack of identity among occupational therapists. Students generally find the history a helpful way of making sense of the wide range of facts they must learn as part of their training. Since the field is a dynamic and changing medium, the history provides the best possible definition of occupational therapy—not only what it is, but what it has been in the past and where it seems to be headed.

GK

All probably agree that each occupational therapy generation seemingly acquires a sense of self-sufficiency. It is true that we of the present occupy the positions that once were filled by others.

It is, however, of great importance that we realize we are influenced by those who came before us more than we can truly know. Who they were and what they did has immeasurable bearing upon what we are and what we do. No generation is capable of isolating itself from its past. The past, plus what we are and what we do, greatly assists in fashioning our future. (Bing, Occupational Therapy Revisited: A Paraphrastic Journey)

The history of occupational therapy as an organized discipline is a relatively short one. After several years of intense interest and application of the principles of using occupation as therapy, a national association for the promotion of occupational therapy was formed in 1917. When the field established its first journal in 1922, several books on occupational therapy had already been written. Formal education of occupational therapists was initiated at this time. These activities signaled the beginnings of a new field which has since rapidly expanded into a multifaceted profession.

Through its sometimes exponential growth and change in knowledge and practice, occupational therapy has arrived at what appears to be a critical juncture in its development. Surviving its own internal metamorphosis and holding its own in a turbulent and often unpredictable health care system are current challenges to the ingenuity of the profession. Underlying and augmenting the uncertainty of the future are the absence of a unifying theoretical basis for occupational therapy,[60,89,159] a concomitant lack of identity in the field's clinical service and among occupational therapists,[44,146] and the dilemma of maintaining cohesiveness while allowing specialization in practice.[72,95] Each of these, separately and in combination, bear on the viability of the field, its service and its survival as a single profession. The consequences of the current situation are felt by therapists who cannot define their service or articulate its basic worth, by students lost in the seemingly unconnected bodies of knowledge and practice techniques that must be assimilated, and by educators whose curriculum is long on content but short on integration.

Our thesis is that the circumstances which confront occupational therapy are not unique, nor are they signs of a hopeless situation. Rather, they represent the underlying dynamics that characterize any discipline as it seeks to survive, collect, and refine knowledge, and develop a service valuable to society. Further, this process is fundamentally socio-historical, and understanding it will lead to the resolution of current problems and provide a means of charting directions for the future.

This chapter presents an historical analysis of the development of occupational therapy with an eye toward the problems of generic theory, the identity of practice, and the need for unity among practitioners. Thus, the purpose of this account is to chronicle the emergence and shifts of ideas and applications that constitute the mainstream of occupational therapy theory and practice. Its goal is to identify the roots of the current situation in occupational therapy's evolution and to determine possible solutions to problems facing the field.

HISTORICAL METHOD

Historical research requires careful selection of the data, analysis, and synthesis that comprise an account.[73] The data for this study are the formal writings of the field. A wide array of books and journal articles from the turn of the century to the present are sources for this account, especially those writings which reflect theoretical knowledge and the organization and nature of practice. In addition to these primary sources we have consulted secondary analyses of occupational therapy's history, so as to build upon previous work.

GUIDING ASSUMPTIONS

All data analyses, especially qualitative historical analyses, are guided by assumptions which dictate the arrangement and interpretation of data and the conclusions drawn from such data. Thus, it is important to note the concepts which underlie the present analysis.

Major influences on this work are themes and concepts from the sociology of knowledge. This conceptual perspective argues that all organized human activities involve the maintenance, application, and revision of a local universe of knowledge.[16] Professions, cultures, craft guilds, organizations, and any organized collection of human beings engaging in coordinated and interactive lines of action share some universal information which defines, informs, and limits their actions and shapes the history of their collective enterprise. Science takes its place along with other human activities as a process of humans interacting in a common purpose.[28,173] That scientific knowledge is a socio-historical phenomenon subject to political forces, human bias and conviction, and upheaval has been most aptly documented in Thomas Kuhn's[97,98] extensive analysis of the physical sciences. His findings concerning scientific development have challenged traditional views and offered a new vision of what the development of knowledge entails. The most important of Kuhn's propositions are his concept of paradigm and his explanation of knowledge development as a revolutionary process. Both are interrelated; however, the concept of paradigm facilitates an understanding of what he means by revolution in science.

The paradigm is a consensus-determined matrix of the most fundamental beliefs or assumptions of a field. It defines in the most fundamental sense what the practitioners will see when they view the world as scientists, and what kinds of puzzles they will seek to solve in their work. The paradigm includes the relevant universe of knowledge that serves as the interpretive framework for the group's activities. It is what they know and do.

In time the group may find reason to reject the guiding principles of the paradigm and to accept a new paradigm that completely restructures all previous knowledge. When the paradigm changes, the world that is "out there" to be studied and acted on changes; it becomes fundamentally different. Kuhn refers to this conceptual shift as the process of scientific revolution. When a science has given up one way of seeing the world for another, it has undergone revolution—a term intended to convey the drastic nature of the conceptual restructuring that takes place.

OCCUPATIONAL THERAPY: AN APPLIED SCIENCE

Before detailing how Kuhn's work was used for this analysis, some discussion of the relevance of his ideas to occupational therapy is needed. Kuhn's analysis of scientific revolutions was derived from his historical study of the physical sciences. It may be questioned whether similar circumstances and processes exist in other sciences, and especially in applied science such as occupational therapy. Kuhn's schema has been applied in sociology,[138] suggesting that it is relevant for the behavioral and social sciences. Filstead[63] used the concept of paradigm as a means of contrasting qualitative and quantitative methodologies in evaluation, suggesting its further relevance in areas besides pure science. Finally, use of Kuhn's concept of paradigm is found in analyses of medicine.[68] These examples suggest the appropriateness of a wide application of Kuhn's concepts.

Extension of Kuhn's work into applied arenas requires acknowledgment of the similarities and differences between purely scientific and applied disciplines. The former serve to justify the use of the paradigm concept and the latter to set boundaries on its applicability, or to point to ways in which the concept of paradigm must be altered for application to occupational therapy. In fields such as physics, from which Kuhn's historical analysis first yielded the concept of paradigm, the activities of practitioners center on the generation of knowledge; however, such fields are not devoid of application. What differentiates scientific fields from the applied fields such as occupational therapy is the primacy attached to knowledge generation in place of application. In applied fields the raison d'etre is application of knowledge; knowledge generation may be only a small part of the field's overall activities. In pure science a paradigm is a conceptual structuring of the world that sets the stage for inquiry. The paradigm defines the phenomena scientists seek to investigate and reveals practical puzzles which can be solved. In occupational therapy, the activity of practitioners is not primarily directed to the solution of a knowledge gap (scientific puzzle), but rather to the solution of practical problems that disabled human beings face. While the scientific puzzle demands explanation, the applied field's puzzle requires action. However, such action eventually demands explanation if the field is to provide a rationale for its puzzle-solving capacity. The occupational therapy paradigm would thus be the field's means of defining human beings and their problems in such a way as to provide a rationale for a course of action to solve them.

These differences are no doubt reflected in the organization of knowledge and action in purely scientific versus applied fields. The applicability of the concept of paradigm and scientific revolution rests in the degree to which a similar pattern of knowledge organization and change can be identified in occupational therapy's activities. To determine whether Kuhn's concepts of paradigm and scientific revolution were relevant we searched for the existence of appropriate fundamental conceptual gestalts and gestalt switches in the literature of occupational therapy. We attempted to locate and identify periods of consensus or disagreement with respect to fundamental views. We found that there are periods in the literature of occupational therapy that clearly demonstrate features similar to Kuhn's concepts of paradigm and scientific revolution. However, our use of Kuhn's schema should not be interpreted as a judgment that occupational therapy has achieved the status of a mature science comparable to physics or chemistry. Occupational therapy is an infant discipline compared to the centuries of development in the physical sciences. In the final analysis, the schema borrowed from Kuhn's work is useful because it casts the history of occupational therapy in a framework that is uniquely revealing and aids our attempt to explain changes that have taken place in the past 80 years. Thus, concepts of paradigm and scientific revolution are employed for their heuristic value in analyzing the evolutionary patterns of knowledge and practice in occupational therapy.

COMPONENTS OF A PARADIGM: APPLICATION TO OCCUPATIONAL THERAPY

Kuhn's writings[97,98] suggest that a paradigm can be identified in several features of a science. These were translated for use in occupational therapy (Fig. 1). During the stages of the paradigm, members of a discipline share a common set of perspectives or consensus concerning the basic nature of the phenomena they study. Since occupational therapy concerns itself with service to persons, its paradigm would be reflected in a consensus concerning the nature of human beings. Thus, the first question we investigated was whether and during what periods the literature reflected such a unified perspective.

Elements of Paradigm	Categorical Questions
View of the Phenomena:	Does the literature demonstrate a unified conceptualization of human beings?
Puzzles:	Does the literature identify clinical puzzles which flow naturally from a view of human beings?
Methods of Solution:	Are clinical methods and their rationales articulated in a fashion consistent with the previous two elements?
Goals:	Are goals for the field proposed? Do they reflect consistency with the previous elements?

FIGURE 1. Questions for historical analysis.

A consensus-determined view of a phenomenon offers scientists a common set of puzzles within which to conduct their investigative enterprises. This puzzle solving is called normal science.[97] While the puzzles of science are basically gaps in knowledge and phenomena requiring explanation, the puzzles of occupational therapy are patient problems. As noted above, occupational therapy puzzle solving requires change-making in human beings. In occupational therapy, the existence of a paradigm is reflected in clinical puzzles revealed by a unified view of human beings. That is, the medical or psychologic problems of people are translated into common puzzles for practice according to fundamental paradigmatic views of the field. Thus, our second question was whether common puzzles existed and reflected an articulated view of humans.

The paradigm not only reveals puzzles, but also suggests the methods of puzzle solution to be followed. The rationale for these methods is located in the accepted definition of the phenomena. Thus, our next question concerned the methodologies employed in patient care and, importantly, the rationale for the efficacy of those methods as reflected in the literature.

The paradigm also determines certain goals to be of paramount importance for the field. Such goals set direction for the group, specifying what kinds of efforts will be highly regarded and what kinds of achievements recognized.[98,138] In occupational therapy such goals are reflected in the kinds of effects occupational therapists wish to have on patients (i. e., clinical goals).

In summary, the elements of Kuhn's thesis concerning the features of a field in paradigm were examined to generate a set of categorical questions for study of the history of occupational therapy. By applying these questions to the literature year by year and asking whether the writings reflected consensus, it was possible to identify the paradigm status in occupational therapy writings of the past 80 years. By examining the literature of the field historically we identified periods reflecting the paradigm state and times during which no consensus existed in occupational therapy literature. This indicated that there was paradigm change and that an historical analysis should include explanation of these changes.

THE SCHEMA OF PARADIGM CHANGE

Kuhn's schema of paradigm change, scientific revolution, is a process of building, articulating, and eventually rejecting paradigms. The stages of this process are: (a) pre-paradigm, (b) paradigm, (c) crisis, and (d) return to paradigm. The pre-paradigm stage occurs (see Figure 2) prior to the formalization of a discipline. During this period, several schools of thought may have an interest in the same phenomenon, but define it differently and propose different sets of related problems and methods for its solution. Since some schools have their roots in other movements or disciplines, the pre-paradigm stage of a field may reflect the internal struggle of another group.

Ultimately, as one school of thought predominates or breaks off from the larger group to form its own collective, it becomes the paradigm of the new field. Now in paradigm stage, the discipline subscribes to a common definition of the phenomenon it confronts, the puzzles to be solved, and the ways of reaching solutions. The major activity of the field is then aimed at fact finding and puzzle solving within the boundaries of the paradigm. In science, problems called anomalies eventually arise that cannot be handled within the boundaries of the paradigm. When the paradigm cannot explain or guide efforts to deal with these anomalies, the profession enters a period of crisis. In pure science anomalies are generally scientific problems which cannot be solved. In applied fields anomalies may be other issues which influence questioning and eventual rejection of a paradigm. Kuhn also points to the importance of outside influences on the discipline, noting that external pressure may also contribute to a field's crisis.

During crisis, the old paradigm is criticized, and new competing schools of thought arise in an attempt to deal with the anomalous problems. The scientific revolution is completed when one of these competing schools successfully deals with the problems. The new state is a return to paradigm. This shift to a new paradigm necessitates a reorganization of the field, its phenomena, related puzzles, and its methods of solution and goals. Although this reorganization requires realignment of the field's perspective, it retains the knowledge and technology accumulated under the old paradigm. Figure 2 illustrates the ongoing cycle of paradigm, crisis, and return to paradigm that is the basic sequence of how knowledge and technology evolve within a field. We have used it as a schema for examining the history of occupational therapy and as an organizing analytic device allowing events and trends to be labeled and placed within a coherent framework. Therefore, in sections that follow, the history of occupational therapy has been organized to demonstrate its own passage through the stages of pre-paradigm, paradigm, crisis, and return to paradigm. Each stage is presented according to the questions identified above.

THE PRE-PARADIGM STAGE OF OCCUPATIONAL THERAPY.

Since formalization of the field of occupational therapy and its entry into paradigm occurred in roughly the second decade of this century, the pre-paradigmatic period should precede this time. Modern historians and early chroniclers of occupational therapy locate its roots in the moral treatment movement.[19,24,48,105] Moral treatment was the

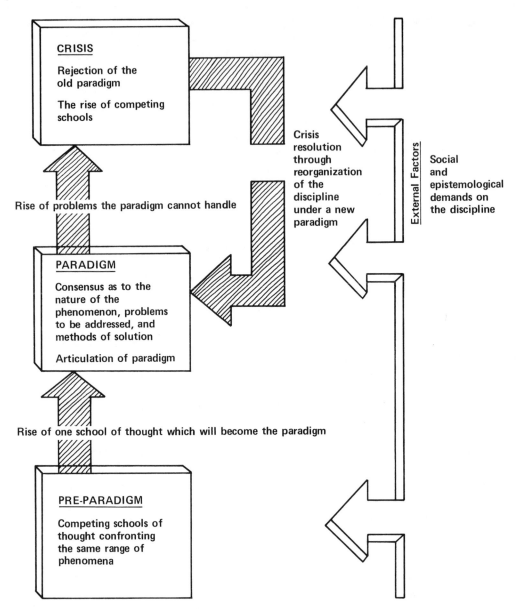

FIGURE 2. Stages of scientific revolution.

dominant treatment for the mentally ill in the 18th and 19th centuries, and early occupational therapists borrowed their most fundamental concepts from the writings and tradition of this mode. Examination of early occupational therapy literature reveals the pervasive influence of moral treatment ideas on the new paradigm. Consequently we propose that occupational therapy's pre-paradigmatic stage was the moral treatment movement of the 18th and 19th centuries.

THE HUMANISTIC APPROACH OF MORAL TREATMENT

The humanitarian philosophy of the 18th and 19th centuries held promise that science could produce therapeutically effective measures for the mentally ill.[109] All men were seen as equal and governed by natural universal laws. Bing proposes that:

> Moral treatment of the insane was one result of the *Age of Enlightenment*. It sprang from the fundamental attitudes of the day: a set of principles that govern humanity and society; faith in the ability of the human to reason; and the supreme belief in the individual.[19]

Moral treatment of the mentally ill emerged out of this philosophical and scientific framework.[19,24] According to moral treatment the mentally ill had merely succumbed to external pressures, and society had an obligation to help them return to the mainstream of life. One of the foundations of moral treatment was the belief that:

> most insane people retain a considerable amount of self-command. Upon admission, the patient was informed that treatment depended largely upon one's own conduct. Employment in various occupations was expected as a way for the patient to maintain control over his or her disorder.[19]

The physical, temporal, and social environment was engineered to correct faulty habits of living and to generate new ones. Engagement in normal daily activities within a cheerful and supportive environment was considered essential. Moral treatment was a grand scheme which placed the patient in a total program of daily living. It employed the remedies of education, daily tasks, work, and play as therapeutic processes for normalizing the disorganized behavior of the mentally ill.[24]

THE PATHOLOGIC APPROACH TO MENTAL HEALTH

There was a competing scientific school of thought based on the scientific methods of the physical sciences at the same time that the humanistic approach of the moral treatment school enjoyed its heyday.[36] The human brain, rather than the environment, was the center of focus in the explanation and treatment of mental illness. Mental illness was seen as a disease, with its etiology in brain pathology, and its curability was seen with pessimism. This approach served to designate the mentally ill as incurable, resulting in custodial care in large, crowded institutions. This school eventually evolved into a model for psychiatry, and out of it developed psychiatric treatment with chemotherapy and surgery.[24]

Social and ideological currents in the 19th century ultimately led to the demise of moral treatment and predominance of the pathologic school in the area of mental illness. The rapid growth of the American population and the influx of European immigrants led to overcrowding in state hospitals for the insane. Additionally, prejudiced views toward the so-called "insane foreign immigrant" fostered neglectful social attitudes toward the mentally ill.[24] The philosophic tone of the culture was changed also by the impact of growing technology. Social Darwinism and its survival of the fittest ethic was the dominant attitude of the public.[109] Rugged individualism and accountability for one's own welfare replaced the humanitarian philosophy that had supported moral treatment. Without a strong social commitment to treat the mentally ill and with overcrowded facilities, moral treatment declined.[24] However, a number of energetic and dedicated individuals eventually reapplied moral treatment in several areas of caring for the ill and disabled, generating a new profession that came to be known as occupational therapy.

THE PARADIGM OF OCCUPATION

Our conclusion that a paradigm existed in roughly the first four decades of this century is based on the striking degree of consensus in the literature among supporters and practitioners of occupational therapy concerning its most fundamental assumptions and principles. Moreover, this confluence of basic concepts is reflected across a spectrum of practice for the physically disabled and the mentally ill. The original development of the paradigm was within mental health, but its principles were rapidly applied to physical disabilities.[48,147]

VIEW OF HUMANS

The paradigmatic view of humans can be summed up in the statement that human beings were seen as having an *occupational nature.* Meyer articulated this concept in the new *Archives of Occupational Therapy* claiming that:

> Our body is not merely so many pounds of flesh and bone figuring as a machine, with an abstract mind or soul added to it. It is throughout a live organism pulsating with its rhythm of rest and activity, beating time (as we might say) in ever so many ways . . . . Our conception of man is that of an organism that maintains and balances itself in the world of reality and actuality by being in active life and active use, i.e., using and living and acting its *time* in harmony with its own nature and the nature about it. It is the *use* that we make of ourselves that gives the ultimate stamp to our every organ.[114]

The occupational nature of humans referred to an essential unity of mind and body and the integrated and balanced nature of the organism which maintained itself through acting in the world. Healthy human existence thus required being occupied. Occupation was a fundamental dynamic. The organization of the human organism—mind and body—was proposed as a function of habits which the individual acquired in this acting on and in the world.[114] Personality and competent behavior were seen as habit functions that were maintained through occupation.[147]

THE DYNAMIC BALANCE OF OCCUPATION. Rhythm and balance referred to the human alternation between modes of existing, thinking, and acting. Meyer[114] postulated work, rest, play, and sleep as the four major rhythms. Similarly, Dunton[49] proposed work, sleep, and leisure as the basic rhythms of occupation. He attributed considerable importance to leisure time and the cultivation of creative instincts. Indeed, the early writings of occupational therapy resonated with the theme that creativity, leisurely diversion, esthetic interests, competition, and celebration were essential to health. For example, Kidner[92] proposed creativity as a basic human need with biologic roots, "a concomitant of our having been born with hands, controlled by the brain." Slagle and Robeson identified creativity as a primitive evolutionary instinct:

> We have only to glance back through the ages to see that necessity demanded the invention of tools and equipment required for daily living. Then, with the artistic and creative urge inherent in men, came the beautifying and decorating of these crude utensils, the development of pottery, fabrics, and the resulting dignity and recognition. [149]

This inventiveness, competition, and leisurely self-enrichment were postulated as components of a play spirit in humans. [92,114,147] Play was proposed as a fundamental human trait, as primitive and important for health and survival as work. Kidner[92] argued that the play spirit should reign even in work, and that many human problems emerged from the monotony and drudgery of modern work; the craftsman epitomized true work that allowed control, creativity, and satisfaction from its results. Dunton[49] envisioned play as a necessary antidote to work, and that play be mental if work is physical, and vice versa. The creative, esthetic, playful, and leisure sides of human nature were viewed as essential tempering of the necessity for work. They complemented work and balanced its demands with self-chosen pursuits. Occupation was not considered just a compendium of work, rest, and play, but a necessary dynamic and delicate balance of daily human activities.

THE GOVERNANCE OF MIND. In addition to the recognition of an essential mind-body unity it was postulated that the mind governed and profoundly affected the body. Meyer proposed this as a feature of evolution in which the hierarchical arrangement of emergent phenomena constituted the latter as ruling or governing entities:

> In the great process of evolution there is a great law of unfolding which shows up in every new and higher step what we call the *integration* of the simpler phases into new entities. Thus the inorganic world continues itself into the plant and animal world. The laws of physics and chemistry expand into laws of growth and laws of function, still physical and chemical, but physical and chemical in terms . . . of more or less highly gifted man, with all that capacity to enjoy and to suffer, to succeed and to fail, to fulfill the life-cycle of the human individual happily and effectively or more or less falteringly. The great feature of man is his new sense of time, with foresight built on a sound view of the past and present. Man learns to organize time and he does it in terms of *doing* things. [114]

The sense of time that Meyer referred to was the basis of human morale and will, two fundamental traits of the mind. Morale, a concept from the moral treatment era, referred to the ability to see the present and future with a sense of interest and commitment. Will referred to the ability to make decisions based on a clear sense of value and desire. [14,163] The maintenance of morale and will were made possible by engagement in everyday life and its features of interest, value, sense of accomplishment and challenge. [49,114,147]

When morale was good the mind was centered on the reality of the world. [114] However, if morale was affected by a failure of normal daily occupation, the mind might focus on morbid or unreal thoughts. [49,92] This could lead to a breakdown of daily life habits and degeneration of the body. [92,147] Thus, if the properties of mind were disorganized, dysfunction reverberated throughout the organism. The mental status of being engaged, having interests and values to pursue—the morale for everyday living—was a key organizing feature in healthy human existence.

SUMMARY

The paradigm of occupation was based on the dogma that humans had an occupational nature. This included the tenet that the mind and body were linked in unity in which the mind governed the organism. Important features of the mind were awareness of time and morale that stimulated interest and commitment to one's daily occupations. Occupation was conceived as a dynamic rhythm and balance that included alternation between the essential components of work, play, and rest. Finally, the whole organization of the organism was seen as structured in human habit and maintained through ongoing engagement in everyday occupations.

CLINICAL PUZZLES

When a field is in paradigm, its view of the phenomena it addresses determines what kinds of puzzles it will attempt to solve.[97] The puzzles which early occupational therapists identified for clinical practice directly reflect their view of humans. These puzzles were breakdowns or dysfunctions of normal occupation.

IDLENESS. The most frequently discussed puzzle was *idleness*. Since it was human nature to be engaged in occupation and since occupation maintained the mind and body, a lack of occupation threatened the entire organism. The occupational therapist attempted to intervene immediately "before enforced idleness has started to do damage to the mind and to the body of the ill person."[149] Idleness was differentiated from leisure:

> There is a world of difference between leisure and idleness. Leisure is well-earned repose, in every way desirable. Idleness, at any rate the kind which is forced upon us in long illness, or in delayed convalescence, too often means degeneration, and in the end, increased suffering.[76]

It was also pointed out that idleness could prevent needed rest since it created tension:

> It was formerly supposed that a patient rested if he merely remained inactive; but it is now recognized that worry of mind, discontent, boredom and irritability often counteract the good that might result from complete rest of the body. This has led to a great increase in the use of occupational therapy in the sanatoria for the tuberculous in recent years.[92]

The effects of idleness on both mind and body revealed many related problems which also constituted puzzles for the early paradigm. One effect was the *demoralization* of the individual, that is, loss of temporal perspective, disengagement from daily life, and his possible acceptance of an invalid identity:

All victims of disease, either acute or chronic, suffer from a sense of a loss of time. They feel that they have been interrupted in their work. Even the child, whose work is play, feels this. Some accept this philosophically, others chafe constantly, still others are deeply depressed, while a fourth and, perhaps, most pitiable class seem to take a certain pride in their disability. All these mental attitudes aggravate existing conditions and retard recovery.[162]

Idleness could also result in a preoccupation with *morbid thoughts* and a breakdown of the faculty of attention. Persons simply lost interest in the world and consequently, their ability to attend, respond, and adapt to that world.[49,76,147]

THE BREAKDOWN OF HABITS. A second major puzzle of the paradigm was the breakdown of habits. Mental illness was considered largely a function of degeneration of habits of everyday life. Along these lines Slagle wrote that:

Our lives are made up of habit reactions . . . . Habit building for dementia praecox patients is highly important . . . since the disorganization of habit is basic with this type.[147]

Kidner[92] noted a similar breakdown of habits in tuberculosis where long periods of convalescence were to blame. Habits organized behavior for the demands of daily living. When habits deteriorated patients lost their ability to perform competently in daily life. Extreme habit degeneration resulted in total withdrawal from everyday occupation.

FAILURE OF BALANCE. Another major puzzle was the failure of balance in daily life; for the most part, this referred to a loss of the play spirit. For instance, Slagle linked the problems of many psychiatric patients to a loss of playfulness which led to breakdown of morale and then of habits:

How many here present have lived in a congested part of the city and watched children day after day in their vain pursuit for continuity in their play. While traffic on street or alley is momentarily suspended the game starts—an automobile whisks along and the game stops. And while the flow of traffic goes on, the play spirit goes out, and we get what Jane Adams so clearly described as "the fatal passivity that leads to social deviations, all too many of which lead to state institutions of one kind or another."[147]

Psychiatric illness was similarly linked to a suppression of play instinct in adulthood:

As many of the patients are men and women who have broken down because of too close application to business, or housekeeping, or care of a family, it is an excellent plan to develop the play-instinct which has been too much suppressed, this frequently being responsible for the breakdown.[49]

The importance of leisure in the balance of occupation was also apparent in persons without sufficient leisure interests. Dunton[49] pointed out that many successful persons who worked mightily also lacked leisure interests and, as a consequence, were frequent candidates for chronic boredom and depression. He advocated training such persons "how to live"—that is, how to strike a balance in their work and play lives. It was the lack of balance which brought on the psychologic problems.

THE ROLE OF THE MEDICAL DIAGNOSIS

Characteristically, clinical problems focused on disorganization of occupational life rather than on medically termed diseases or dysfunctions. Concentration on such puzzles of occupational dysfunction did not mean that medical diagnoses (i.e., psychiatric problems or physical injuries) were ignored. Rather, these problems were generally recognized as *part* of the occupational dysfunction. However, in a statement characteristic of most views, Slagle and Robeson[149] made clear that the psychiatric diagnosis was of secondary importance, noting that "it is immaterial whether the patient has been diagnosed dementia praecox or manic-depressive psychosis." The therapist's primary problem was to understand how habits had degenerated, for this was the focus of the occupational therapy problem in psychiatry. The problems of physically disabled patients were considered to be important as they contributed to the picture of the whole person. It was therefore argued that the occupational therapist needed a thorough understanding of the principles of physical function and dysfunction. These problems were integrated and attended to in the context of the occupational dysfunction as it was revealed in the patient's idleness and demoralization.

> In every functional disturbance, in addition to disorders of the central nervous system, there is a mental reaction. Pain, anemia, impairment of circulation, and sense impressions and emotions, such as anxiety and depression, are all communicated to the brain, which may be either highly sensitive or dull and apathetic, often showing such extreme symptoms as ennui, melancholia, restlessness, morbid introspection, discouragement, and fear. In ennui the tonicity of the muscles is affected so that they actually contract less strongly and develop less force. In melancholia the general physique, and especially the heart, is acted upon. Restlessness, or so-called nervousness and lack of concentration, is muscular activity of a wasteful type and gives rise to harmful fatigue. Morbid introspection produces a particularly vicious cycle of thinking, since continued attention focussed on any particular part of the body may actually increase its morbid condition. Discouragement and fear have a tendency to impair circulation, which may produce serious results upon the heart, digestive apparatus, and muscles.[163]

This integration of physical problems under the mental dimension of occupation was a natural consequence of the view of human beings in which mind-body unity was fundamental. Similarly, all pathologic states were seen as part of a larger occupational problem.

SUMMARY

The puzzles of occupational therapy practice during the paradigm of occupation were in the dysfunction of human occupations. Three major puzzles were idleness, habit dysfunction, and breakdown of the balance of occupation. Idleness led to demoralization, the degeneration of attention, preoccupation with morbid thoughts and assumption of an invalid identity. The breakdown of balance in daily life occupations emanated primarily from a loss or failure of playfulness. Loss of habits could accompany both mental and physical illness and threatened competent performance. These fundamental puzzles de-fined the need for occupational therapy intervention. Medical diagnosis and associated pathologic states were legitimate but subsidiary concerns. Consequently, the methods of puzzle solution used under this paradigm addressed problems of occupational dysfunc-tion.

RATIONALE AND METHODS OF TREATMENT

The principles of occupational therapy intervention during the paradigm of occupation were well articulated, and the coherence and systematic nature of treatment programs described in the literature are striking. A thorough rationale was developed to justify the use of occupation as therapy.

RATIONALE OF TREATMENT. The rationale of treatment was that since occupation was a natural means of maintaining the body and mind, it was also best suited as a method of regenerating lost function. This rationale included the recognition that occu-pation was a successful organizing force because it required an exercise of function in which mind and body were united. The theme of integrated use of mind and body and their mutual effects was paramount.[49,92,149]

The major reasoning that justified treatment was the beneficial effects of occupationally-derived mental experience on the regeneration of the mind and body:

> It was frequently observed that, while the patient's mind was absorbed in mastering an occupation in the hospital workshop, his interest was awakened, his ambition stimulated, his morbid and brooding thoughts eliminated, and his hope and self-confidence were restored. More recent analysis of the function of occupational therapy discloses the fact that, in addition to producing mental changes, it may also impose certain bodily changes.
>
> Although the fields of the mind and the body are fundamentally related, occupational therapy may be considered from the point of view, first, of psychological functions and, second, of physiological functions.[163]

Sheer activity was deemed insufficient for therapeutic benefits. Occupation was an exercise of both mind and body critical for regeneration. Kidner offered a rationale for the benefit of purposeful and interesting activity over exercise:

> The patient feels a psychic urge to exercise when he is producing some useful object, and when thus occupied is much more likely to overcome his sub-conscious inhibition to move a hand, an arm or a leg that has been injured, than he is when performing, by direction, exercises of a non-productive kind.[92]

It was also hypothesized that occupation provided a mechanism of subconscious learning which enhanced the regeneration of motor capacities. Along those lines Dunton noted that the crafts value was that "the patient's attention is directed to an object and away from himself, and he learns motion unconsciously and naturally".[49]

The same theory of the importance of occupations for centering attention away from the disability and on the activity was supported by Hall.[76] He argues that in some cases it may be preferable to prescribe a more general activity than one which brings attention to the pain or lack of function of a given joint or limb. Hall offers the following case illustration:

> I had as a patient once a girl who had received a bad cut across the palm, severing the tendons. After the necessary surgery, the fingers became contracted, and the slightest attempt to straighten them caused pain, and what was worse, the fear of pain. Massage and hydrotherapy had little effect. It looked as though the hand would be permanently crippled, for the longer the fingers remained unused, the more difficult became the recovery. The girl was given work to do with the other hand. She found presently that she could use the bad hand to steady her work, and after awhile, because she could control the amount of pain, she began to use the affected muscles and joints more freely, so that there was finally a complete recovery.[76]

Similarly, Slagle and Robeson note:

> Let our minds be engaged with the spirit of fun and competitive play and leave our muscles, nerves and organs to carry on their functions without conscious thought—then our physical exercised will be correspondingly more beneficial and we can readily picture the effect exerted on the mood of the sullen, morose patient by the genial glow which suffuses the body following active exercise.[149]

The latter writers proposed a neurologically reasoned theory as the explanation for this effect, noting the ruling influence of higher brain functions over the lower. They reasoned that any improvement in lower centers had to be accompanied by the higher centers that functioned as parts of the attentional process of the patient in occupation.[149]

All early writers were in agreement that occupations, when arranged to be meaningful and interesting to patients, could exert a stronger organizing influence on the total function of the person, making possible more complete and efficacious recovery from a specific dysfunction. The implication of these perspectives on therapy is reflected in the statement that "therapy to be of a successful physical nature, must originate with the individual in his mental attitude toward it."[52]

Because the mental impact of the occupation was paramount, every care was taken to provide occupations that would have favorable mental effects. The understanding of activities and their special characteristics for influencing the patient's experience was stressed as a major requirement for effective occupational therapy.

> It must not be inferred . . . that occupation can be used successfully in a haphazard manner. Not only must the nervous and physical strength be carefully estimated, but the temperament, natural tastes and disposition have to be taken into account in the kind and amount of occupation suggested, as well as in the manner and place in which it is presented.[69]

Slagle & Robeson also point out that:

> Crafts can also be easily graded and selected to meet the mental capacity of either a mental defective or an intellectual; the interests of a day laborer and a genius. The crafts can supply all physical movements required in restoration of impaired function of joints and muscles,

etc. To these may be added the less tangible (but not the less useful) psychological value of that peculiar pleasure derived from work accomplished with one's own hands.[149]

Activity analysis was advocated as a means of anticipating how occupations would affect patients. Activities were classified according to their sedative, exciting, mirthful or other characteristics to be considered in assigning a particular occupation to a patient. For instance, Kidner offers these guidelines:

> The precise type of work to be given to a mental patient at this, or at any stage, of treatment will depend largely on the patient's condition. The manic, or excited type of patient whose condition is characterized by elation, weak attention or distractability, . . . and motor activity, should be given a sedative occupation; that is, an occupation which involves a repeated, rhythmic movement which has a lulling effect.[92]

Thus, not only were occupations indispensible as therapeutic agents, but their application required careful study of their inherent qualities for eliciting emotion, attention, satisfaction, and a whole range of other effects. The experience of the patient engaging in therapy was paramount in this existential-like approach to the patient's self-healing.

METHODS OF TREATMENT

Emphasis on the mental process in therapy meant that the occupational therapy had to be one which elicited the most favorable mental reactions.[48,76] There were three reigning methods for organizing the impact of therapy on the mind: the method of regression and graduation, the method of attention, and the method of socialization.

REGRESSION. Both Slagle and Hall formulated the regression approach. Hall[76] noted that physically disabled patients were reduced to the helpless position of a child and observed that they would best benefit from occupations resembling the play of children. Slagle, recounting that both the physically disabled patient and the psychiatric patient regressed to a lower level, designed therapeutic programs to organize patients through the continuum of development.[147,149] In her habit training programs for dementia praecox patients she replicated the conditions of childhood. Strict schedules of self-care and normal occupation were provided under the direction and supervision of hospital staff. Next, Slagle employed games, music, colorful atmosphere, and other modalities which she proposed stimulated the senses.[147] Slagle and Robeson reasoned that the success of crafts in occupational therapy also came from the satisfaction of a more primitive or regressed need:

> In all sick persons the normal mental and physical functioning is in abeyance and the primitive instincts usually come to the fore. The "censor" is off duty, and inhibited tendencies of primitive man's creative mind . . . stir voluntarily . . . at this time especially, handicrafts have an appeal.[149]

GRADUATION. Together with the principle of regression was the principle of graduation in therapy. As the patient progressed from a regressed and disorganized state toward a regeneration of mind and body, demands and challenges had to be graduated both to provide optimal stimulation and to restore everyday functioning. In habit training, psychiatric patients were directed through programs which emphasized sportsmanship and craftsmanship as the basis for later progression toward workmanship and citizenship in the community.[50,75] Bryan[32] and Marsh[110] proposed industrial therapy as the next phase to prepare the advanced patient for the world of work. In this step, the occupational therapist analyzed jobs and trained patients for work. Patients were placed in occupations matched to their interests, experience, and aspirations.

In physical disabilities the occupational therapy program began with bedside games and crafts that required little physical stress and were within the capacity of the patients. Recovering patients then proceeded to shop work. Finally, they were employed in industrial work within the institution.[12,92]

Treatment progressed from acquisition of skills and habits of self-care and the nonserious business of play to the more demanding tasks of arts and crafts, and finally to the serious activity of work. The graduated program began in the homelike atmosphere of the ward, progressed to the moderate school-like challenges of the workshop, and culminated in the industrial setting.

ATTENTION. The method of attention was related to regression and gradualism. A major theme throughout the early literature was the idea that occupation functioned by diverting attention from morbid thoughts or from attending to one's disability rather than to the world:

> Occupational therapy aims first to create a wholesome interest in something outside the patient's morbid interest in himself and his symptoms; second, to fill the unoccupied portions of the patient's day; third, to prepare his mental attitude so that he may adjust himself to normal demands and environment after the hospital discharge.[163]

Diversion of attention was also used as a preventive measure; it kept the patients from beginning to brood over their disabilities.[49] Based on the principle that "but one idea can occupy the focus of the attention at a given time,"[48] attention was substituted for morbid thoughts.

Since the need to occupy the patient's mind and prevent or reverse demoralization was a central theme, it was natural that therapists thoroughly considered the problem of motivation in therapy. The following is a typical proposal for motivating even the most recalcitrant patients:

> It is easier to find something that the patient can do than to find something he will do. One needs to be resourceful, with a large variety of appeals, for it goes without saying that even in health what appeals to one person will not to another. The difference is even more marked among the insane. Appeals may be made through praise, competition, rewards; to the sense of the beautiful or of the useful; through affection for relatives, home needs, gifts to friends, or more diffuse altruism, as helping other patients, making preparations for special entertainments, such as Christmas gifts and decorations, or work for children. . . .[162]

Similarly articulated methods for motivating the patient ranged from the manner of introducing the patient to the therapist and the workshop to the carefully arranged physical and social atmosphere of the occupational therapy setting. Slagle[147] advocated a wide variety of games, crafts, music, and other occupations and the maintenance of an atmosphere of cheerfulness, playfulness, interest and value. To these ends the therapist needed to show wholesome interest and competence in the occupations used as therapy. Tracy,[162] Dunton,[49] and Hall[76] stressed that the occupational therapist be a craftsperson, sportsperson or artisan who had genuine interest and mastery of the occupations used as therapy. Only then could one inspire persons who had lost interest and hope. The therapist was to be a model for the pleasure of living; a cheerful and confident attitude was required.[49,76,162] Therapists used these attributes artfully to lead patients into participation in therapy, recognizing that the problem of attention in therapy required a close observation of patients and their reactions, and an inventive orchestration of the circumstances optimal for each person.

SOCIALIZATION. In addition, the therapist organized treatment to give the patient an implicit message that performance in the occupational therapy clinic was expected and valued. This was the socialization function of therapy. While patients were allowed choice whenever possible, idleness or unwillingness to perform was not an option.[49,147] Patients were not allowed to use their disabilities as excuses for not participating. Fuller[69] further recommended the strict rule that patients were not allowed to talk about their problems in therapy. People were expected to be involved in the task at hand.

To assure proper socialization the therapist sought to provide a normalized environment in the hospital. Slagle and Robeson proposed:

> Work, exercise and play are factors in every well-balanced life and are essential to health. In the pressure of the times, the last two are often neglected. In our aim, therefore, to normalize hospital life, or in any program of rehabilitation, physical activities and recreation must find a place.[149]

Natural rhythms of time use were seen as essential to the regeneration of habits in patients.[114,147] Such an environment conveyed to the patients the manner in which they would be able to lead meaningful and more normal lives. Occupational therapy clinics required the presence of persons (usually therapists) who demonstrated interest and a high level of competency in these occupations:

> Much importance was placed on the occupation room, wherein opportunity was provided for various forms of interesting and useful work. Weaving rugs and finer fabrics, basket work, bookbinding and clay modeling were employed at the start. Fortunately there was secured an excellent leader, trained in teaching, conversant with the work to taken up and interested in it. The room was open at definite hours each day, but at other times those who wished could work without the presence of the teacher if their condition permitted . . . . The atmosphere of interested activity prevailed. The work became the source of new purposes, of changed avenues of thought and of stimulated ambitions. Other kinds of work were introduced from time to time, such as leather work, brass work, free-hand drawing, chair caning, the manufacture of photograph albums, notebooks, etc. The department was a success.[69]

In short, the occupational therapy service was the curator of everyday life in the hospital and of the demands and satisfactions which went along with daily living.

SUMMARY

The rationale for occupational therapy as an efficacious intervention began with its property of unified action of mind and body. The ultimate focus in therapy was always the provision of an occupation which would elicit positive mental experiences and thus benefit the entire person. This required careful attention to the details of occupations and their properties. Simple crafts, games, and self care were designed to reorganize the regressed patient; treatment was graduated to bring the individual through a continuum to full and direct participation in occupational life. Further, occupations were designed to capture attention and influence the positive morale of patients (a critical variable for their recovery). Finally, occupational therapy served as a socialization process where patients were brought to an appreciation of the satisfaction and control they could experience, the worth of occupations, and the continued social expectation for their performance. All successful therapy centered on the artful use of occupations and the orchestration of material and social circumstances which surrounded the occupations. Occupational therapy served as a carefully arranged environment in which patients could find support, opportunity, value, and expectation for performance matched to their limitations and natural inclinations. In such an atmosphere patients could muster the will and effort needed to begin the process of self-regeneration through occupation.

GOALS

In the early literature, the goals pertaining to patients are broad in range yet recognizably interrelated. For instance, Slagle and Robeson proposed the following aims:

> . . . to reconstruct, to rebuild or re-educate the patient, (a) mentally; (b) physically, and (c) socially according to the individual need and to the highest capability of the patient.[149]

It is not surprising that such goals should be articulated, since the patient's body, mind, and social position were seen as intricately related:

> Remember that restoration of physical capacity without the will to do is a futile thing. Good medical practice demands healing of mind as well as of body or organ and a cure is not completed until it has re-established habits of work, if they have been destroyed through long convalescence and illness.[149]

Examination of the literature suggests that the proposed goals of therapy can be adequately characterized as restoration or reorganization of skill, habit, and occupational role and the enrichment of the latter. The patient's increased ability to move a disabled limb in some purposeful activity was a frequently articulated goal. Notably, movement itself was not the goal, but movement in the context of some actual occupation. Dunton presents a typical argument along these lines: "The clumsy fingers become nimble, in typewriting, weaving, splicing or modeling and the practice of these trades must be regarded as important parts of one general and progressive system of treatment."[49] Similarly, Slagle notes, "of highest value to the patients receiving physical-curative exercises is the *psychological* fact that the patient is working for himself."[148] The early literature further specified that discrete function alone was not sufficient, but that patients needed to have regenerated habits. In Slagle and Robeson's words[149] this meant substituting better habits or building new habits to replace those which were lost.

Finally, the importance of being able to return a patient to some useful and satisfying occupational role was acknowledged. This process was conceptualized as a continuum of rebuilding capacity and organizing morale in order to help a person gain occupational competency, thus a variety of subsidiary goals such as stimulating interest,[76] increasing self-confidence,[49] and focusing thoughts on external reality[114] were included. Since the ultimate return of a person to occupational functioning was a problem of overall organization of the body and mind into a rhythm of daily life,[76,114] these goals were part of a larger aim of preparing for the occupational role.

While the occupational role—which meant work, play, and routine behaviors—was the target of occupational therapy practice, direct vocational preparation was not one of the aims of therapy. The latter consisted of actual training for a job. It was the role of occupational therapy to give individuals opportunities to discover aptitudes and interests that might ultimately result in a new occupation.[49,76] Actual training for a job occurred fortuitously only if a marketable interest or aptitude was discovered or pursued.

Notably absent from the early literature are claims of directly influencing pathologic processes. Occupational therapy was proposed as a means of enhancing convalescence and healing;[76,92] as a means of rebuilding motor and mental capacity;[48,147] and as a way of restoring the habits of daily life and the natural balance of work and play,[114] but disease was clearly not the direct target of therapy. Hall aptly illustrates the thinking of the time:

> The therapeutics of occupation is a curiously complex matter. No one claims that prescribed occupation can, as a rule, of itself, cure anything. But it is beyond controversy that the patient pleasantly and usefully occupied is a better subject for medical treatment of any kind that one who is discouraged, introspective, and idle. In many people and in many disabilities, the fatigue point, the breaking-down point, is so easily reached that life is hopelessly ineffective. By means of manual work carefully prescribed, it is often possible to push this point along, to build up a degree of resistance which is in itself worth while. Such gains may tip the scale toward recovery, may develop a morale, a courage, which is of more value than medicine.[76]

It is not surprising that there should be a lack of articulated aims for directly influencing pathologic processes, since the puzzles of occupational therapy were not diseases, but the disorganization of daily life behavior. It was recognized that the course of recovery from disease was enhanced when occupational deprivation was minimized. However, the occupational dysfunction and its remediation were the focus and aim of therapy.

SUMMARY

The goals of occupational therapy included increasing function in the mental, physical, and social domains. These were seen as part of the interrelated makeup of the individual. The goals focused on this organized wholeness, rather than on discrete changes in partial functions or modification of pathology. The ultimate goal was return of patients to satisfying and socially useful occupations.

THE PARADIGM IN PERSPECTIVE

We have noted that the early paradigm of occupation is found in the field's literature in the period from the turn of the century into the 1940's. There was a unified conceptualization of occupational therapy which included application in two main areas, mental illness and physical disabilities. While our earlier discussion incorporated elements of writing and practice from both areas in order to illustrate the coherence of the paradigm, it is useful to note that the single paradigm was established and utilized in the diverse areas of physical disabilities and mental illness. It is remarkable that the idea of occupational therapy found its way into such apparently discrete areas of practice. Examination of the principles applied in each of these two areas reveals a single matrix of ideas which underlies both. Figure 3 summarizes the elements that distinguished concepts of practice in physical disabilities and in mental illness. Both applications share the same view of persons; their puzzles, methods of solution, and goals are similar and flow from the larger paradigm.

It is also important to recall that this paradigm was empirically successful. Early writings are replete with observations of the positive effects of occupation on a vast array of patients and in a variety of settings. Indeed, it was frequently observed that occupational therapy was the most efficacious treatment for patients. An overwhelming enthusiasm for occupational therapy as a great asset to modern medicine is found in this literature.

While the early paradigm was primarily a set of concepts for direct patient care, we share the convictions of Reilly[133] and Johnson[89] that an important scientific discovery was involved. The hypothesis that humans maintained and could restore their function through occupation was rich in its implications for theory and research.

Early writers, along with their *primary* concern for clinical application, espoused the advancement of this science of human occupation. Many therapists advocated a more detailed study of the crafts and their properties—a science of activity analysis which would entail investigation of both the psychologic and physical impact of various crafts.[49,75,76] Such studies would determine the kind of atmosphere a craft created (e.g., competitive, sedative, demanding, soothing); the kind of capacities it required; and the cultural meaning or value it was likely to communicate. Descriptive studies would enhance the prescription of occupational therapy with precision.

Many persons saw the need for a more thorough study of occupation in everyday life. Meyer[114] advocated a deeper understanding of the natural rhythms of occupational life and the role of the environment in maintaining them. Dunton[49] and Hall[76] both proposed that the understanding of work and play and their interrelationships was important knowledge to be developed. Finally, it was proposed that the study of how occupation impacted and affected the disabled person should be undertaken.[48,76] Many early proponents of occupational therapy did attempt systematic study of the effects of occupation.

To reach these goals, early research in occupational therapy was largely descriptive, and hospital and individual case studies were the investigative work most frequently reported. In addition to this empirical approach, phenomenological studies were also used. Many of the early proponents used self-study and self-reflection as a means of deriving principles for theory and practice. Dunton often wrote of the nature and impor-

	VIEW OF HUMANS	PUZZLES	RATIONALE AND METHODS OF SOLUTION	THERAPEUTIC GOALS
PARADIGM	Occupational nature of humans: -Mind-body unity with mind (temporality and morale) governing the organism -Rythm and balance in work, play, and rest structured by habit and maintained through engagement in occupation	Occupational dysfunctions: -Idleness leading to the degeneration of mind & body -Demoralization and aquisition of an invalid identity -Habit deterioration -Disruption of the balance of daily life	Use of occupation as therapy: -Maintain a normalized work and play atmosphere which motivates and expects participation -Engage patient in occupations to regenerate morale and attention and positively influence entire organism -Allow regeneration of regressed behavior and damaged body through graduated exercise of capacity	-Restore required skills, habits, and roles -Prevent invalidism from replacing occupational role
PHYSICAL DISABILITIES	Same view of the occupational nature of humans	Occupational dysfunctions: -Imposed idleness during convalescence resulting in demoralization and loss of physical capacity -Atrophy of habits during institutionalization -Physical problems leading to loss of capacity for work and play behaviors	Use occupation to: -Fulfill the primitive needs for activity and prevent breakdown of morale -Engage patient in graduated occupations with progressive motor and social demands for performance -Divert attention from physical problems to the external world -Enable patient to discover new aptitudes for modified occupational life	-Restore motor skills -Reorganize habits of daily life -Prepare for new or altered occupational roles -Prevent enforced idleness, demoralization and invalidism
PSYCHIATRY	Same view of the occupational nature of humans	Occupational dysfunctions: -Idleness resulting from disengagement from daily life -Faulty habits or the failure to build habits through life experience -Loss of play spirit and imbalance of work and play	Use of occupations to: -To elicit primitive play instinct and develop leisure capacity -Divert attention from morbid thoughts to external reality -Learn new habits of self-care and work in a normal environment	-Restore morale, work, and play, skills and habits of daily life for a productive role

FIGURE 3. The paradigm of occupation and its treatment applications.

tance of occupation from his own experience. Barton epitomized the phenomenological approach. He was at one time seriously disabled, and studied the effects of occupation on his own recovery.

Dunton summarized the sentiments of early writers and researchers concerning how knowledge of occupational therapy should be developed as follows:

> It must be understood that I am in complete sympathy with scientific research, but we must not despise empiricism . . . the scientific investigation of occupational therapy will be most heartily welcomed, but in the meantime let us continue to welcome the "casual observations" of the subject, hoping that they will eventually be corroborated by scientific observations.[49]

The development of a systematic body of knowledge and therapeutic techniques was an articulated goal of early occupational therapy. Scientific investigation was seen as an objective to be accomplished through the building of a descriptive body of knowledge.

Our examination of the early literature left us with a deep respect for the ideas and accomplishments of the fields' first generation of therapists. Both a science of occupation and the art of using occupation as a medical therapy were conceived, clearly articulated, and applied. As therapists we were struck with the feeling that something had been lost in the interim. A sense of confidence and enthusiasm for occupational therapy seems to have waned, and today we seem bewildered in the face of clinical problems which early occupational therapists readily embraced. Furthermore, our confusion over the identity of occupational therapy seems inexplicable compared with the unified view of early occupational therapists concerning the nature of their service. These issues are what make the period from that paradigm to the present most intriguing for us. No doubt some important gains have been made. We are technologically superior to our predecessors in many ways. However, the apparent losses concern us. We felt compelled to ask why some of these seemingly timeless ideas of the early paradigm are weak or absent from current practice. The following section outlines the answers we found in the literature of subsequent years.

CRISIS IN OCCUPATIONAL THERAPY

As noted above, a paradigm can be brought into question when problems arise that it cannot encompass. When competing points of view begin to affect the paradigm and offer alternative explanations, principles, methods, the paradigm may be rejected and replaced by another. This is often a gradual process which takes place over generations of practitioners.

Examination of the occupational therapy literature of the late 1940s and 1950s reveals such questioning of the dominant paradigm of occupational therapy. During the 1940s the literature attests to the continued dominance of the paradigm of occupation. Applications of industrial therapy[1,127,144] and habit training[35,156] continued. The use of art, games, recreational activities, and a variety of crafts was regularly reported with the same principles and objectives of the earlier decades articulated. Writings from the moral treatment were reprinted in the field's journal, suggesting that these ideas continued to strongly influence occupational therapy.[54,101,129,142] Additionally, Licht published the *Occupational Therapy Source Book*[105] which recounted the field's connection to moral treatment and reprinted writings from that era.

COMPETING SCHOOLS OF THOUGHT

During the 1940s there was a growing articulation of kinesiologic principles by Licht[102,103] and Hurt[81,82] and Spackman,[153] all of whom attempted to integrate them into the concepts of the paradigm of occupation. Neurophysiologic principles of treatment for nervous system disorders were also articulated in this period.[21,31] Some of the first writings suggesting application of psychodynamic principles to occupational therapy also appear.[77,124,152]

Haas[75] published his second book on occupational therapy in which he attempted to incorporate principles from the therapeutic community and kinesiology. Principles from psychiatry, kinesiology, and neurology were still seen as part of the larger occupational therapy purpose.[112,164]

In general, the field appeared in the 1940's to be continuing normal science under the paradigm of occupation. Concepts of occupation were being further articulated while knowledge of the nervous system, kinesiology, and the personality of the mentally ill was imported to advance knowledge of how occupations could be adapted to the particular needs of individuals with various disabilities.

However, in the latter part of this decade and in the 1950s there was growing pressure on occupational therapy to establish a scientific rationale for its methods and to engage in research to support its claim to efficacy. Licht[103] pointed out that physicians openly criticized occupational therapy for lack of a scientific rationale and called for research in the field.

In addition, the Depression of the 1930s had brought concerns for job security and professional survival and led occupational therapy to seek a closer alliance with medicine. An alignment with the American Medical Association to credential schools of occupational therapy was followed by a narrowing of occupational therapy thinking to conform more closely to the medical model.[136] To understand the effects of occupational therapy's alliance with medicine during this period requires some appreciation of what was happening in the latter field.

MEDICINE'S REDUCTIONISM

Early in the 20th century medicine committed itself to becoming a scientific discipline.[137] At the time this meant that medicine would import the concepts, methods, and techniques which had been successful in the physical sciences. The term for this brand of science is "reductionism."[96] Reductionism is defined as an effort to reduce the empirical world to its most elementary constituents and relationships in order to understand and influence them. It is founded on assumptions that the world operates basically as a *mechanism* with cause and effect laws governing the interrelationships of its parts.[17] It followed that the most efficacious method of studying the empirical world would be to discover those elementary parts and their effects on each other. Thus, phenomena studied by the scientist were to be reduced or divided into discrete or measurable units whose relationship to other units could be specified through study. Ultimately, the hope was that when all the units and relationships had been described at the micro level, they could be reconstructed to achieve an understanding of the whole and its functioning.[17,168] Reductionism ushered in great achievements and became the dominant method of all science. However there were tradeoffs; in reductionism "breadth is given up in favor of depth, and universality and versatility are traded for the thrust of concentrated effort."[168]

In order to achieve a scientific status, medicine drew upon the methodology of reductionism[100] which yielded a medical model that embodied the principles of biophysics and biochemistry and the psychoanalytic perspective of psychiatry. Through the medical model physicians came to view human beings via the concepts of homeostasis and disease.[17,33] Homeostasis refers to the equilibrium of the physical or psychic forces within the organism. In this schema, disease is an imbalance of these forces precipitated by some stressful or traumatic agent. Medicine came to understand humans vis-a-vis their *internal mechanisms*, or literally, that which could be seen by means of the microscope or x-ray and by the scrutiny of psychotherapy. Because of its new brand of science, medicine did not recognize as scientific the holistic concepts which characterized the paradigm of occupation. The new focus in medicine was the understanding and manipulation of internal mechanisms. The importance of humans acting within their environment was largely forgotten.[46]

It is important to recognize that medicine's focus on reductionism was a choice to embrace the most successful way of doing science available at the time. While reductionism is still acknowledged to have efficacy in science today, there is also recognition that other approaches to science are possible.[28]

By aligning itself more closely with medicine, occupational therapy brought its early paradigm into a confrontation with the concepts of reductionism in medicine. The expanding concepts of kinesiology, neurology, and psychiatric pathology, which had been incorporated under the paradigm, now competed as primary concepts for occupational therapy, and these areas of knowledge more readily complemented a reductionist mode of thinking.

Under the influence of these factors occupational therapy developed into a state of crisis by the 1950s. In this period several competing approaches can be found in the literature of the field. The first is a continuation of ideas from the paradigm of occupation, represented primarily in industrial therapy,[37,55,70] prevocational efforts,[42,166] together with continued applications of games, music, dance, and so forth.[41,128]

A second school of thought in psychiatric occupational therapy was the psychodynamic approach based on Freudian principles.[10,11,57,67] Proponents of this perspective were often the most vocal opponents of the earlier paradigm of occupation. The third perspective was a neurologic approach.[2,3,4,90,126,141] The fourth approach was based on kinesiologic principles and included concepts such as joint mobilization, prevention of deformity and increasing function through exercise, splinting, and adapted equipment.[15,20,26,51,66,80,86,158] Daily living activities for the physically disabled came to be viewed almost solely through this perspective of kinesiologic principles.[29,53,85,108]

In the years 1950-60, criticism of the paradigm of occupation increased amid further articulation of other approaches, and fewer references to universal principles of occupation. Throughout this period the concern for scientific rationale or theory in occupational therapy grew increasingly stronger.[27,79,125,140] The following statement sums up the dilemma:

> No one who has seen a good occupational therapy program in action can doubt that it seems to result in great help for some patients, and some help for many. There appears, however, to be no rigorous and comprehensive theory which will explain who is helped, how, by what, or why; and there is little objective evidence that occupational therapy is actually effective.[115]

In her call for occupational therapy to become more scientific, West echoes this theme:

> Much of the "common sense" according to which we have traditionally operated is more in the nature of a collection of information than a system of sound, interrelated theories and procedures that is the ideal of science.[169]

Growing pressure from medicine for the field to define its theory was evidenced in the literature:

> Medicine is asking occupational therapy to be more aggressive in thought. It is asking us to grow with clinical practice. The doctor expects the occupational therapist not only to receive the prescription for what is written on it, but for what is inferred in it. He must count on the depth and breadth of concept before he refers an individual case . . . .[113]

The quote reflects the pressure on occupational therapy for importation of knowledge from medicine. McNary presaged what would become the next paradigm of occupational therapy in the following words:

> Occupational therapy is not enough of an isolated science to select a formula, learn it by heart, and just apply it. As we talk techniques let us think of underlying principles and build procedure on scientific fact. The clues lie in the basic concepts of psychology, physiology and anatomy. We must turn to bodies of knowledge that have established principles known to be true. It is on these principles techniques can be built.[113]

With principles adapted from psychodynamic, neurophysiologic and anatomic perspectives a new paradigm was constructed. As each of these views achieved a stronger position and found problems with the earlier paradigm's lack of science, the field moved further and further from the paradigm of occupation. By the end of the decade articles supporting its concepts were rare. Near the end of the decade, Reilly, noting the growing loss of concern for occupation, called for occupational therapy to "liberalize . . . understanding of activity and the central role it plays in human behavior."[130] It was a call that went unheeded.

Psychiatric occupational therapy was besieged with propositions from psychiatry that psychodynamic concepts should underlie occupational therapy practice. Solomon[151] typified this perspective in his criticism of occupational therapy as a humanitarian enterprise instead of a scientific treatment. Similarly, Azima and Azima criticized the concepts of the earlier paradigm:

> According to our point of view occupation is neither the aim nor the mechanism operating in this field which uses the media now in operation in an occupational therapy situation. Hence, occupational therapy taken as such is undefinable if the framework within which it seeks theoretical clarification is psychodynamics.[10]

Azima and Wittkower[11] directly attacked several concepts from the paradigm of occupation. They found fault with the therapeutic ideas of diversion from morbid thoughts, providing satisfaction, and the re-education of mental functions.

Arguments from the physical disabilities perspective faulted longstanding concepts of the first paradigm as unscientific and insufficient:

> A commonly accepted justification of the use of crafts and games as therapeutic media is the emotional value to the patient of an interesting and creative experience. The reasoning is accepted as a basic and important assumption empirically but not scientifically demonstrated. *While the interest and pleasure of a creative activity are important, they do not provide the most fundamental and vital concept underlying occupational therapy of physical disabilities* . . . (emphasis added) Realization of the importance of neurophysiological mechanisms in the treatment of the motor system is increasing. A study of them increases understanding of how the neuromuscular system operates in terms of purposeful function.[3]

In this emerging viewpoint the primary value of activities was their ability to affect neurophysiology. The concepts of humans' occupational nature, the rhythm and balance of occupation, and other ideas which were part of the earlier paradigm were being replaced by narrower concepts of purposeful activity and function. This perspective reversed the earlier view which saw neurophysiology in terms of occupation; occupation was now seen as a means of affecting neurophysiology. The understanding of function was narrowed to focus on the nervous and musculoskeletal systems. In sum, these arguments called for a new orientation in occupational therapy toward the understanding and modification of *inner mechanisms*. Concern with these neurologic, kinesiologic and intrapsychic mechanisms developed into the new mode of viewing patients and their problems, gradually replacing the view of humans maintaining themselves in the balance of daily occupation. Mosey summarized the shift as follows:

> Occupational therapists were uncomfortable with their simple operating principle that it was good for disabled people to keep active and busy doing things they enjoyed. Rather, the occupational therapists borrowed techniques from other disciplines. . . . Like other workers, occupational therapists were oriented to the rehabilitation of specific disease or disability categories. Underlying or common principles were not recognized.[120]

Because the reductionist thinking of medicine focused on cause and effect chains and the relationships of discrete variables, the ideas of connectedness of phenomena (mind and body) were less viable. Moreover, the recognition of hierarchical arrangement of phenomena (mind as a ruling influence over the body) and of the dynamic maintenance of systems (occupation maintaining function of mind and body) was not accommodated by the reductionist perspective. And as the knowledge content of the new perspectives of neurology, kinesiology and psychodynamics grew, the balance of information in occupational therapy became disproportionate. As the understanding of occupation and its holistic healing influence slowly eroded, phenomena of the neuromuscular and nervous systems and intrapsychic dynamics became more plausible theoretical explanations for what occupational therapy did.

While the transition was gradual and subtle, it did revolutionize occupational therapy's view of human beings with a consequent reconstitution of other paradigm variables. The literature suggests that by the end of the 1950s a new paradigm was firmly entrenched in the thinking and practice of occupational therapy.

THE EMERGENCE OF A PARADIGM OF INNER MECHANISMS

That a single paradigm would include the diverse concerns of psychoanalysis, kinesiology, and neurology may seem unlikely. However, a detailed examination of these bodies of knowledge and their use in occupational therapy in the 1960s reveals a common underlying pattern. Each perspective offered the possibility, in its respective specialty, of achieving a more acceptable scientific explanation for occupational therapy, thus resolving the problem which brought the field into crisis. These three approaches also gave the field a singular way of viewing human beings: the view of their inner mechanisms. The internal workings of the intrapsychic, neurologic and kinesiologic systems of the person thus became the primary mode of viewing patients. The unity of these perspectives is aptly described in the following passage which compares the neurologic to the psychodynamic approach in therapy:

Much of the time both the sensory and the psychotherapeutic situation are dealing with semi- or nonconscious experiences. The psychotherapist thinks in terms of subconscious psychic complexes and dynamics; the sensory integrative therapist includes many subcortical integrative mechanisms in his thinking and treatment planning. While one therapist is considering the Oedipus complex, the other is considering brain stem integrating processes. In both cases the underlying mechanisms are recognized, their effect on behavior analyzed, and methods of dealing with them contemplated.[8]

Similarly, the kinesiologic approach is compared with psychodynamic principles:

As the give and take of shortening and lengthening reactions of muscles is necessary for the health of both, so the giving and receiving of love and of stress is necessary for healthy emotional reactions, and these must be in the sequence of normal development.[141]

Since the view of human beings refocused on inner mechanisms, the puzzles and methods of therapy similarly shifted. Each of the three approaches addressed the common puzzle of modifying these internal mechanisms. In psychiatry it was modification of intrapsychic dynamics. In physical disabilities and pediatrics it was the modification of movement patterns and neurophysiology. The paradigm embraced the idea that focus on such modification of internal mechanisms would bring occupational therapy into its own right as a demonstrably efficacious service with an acceptable rationale.[6,57,141] In addition to its scientific respectability, it gave practitioners discrete, tangible objectives of modifying dysfunctional parts. Eventually, formulated approaches allowed therapists to follow a specific schema of identifying internal deficits that were to be addressed with a predetermined course of action.

Commenting on the change in occupational therapy's underlying base, Conte labeled it "evolutionary rather than revolutionary."[40] While the process of change may have been gradual and incremental, its effect was a radical departure from earlier concepts. Most significantly, the fundamental perspective of the field with respect to human beings had been radically altered. The early paradigm began with a broad appreciation of the occupational nature of human beings, their mind-body unity, their self-maintenance through occupation, and the dynamic rhythm and balance of their organized behavior. The new paradigm achieved a depth perspective. It shifted from gestalt thinking to a reductionist focus on the inner workings of the human psyche and body. The latter perspective was not simply added to the original paradigm; it *replaced* that paradigm and relegated its tenets to a position of unimportance or secondary significance. In a similar vein the therapeutic rationale drastically changed. The reductionist perspective of the new paradigm recognized neither mind-body unity nor the wholeness of the human being. In order to achieve its specific focus on modifying internal mechanisms, it necessarily abandoned the more ambiguous concept of organizing the whole. The earlier rationale of therapy, which had recourse to concepts such as diversion, morale, habit regeneration, and stimulation of interest as central explanatory principles, was now replaced with psychodynamic, neurophysiologic, and kinesiologic rationales which relegated the former perspectives to *considerations* in therapy. The price of this shift was a loss of critical ideas from the earlier paradigm. Jantzen summarizes it as follows:

The factor of creativity available to patients through occupational therapy was recognized early in our history and is a major theme in the writings of the pioneers of the field. As we have competed for status in a medical group with a highly developed technological competence we have lost this qualitative aspect of patient care.[87]

In our estimation these changes merit the name revolution; they reflect the underlying dynamic of paradigm shift which Kuhn[97] describes. The literature suggests that therapists viewed the change enthusiastically with good reason, for the problem of being seen as unscientific had been resolved. Therapists felt a greater sense of control over the processes they managed in therapy because procedures could be clearly articulated. There were important technologic gains for the field as new uses for activities and other therapeutic means were generated. The neurologic, kinesiologic and psychodynamic approaches developed into coherent bodies of knowledge and practice techniques. The sections that follow provide a brief description of each approach, its view of humans, puzzles, methods of solution, and goals.

THE NEUROLOGIC APPROACH

VIEW OF HUMANS. The neurologic approach developed with emphasis on several areas associated with neurophysiology, including cognitive perceptual motor skills and sensory integration. The person was seen as a complex network of neurophysiologic impulses that had important guiding and coordinating functions in movements. This approach employed the principle that in order for a person to develop normally, sensory and motor systems needed to be functioning and focused on the important role of sensory stimuli in positioning and moving the body.[6,22,141]

Coordinated movement was seen as governed by inherent patterns of motion. When these patterns were atypical, as in the case of the child with cerebral palsy, the therapist utilized sensory stimuli to elicit and shape more adaptive patterns.[22,43,141] In addition, purposeful movement was recognized as a useful means of remediating many neurologic problems. However, the concept of purposeful activity was a much narrower concept than the earlier paradigm's concept of occupation, for it referred only to the idea that effort was applied toward an objective, rather than toward the movement itself.[43]

The view of humans that emerged from this perspective perceived them as receptors of sensory stimuli, with programmed response patterns. By reducing occupation to purposeful activity defined in terms of goal-seeking, the perception of human performance became more mechanistic. The most efficacious way of viewing persons was as cybernetic, goal-seeking mechanisms that received sensory information and encoded it for motor output. While its proponents admirably espoused humanistic approaches to treatment,[8,83,117] the knowledge base of the neurologic approach created a mechanistic view.

PUZZLES. The clinical puzzles to be solved by the neurologic approach were those stressing breakdowns or dysfunctions in the central nervous system. Neurologically based diseases and disabilities such as the results of brain damage, cerebral palsy, and cerebral vascular accidents were included among the puzzles of this approach.[23,30] Clinicians and researchers also began to test and treat individuals experiencing behavior and learning problems as they sought neurologically based answers to these puzzles of dysfunction.[9] The approach also stressed the intimate link between the nervous system's maturation and readiness to learn a new skill.

WHAT THE PRACTITIONER MUST KNOW: THE KNOWLEDGE BASE OF OCCUPATIONAL THERAPY

The growing efforts of clinicians and researchers translated the neurologic puzzles with greater precision. Details of differing dysfunctional states and their neurologic bases became the points of scrutiny for the occupational therapist. Consider this excerpt from a paper discussing the neurophysiologic considerations of cerebral palsy:

> According to the neurophysiologically based view, cerebral palsy may be seen as the reflection of a lesion which manifests itself, to a large degree, by phylogenetically older postures and movements in association with abnormal muscle tone.[121]

In order to formulate treatment strategies for specific dysfunctions of the nervous system each problem was reduced to its elementary cause and effect relationship. For instance, in addressing the puzzle related to the development of body schema Ayres wrote:

> When a child does not learn through the normal course of development to synthesize impulses into a body schema, training procedures are based on increasing the flow of sensory impulses, developing a conscious knowledge of the construction and basic movements of the body, and associating the sensation and conscious knowledge through simple gross meaningful tasks.[5]

Thus the attention of this approach centered on precision in determining exactly what neurologic structures and processes were involved in a given problem. The puzzle was to isolate, identify, and attack the particular problem.

RATIONALE AND METHODS OF TREATMENT. The rationale and methods of treatment of the neurologic approach were grounded in developmental theories of growth and maturation of the nervous system. The principles of therapy included the proposal that sensory abilities develop in a definite sequence of learning to understand sensation, increasing ability to discriminate intensities, durations, and locations of sensation, and knowledge of sensation conceptualized to understand complex sensory inputs. As the sequence of development proceeds, higher level cortical functions are required to process the information.[6,8] Motor development follows a similar pattern of unfolding, with lower level centers controlling initial movements.

Methodologies developed from the traditions of Rood[141] and Bobath and Bobath[22] stressed inhibition of abnormal and facilitation of normal movement by the use of reflex-inhibiting patterns of posture and movement and by stimulating appropriate sensory channels. Reflex-inhibiting positioning and passive movement, verbal attention, duplicating of observed motion, sandbags to increase proprioception and brush stroking were among the methods of treatment used to improve central nervous system functioning.[22,157] The sensory-integration tradition based on the work of Ayres[8,9] stressed self-directed, purposeful, and playful activities, and the use of specialized equipment (especially for vestibular stimulation) for stimulating the sensory input to the child. While the importance of the patient's active participation and goal-directedness was emphasized in this latter framework, the basic rationale for the efficacy of therapy was, as with the other methodologies, based on neurologic principles. Thus it was with an understanding of the nervous system and the operation of its various components that occupational therapists began to treat the discrete parts that influenced the functioning of a person in everyday life.

GOALS. Proponents of the neurologic approach stressed the goals of careful evaluation of motor patterns and identification of underlying neurologic disorganization via standardized testing.[8,22,141,157] Patient goals were based on therapists' ability to analyze the level of reflexive maturation, to design reflex inhibition postures to normalize muscle tone, and to activate higher integrated movement reactions by facilitation.[8,22]

Progress toward these goals was measured through testing and observation. Functional activities were used to stimulate interest of the patient and ultimate movement. The central principle guiding therapy was to provide a "planned and controlled sensory input" for the purpose of "eliciting a related adaptive response in order to enhance the organization of brain mechanisms".[8]

Therapists using the neurologic approach sought to enhance the organization of the nervous system and to improve perception and motor capacity. Ayres[8,9] also included goals of increasing the patient's functional performance, ability for purposeful activity and self-esteem.

THE KINESIOLOGIC APPROACH

VIEW OF HUMANS. The kinesiologic approach provided a view of humans based on information about normal structures and functions of the musculoskeletal system. Thorough knowledge of movement was considered essential to understand the effects of disease and injury and resultant abnormal movement. Knowledge about mechanical concepts, the effects of exercise, the function of muscles during activity, the types of muscle contractions that occur during activity, and the influence of gravity and resistance on movement during the performance of a task was included in this model.[150]

Purposeful activity was used to analyze a body part in motion to determine the role of each muscle in performing the task. Once more, emphasis placed on movement qualities of an activity diminished the importance of the task's significance to the person. Therapists concentrated primarily on motions produced as the person participated in the task:

> Synergistic muscle may be used to prevent an unwanted movement, thus assisting in the performance of a task. Forcefully gripping a tool is used to illustrate this concept; the long finger flexors cross more than one joint and have the potential to act on each joint they cross. Forceful gripping of a tool would cause the wrist to flex if the wrist extensors did not contract synergistically to prevent this unwanted motion.[150]

Secondary significance was given to presenting interesting activities to the patient. The use of the term "functional activity" replaced the notion of purposefulness when selecting a task for a patient. A functional activity was defined by its distracting effect on individuals, permitting them to "focus on the activity instead of the goal of specific muscle or extremity function."[155]

This view of humans sought to understand movement as it influenced adaptive behavior. A person had to be able to perform daily activities that required motion. With attention concentrated on the details of motor performance, the importance of occupational behaviors and the satisfaction derived from them were diminished. The view of humans as motor mechanisms occasionally led to complete abandonment of meaningful occupations in therapy. For instance, Spackman[154] decried the common practice of therapists using sanding as a progressive resistive exercise without incorporating the activity into a woodworking project.

PUZZLES. The puzzles to be solved under the kinesiologic model were failures of movement. Observation, analysis, and testing of muscle groups gave information about how motion was limited or distorted. Polio, hemiplegia, rheumatoid arthritis, and other conditions affecting movement were the focus of clinicians. Muscles were classified according to their performance as prime movers, assistants, agonists, and stabilizers, and their status after trauma carefully examined.[30]

Occupational therapists also became interested in the role of proprioceptors in the joints, tendons, and muscles. From this perspective puzzles of altered and dysfunctional movement and perceptual patterns were noted. The study of how deficit motion disallowed performance of daily activities grew, and the gaps between movement and required life tasks also became puzzles of this perspective.

Energy conservation and efficiency of movement provided further puzzles to be solved by the occupational therapist. Consideration was to the everyday energy needs of the handicapped person returning to responsibilities outside of the hospital.

RATIONALE AND METHODS OF TREATMENT. Treatment programs were based on knowledge of the etiology of disease, prognosis, and potential side effects from prescribed drugs.[150] A wide range of treatment methods was available to the therapist for treating musculoskeletal deformities and dysfunction. The use of splinting for stabilizing a joint during active use, proper methods for positioning a patient for optimal performance, passive and active range of motion to affected extremities, and resistive exercise to develop muscle strength and coordination were primary methods used in therapy.

These methods were grounded in knowledge concerning the facilitation, stimulation, and re-education of muscle mass. This information was then integrated with activities so that a person could be engaged in a craft or art project while receiving stretching and conditioning of an affected arm or hand. The therapist became an expert in activity analysis, as indicated by the following:

> Sensory stimulus is developed through adapted cutaneous contact with tools, the beater of a loom, or the handle of a sander. . . . Gross motor reaching and throwing activities stimulate proprioception and kinesthetic awareness. . . . Use of a skateboard attached to the forearm for directed range of motion activities stimulates upper arm active movements.[155]

In addition, therapists became proficient in the manufacture and prescription of adaptive devices which bridged the gap between patients' limited motion and the tasks they had to perform. Therapists also served as trainers, enabling patients to learn techniques of self-care, dressing, and other performances within the constraints of their remaining motion and with the aid of assistive devices.

GOALS. The goals for occupational therapy intervention were derived from principles taken from pathology, including symptom reduction and disease arrest. For instance:

> The first goal in training is for the patient to acquire ability to perform the basic hemiplegic synergies of flexion and extension, which are the only feasible ones at first. It is believed that

these synergies, once mastered, may serve as stepping stones for more advanced work and that they can be considerably modified to serve various useful purposes.[30]

Different prescribed goals and stages in acquisition were established for each disability group. For example, goals for the patient with arthritis included the use of splints to prevent deformity, and instruction in joint protection measures when the individual engaged in daily living activities.[150] While the overall goals for occupational therapy service included the physical, psychologic, social and economic aspects of patients' lives,[30] they were more frequently articulated in terms of changes of motion or assistive devices which made particular performances possible.

THE PSYCHODYNAMIC APPROACH

VIEW OF HUMANS. The psychodynamic approach was based on Freudian principles as applied in American psychiatry. Human beings were seen as tension-reducing organisms seeking gratification of needs whose development was based on successful need fulfillment at various critical stages throughout life.[58]

The psychodynamic perspective stressed unconscious processes and their role in motivating human behavior,[10,62] while relationship with the environment was seen in terms of the ability to find gratification in objects and persons.[61] Defense mechanisms were ways of coping through which an individual managed to achieve need satisfaction in spite of environmental constraints.[10,123] Successful maturation depended on the ability of the individual to successfully employ defenses and to find gratification in interaction with objects and persons in the environment.

CLINICAL PUZZLES. The psychodynamic approach viewed patients' dysfunctional behavior as a result of internal tension (i.e., anxiety) or of early blocked needs which prevented maturation of the ego. Thus clinical puzzles were anxiety states, inabilities to achieve need satisfaction, and failures of maturation linked to early childhood experiences.[10,61,170] The therapist sought to determine the underlying conflicts or unfulfilled needs that blocked functioning, since these were the mechanisms to be altered in therapy. Activities were often used as a means of discovering patient's hidden feelings and unconscious motives, and therapists interpreted the unconscious meaning of colors, themes, and other characteristics that appeared in patient's creations.[107,170]

RATIONALE AND METHOD OF TREATMENT. The major rationale for occupational therapy was borrowed from the psychodynamic practice of psychiatry and from principles of milieu therapy.[59,107,170] It was believed that if a patient could learn to fulfill needs, and if he or she could recapitulate and satisfy blocked childhood needs, the intrapsychic conflict could be removed and the patient would return to healthy functioning in other aspects of life. Thus, the therapist enabled the patient to function more completely in daily life by directly modifying the pathologic condition that prevented normal behavior. This was accomplished by opening avenues for need fullfillment and ego maturation. Activities were first used as a means of allowing patients to achieve need satisfaction according to their previous level of need deprivation. Therapy thus included regression to stages in development that had not been completed and satisfied:

For the individual who needs to obtain satisfactions at an infantile level the occupational therapist structures and manipulates situations which make possible actual or symbolic gratification of oral or anal needs, dependency needs, infantile aggression, destruction or control and infantile play. For example, some activities which may offer satisfaction for oral and anal needs are those involving eating, preparation of food, blowing musical instruments, singing, et cetera, and those which use excretory substitutes such as smearing or building with clay or paints, preparation of soil, collecting garbage or trash, and others.[57]

A second approach to treatment was the use of activities as an arena for establishing a therapeutic relationship. In this approach the activities themselves held little meaning and the therapist's therapeutic use of self was the real therapy:

The effective therapeutic approach in occupational therapy today and in the future is one in which the therapist utilizes the tools of his trade as an avenue of introduction. From then on his personality takes over.[40]

The personality of the therapist was used in a manner which would permit the patient to develop healthy means of resolving intrapsychic conflict and fulfilling needs. Other methods of treatment stressed the use of group dynamics as a force in facilitating learning and behavioral change. Therapists used methods of facilitating group interaction in activity oriented situations. This task-oriented situation provided a shared work experience where relationships between feeling, thinking, and behavior were explored.[59] Overall treatment strategies were conceptualized as a means of providing pleasurable experiences for patients and for giving opportunity to act out or sublimate feelings.[62] In craft activities patients learned to express and control their feelings, to be less frightened of reality, and to relate to other human beings. Treatment was focused on the feeling aspect of the patient's experience and ability to achieve insight and control over those feelings.

GOALS. The goals of occupational therapy in this approach included the development of ego skills, mastery over feelings, and increased interpersonal abilities.[62,107] Underlying these goals was the broad objective of allowing patients to achieve need satisfaction, thus reducing intrapsychic tension. When this occurred, it was felt that the patient would return to normal functioning.

SUMMARY

We have shown that a paradigm of inner mechanisms (Fig. 4) emerged in the 1960s as a new pattern of thinking and practice in occupational therapy to replace the humanistic and holistic paradigm of occupation. There was a shift in focus from occupation as a basic human trait to viewing persons through internal mechanisms. Along with this shift the puzzles, treatment methods, and goals of the field changed. Figure 4 summarizes the paradigm and its expression in three treatment approaches.

This paradigm of inner mechanisms resulted in both gains and losses for the field. Among the gains was a substantially increased technology of remediating specific dysfunctions. In many ways the potential of occupations to modify pathologic conditions of patients was more clearly articulated. The paradigm also resulted in a deeper understanding of how bodily structures and processes made possible or limited occupational

	VIEW OF HUMAN BEINGS	CLINICAL PUZZLES	RATIONALE AND METHODS OF TREATMENT	GOALS
Paradigm of Inner Mechanisms	Internal workings of the body and mind and their patterns of function and development	Disruptions and failures of an internal order and its sequence of change	Evaluating and modifying internal mechanisms to approximate pre-established criteria of function	Reduce dysfunctions in the internal mechanisms and/or modify their functional roles
Neurologic Approach	Receptors of sensory stimuli with programmed motor responses	Dysfunctions of the central nervous system	Assessing and using patterns of normal nervous system development	Evaluation and facilitation of central nervous system development
Kinesiologic Approach	Motor mechanisms for task performance	Failures of movement and strength	Methods of muscle strenghtening and re-education and adaptive/assistive equipment	Evaluation and restoration or adaptation of functional movement
Psychodynamic Approach	Tension-reducing mechanisms seeking gratification	Anxiety states, blocked needs, and ego immaturity	Need satisfaction and ego maturation through activities and the therapeutic relationship	Development of ego skills, mastery over feelings, and increased interpersonal abilites

FIGURE 4. The paradigm of inner mechanisms and its treatment approaches.

performance. The field acquired a growing technology of adapting devices and environments to the needs of persons with motor impairment. The psychodynamic perspective increased understanding of how emotional pathology might interfere with competent performance and elaborated the role of emotions in behavior.

The major loss of the field under this paradigm was its commitment to the occupational nature of humans. This was the common thread of early practice, and without it, specialties of the field began to drift further apart. The rationale and methods of employing occupation as therapy narrowed, and new concepts of purposeful activity and of activity as a psychotherapeutic medium offered an impoverished rationale for therapy compared with that of early practice. Not surprisingly, the centrality of occupation as therapy faded, and therapists had less appreciation of the importance of the patient's experience when engaging in occupations. Eventually occupations were dropped from the practice of some therapists altogether as they adopted pure exercise, talk groups, and nonoccupational techniques as therapy. Some leaders such as Fiorentino[64] viewed activities as superfluous means of relaxation, proposing that occupational therapy use other methods suggested by growing neurophysiologic knowledge. These and other losses eventually returned occupational therapy to a period of crisis. A new set of problems emerged to challenge the viability of the paradigm of internal mechanisms.

THE PRESENT CRISIS OF OCCUPATIONAL THERAPY

Three circumstances appear to have contributed to the transition from the paradigm of inner mechanisms to a period of crisis. They are (a) general recognition that reductionism was an inadequate scientific framework, (b) growing awareness that the problems of chronically disabled persons could not be handled by medical technology alone, and (c) internal dissatisfaction of occupational therapists at their loss of identity and lack of unifying principles.

BEYOND REDUCTIONISM

In the biologic and behavioral sciences there has been a growing recognition during the second half of the century that reductionism was an inadequate scientific framework. Von Bertalanffy[18] initiated a movement in biology which recognized the need for gestalt principles and scientific methods in addition to those provided by reductionism. This theme was echoed by Koestler,[96] Boulding,[25] and other scientists concerned with human behavior. Since it failed to provide a framework broad enough for the study of human phenomena, there was a call for science to move beyond reductionism. Laslo describes this failure of reductionism as follows:

> Since the time of Galileo and Newton, modern science has been dominated by the ideal of explanation by reduction to the smallest isolable component's behavior in causal terms. Phenomena, however complex, were sought to yield isolated causal relations, and the sum of these were believed to constitute an explanation of the phenomena themselves. Thus two-variable linear causal interaction emerged as the principal mode of scientific explanation, applying to the primitive components of a given complex of events. Explanation in these terms presupposed atomism and mechanism as a general world view. But when contemporary science progressed to the rigorous observation, experimental testing, and interpretation of what Warren Weaver called "phenomena of organized complexity," such explanations no longer functioned.
>
> Complex phenomena proved to be more than the simple sum of the properties of isolated causal chains, or of the properties of their components taken separately.[99]

In the life sciences there was a general call for "emancipation of the life sciences from the mechanistic concepts of nineteenth-century physics and the resulting crudely reductionist philosophy."[96] This proposal was based on the recognition that the reductionist strategy of understanding living processes by examining isolated units of reality and piecing together the information would not work.[25,168] In order to go beyond reductionism, theorists called for a newer view of human beings than that which reductionism yielded. For instance, von Bertalanffy noted:

> I, for one, am unable to see how, for example, creative and cultural activities of all sorts can be regarded as "response to stimuli," "gratification of biological needs," "reestablishment of homeostasis" or the like. . . . Man is not a passive receiver of stimuli coming from an external world, but in a very real concrete sense *creates* his universe.[17]

Reductionism was criticized for having created a passive, mechanistic, and automaton-like version of human behavior.[18] It was proposed that humans must be recognized as conscious, striving, and highly complex beings whose organization involved a multitude of interrelated dimensions. The call for moving beyond reductionism created an intellectual climate in which occupational therapy's reductionist-based paradigm of inner mechanisms appeared incomplete. Reilly introduced this theme, charging that occupational therapy had achieved too narrow a perspective, noting that its mechanistic concepts provided insufficient explanations for the effects of occupation on patients.[135]

TECHNOLOGIC MEDICINE AND THE CHRONICALLY DISABLED

Within the health services arena the reductionistic, homeostatic view of persons accepted by the medical model especially failed to address the problems of the chronically disabled.[46,143] The problems of this group extended beyond deficits of internal mechanisms to their failure to thrive in society. Some critics of medicine suggested that the advanced technology of medicine (a result of reductionism), because of its narrowed approach not only failed in its efforts to help persons, but also created additional problems. Illich[84] labeled technical medicine socially and culturally iatrogenic, charging that it often robbed individuals of their own coping abilities and of those inherent in their social systems. Dubos[46] warned that medicine's promise of health through manipulating internal conditions of the human being was unrealistic. He located true health in the human struggle to adapt to the environment.

It appeared that in its attempts to delve deeply into the inner mechanisms of patients, medicine has lost sight of the humanistic and cultural dimension of its mission. Riley argued that medicine's search for a purely scientific approach was not altogether functional for increasing the health of persons. He notes:

> Indeed, it may be that in some situations the alternative to ostensibly scientific medicine can be *more* effective in ameliorating suffering, as a direct result of not being distracted by a preeminent commitment to scientificness, by being less concerned with the technical, biomedical problems than with the patient's state of mind and feeling of well-being.[137]

Navarro proposed that many persons who turned to consumption of health services (the technologic services of modern medicine) really suffered from loss of control over their work and play lives:

> The most important components in one's life, creativity and worthiness, are not realized in one's daily work. In other words, the worker must spend time at work to get freedom and capacity for development outside the sphere of production and work. Ironically, this hope for fulfillment during leisure time turns out to be an illusion, an illusion that has to be satisfied with the always unsatisfied and never ending consumption. . . . Thus, in the medical care system we also find that (1) the alienation of the individual in his world of production leads him to the sphere of consumption, the consumption of health services; and that (2) the medical care bureaucracy is just administering those disturbances created by the nature of work and the alienating nature of our system of production.[122]

In occupational therapy there was growing recognition of the limitations of technology for practice. Noting that a new focus was emerging in health that focused on intractable chronic conditions, West proposed that occupational therapy prepare itself for a shift away from a purely technologic orientation:

> Health and medical care in the future, then, will emphasize human development by programs designed to promote better adaptation, rather than by technologically oriented programs offering specific solutions to specific difficulties.[171]

Yerxa[175] argued that authentic occupational therapy began with the patient's own experience of meaning in therapy, calling for a more humanistic orientation. Reilly[133] proposed that the occupational therapist's role was as caretaker of the patient's healthy behavior, noting that this process required occupational therapy to function as a social or cultural milieu which elicited and supported competence. She charged that the focus of the current paradigm on internal mechanisms fell short of preparing disabled persons to achieve satisfaction and productivity in their lives. Reilly[132] proposed that knowledge of the nervous and musculoskeletal systems and emotional pathology was necessary, but not adequate for occupational therapy to serve the needs of the chronically disabled.

LOSS OF IDENTITY AND UNIFYING PRINCIPLES

There was a growing recognition in the 1970s that occupational therapy lacked a unifying theoretical base. Gillette[71], Johnson[88], Mosey[120], and West[172] all called for a broader framework which would permit an understanding of humans' ability to function in the environment. Reilly[132] argued that approaches and knowledge borrowed from the medical model would not be sufficient to support the practice of occupational therapy; she called for the field to return its attention to the need for activity and the ability of persons to restore their health through their own efforts.

Mosey[120] charged that occupational therapists had become oriented to specific disease categories without recognizing underlying principles, noting that this condition relegated occupational therapy to a position of technical rather than professional practice. She also questioned the close ties of occupational therapy to medicine, pointing to the field's need for an independent theoretical base. Diasio[45] similarly questioned the centrality of medical knowledge in occupational therapy, supporting a movement toward the behavioral sciences. Rerek[136] charged that occupational therapy had lost its most seminal idea: the importance of occupation as a health restoring measure.

The Task Force on Target Populations noted growing disparity in occupational therapy practice:

> If occupational therapy is to survive as a profession, the schisms within the profession related to diagnostic or disability entities need to be removed by focusing on the essence of occupational therapy rather than a disability or pathological orientation. The disability orientation is actually in opposition to the basic philosophy of occupational therapy which stresses the reinforcement of personal assets through development and strengthening of adapting, coping, and negotiating skills.[159]

The members of this task force also noted that there was a serious blurring of the basic identity of occupational therapy. In a similar vein, Shannon[146] pointed out that there was neither a descriptive nor normative definition of occupational therapy. He charged that the symbiosis of occupational therapy with medicine had diverted the field from its original mission.

The impetus of these issues, the failure of reductionism, the requirements of the chronically disabled, and the loss of identity and unity in occupational therapy, comprise the central problems which led to the current crisis.

DYNAMICS OF THE CRISIS

During a crisis period it is common for several competing perspectives to contest for dominance, and occupational therapy's current status reflects this phenomenon. In the 1960s and 1970s Reilly and her students developed a theoretical base called occupational behavior. The tenets of this base included, (a) a return to the early principles of occupational therapy, including a central focus on occupation;[116,132,139,145,160] (b) the recognition of the human motivation for occupation;[34,65] (c) study of the human sense of time, purposefulness, and personal responsibility for adaptation;[93,165,174] (d) examination of the organizing influence of occupational roles on behavior;[78,111] (e) the importance of the environment in supporting or impeding adaptation;[47,74] (f) the role of occupational therapy as a socializing process in which patients learned competence through exploration and struggle with life tasks;[133,165] and (g) the integration of interdisciplinary knowledge needed for this perspective under a holistic framework focused on the dynamic of human interaction with the environment.[78,94,111,135,139]

Another theme which emerged in the writings of several authors was that of integrating the scope of occupational therapy knowledge under the framework of human development. The work of each of these writers is eclectic, seeking collection of diverse concepts under the perspective of ontogenesis. For example, Mosey[118] proposed ontogenetic schema which included perceptual motor, cognitive, drive-object, dyadic interaction, primary group interaction, self identity and sexual identity skills. In her schema disability was a failure of the individual to develop along the ontogenetic continuum. Remediation focused on acquiring skills in a sequential manner and recapitulating ill-formed stages.[118,119] Llorens[106] used a similar approach, including neurophysiologic, physical-motor, psychologic, psychodynamic, and sociocultural dimensions in her developmental model. Clark[39] attempts to include in her model of development through occupation, occupational behavior together with the biodevelopmental adaptive performance perspective and the facilitating growth and development perspective. She identifies the four approaches in the literature and emphasizes their commonalities in viewing human behavior as a developmental process. Finally, she proposes an integration of these perspectives for clinical practice.[38] Banus, Kent, Norton, Sukiennicki and Becker[13] propose a developmental schema for therapy in pediatrics. Like the writers mentioned above, they include several dimensions of development in their approach to therapy.

All of these writers supported the importance of activities in facilitating and nurturing normal development. However, their eclectic approaches to identifying dimensions of the developing individual did not center on occupation as the earlier group had. They viewed purposeful activity solely for its properties as a therapeutic medium, while the earlier group emphasized that the study of occupation was itself central and required for its effective use as therapy. The occupational behavior school proposed that occupational therapy had a special caretaker role for the human need to master self and the environment and thus achieve productivity and satisfaction. The developmental perspectives proposed no such focus, addressing a wide range of sexual, social, biologic and other needs.

In addition to these two perspectives the neurologic approach gained increasing momentum and support in both clinical practice and research. Spearheaded by the earlier work of Ayres,[7,8] Bobath and Bobath,[22] and Rood[141] neurologic principles were extended into treatment for persons of all ages and a variety of disabilities. The development of this approach has continued along the lines outlined earlier in this chapter.

Occupational therapy continues without a single unifying base. As clinical, research, and theoretical efforts follow separate paths and therapists practicing in one specialty find little in common with those in another. Knowledge and technique accumulate, but not in a coherent fashion, and students, educators and practitioners are left to make their way through a morass of information and procedures which often bear little resemblance to each other.

THE FUTURE OF THE FIELD: RESOLVING CRISIS

The purpose of this final section is not to predict how the field *will* resolve its crisis but to propose a possible route. We begin with a brief review of the dynamics of paradigm change.

A field in crisis is fraught with different perspectives which compete for dominance. This is a transitory state of affairs which results in the *predominance* of *one* perspective. This does not mean that other perspectives are dismissed or that there is no continuity with the pre-crisis paradigm. Rather, the dominant perspective which becomes the focus of the new paradigm is a point of reference for organizing knowledge from other perspectives. It may dictate a reshuffling and redefinition of concepts from other perspectives. It may set priorities of knowledge, puzzles, methods, and so forth. As the leading segment of the field's knowledge base it exerts a ruling influence over other areas of knowledge, a process that occurred when the paradigm of inner mechanisms relegated concepts of occupation to secondary importance.

Because of these features of scientific revolution it would not be realistic to suggest that the future of the field will achieve a simple blending of perspectives. The kind of integration that some writers seek through attaching disparate knowledge bases to the structure of human development does not seem to us a suitable resolution to the present crisis. Moreover, the concept of development does little to resolve problems which brought the field into crisis. The growing neurophysiologically based body of knowledge and practice is undoubtedly an important part of the field's technology, but it also appears to us ill-suited as an overall framework for occupational therapy. It neither defines the unique role of occupational therapy nor does it respond to the irremediable problems of chronic disability. In addition, it remains largely grounded in reductionist principles.

We must agree with Shannon[146] that the best hope of the field is a return to the fundamental principles of the original paradigm. The occupational behavior school has begun this process and the knowledge generated in this perspective has reintroduced the articulation of the occupational nature of humans and the principles of utilizing occupation as therapy.

The focus on human occupation which this approach espouses appears to us the most reasonable rallying point for the field. As Wiemer notes:

> Ours is, and must be, the basic knowledge of occupation. It is that knowledge which permits the occupational therapist to look at an activity of daily living in a unique way, and so determine best how to facilitate the patient's or client's goal achievement. Our exclusive

domain is occupation. We must refine, research, systematize it so that it becomes evident, definable, defensible and salable. The "impact of occupation on human beings" was spelled out as our sole claim to professionalism by our founders in 1917. It is our latent power if we will but keep it as our focus and direction.[167]

While our paradigm must center its attention on occupation, this will not require us to abandon or reject ideas developed in the preceding paradigm that continue to be developed. The emergence of a paradigm calls for a reorganization and priority of knowledge, and this is our proposal.

The most difficult aspect of this process will be the organizational task of integrating knowledge, for it will require more than an eclectic approach that merely gathers a diverse set of concepts under an umbrella theme. Such divergent bodies of knowledge as neurophysiology and role theory are not easily integrated, and their association in human phenomena is a complex process.

Recommitment to the ideas of the paradigm of occupation does not imply a step backward to a prescientific way of thinking. The concepts of the early paradigm must be, as Reilly[134] specifies, modernized to reflect current thinking. This means that we must make use of current knowledge that was not available for the early paradigm. Recommitment to the early focus on the occupational nature of human beings permits us to turn attention to vast stores of contemporary information concerning the evolution of human capacity and its infrastructure and supporting environment—the brain and cultural technology. Because knowledge concerning the work and play behavior of human beings comes from many diverse sources, an interdisciplinary study of occupation within the field will be required. Such knowledge must not be gathered as a composition of eclectic ideas, but as part of a unified perspective that centers on human occupation. The synthesis of diverse information is the challenge of the future.[161] The process will require collecting and integrating knowledge which defines, elaborates, and explains the occupational nature of humans, and that enriches our knowledge of its healing and health-restoring capacity.

For this reason occupational therapy will find it necessary to examine emerging frameworks for integrating interdisciplinary thinking. General systems theory was developed for the explicit purpose of facilitating connections between diverse bodies of knowledge.[25] It is well suited as a framework within which occupational therapy theories may be organized to comprise a single paradigm.

Such a reorganization will not be easy, whether as a cognitive or an emotional task. Currently, individuals in the field are likely to be knowledgeable in a specialty area or in some school of thought. Development of a generic paradigm will require complex negotiation between these points of view and the concerns for theory and practice. The size and complexity of the task is outweighed only by its importance to the integrity, efficacy, and survival of occupational therapy.

SUMMARY AND CONCLUSION

In this chapter we presented a history of the theory and practice of occupational therapy according to a schema provided by Kuhn.[97] In concert with his thesis, scientific and professional development was viewed as a sociohistorical process that is revolutionary,

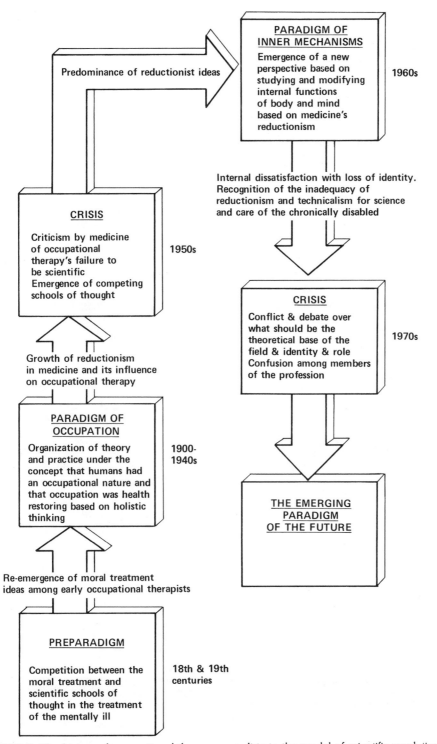

FIGURE 5. The history of occupational therapy according to the model of scientific revolution.

rather than cumulative. The course of change in occupational therapy, as reflected in the literature, supports such a view of its development. Occupational therapy has not merely added knowledge to its stockpile over the past decades, but has undergone profound shifts in its most fundamental orientations and in its clinical technologies.

The chapter identified and documented the following historical events, illustrated in Figure 5: (a) the emergence of a paradigm of occupation early in this century based on moral treatment ideas from the previous centuries; (b) a crisis in the 1950s centered on the failure of occupational therapy to meet the criteria of reductionist science; (c) the emergence of a paradigm of inner mechanisms in the 1960s; (d) a period of crisis beginning in the 1970s precipitated by recognition of the limitations of reductionism for science and of technology for the needs of the chronically disabled and by the internal confusion and incoherence of occupational therapy.

The crisis continues today and creates the need for resolution through acceptance of a new paradigm to unite the field. We have argued that such a paradigm must recommit itself to the early principles of the paradigm of occupation, retain the accumulated technology from the paradigm of inner mechanisms, and center its concerns on human occupation. The paradigm would recognize the special caretaker role of the field for the occupational behavior of ill and disabled persons and a special technology of health through occupation. Finally, we noted that the field's complex body of knowledge will need to be organized under the framework of general systems theory.

Conducting this historical analysis has taught us that examining the past is a much more secure task than planning for the future. However, we remain convinced that both are interconnected and that lessons can be drawn from the past to chart directions for the future. Of all the lessons to be learned, one appears most outstanding. Our heritage is the art and science of healing through occupation, a process which is not simple, nor is it easily grasped or explained. It is paradoxically commonplace yet elusive. It has often been misunderstood and underestimated by those within and outside of the field who seek to describe its essence in narrow or loosely construed propositions. Consequently, it is an idea that requires tough-minded commitment, the struggle of understanding and application, and a measure of vision from its practitioners, researchers, and students. The field has a single yet multifaceted mission: to serve the occupational needs of the disabled and to preserve their health through occupation. The years ahead will show whether occupational therapy will fulfill the greatness of its original ideal and its mission. We know it can, and we believe it will.

REFERENCES

1. ALLEN, W: *Industrial training for the blind.* Occupational Therapy and Rehabilitation, 20:179, 1941.

2. AYRES, AJ: *Ontogenetic principles in the development of arm and hand functions.* American Journal of Occupational Therapy, 8:95, 121, 1954, p 300.

3. AYRES, AJ: *Basic concepts of clinical practice in physical disabilities.* American Journal of Occupational Therapy, 12:300, 1958.

4. AYRES, AJ: *The visual-motor function.* American Journal of Occupational Therapy, 12:130, 155, 1958.

WHAT THE PRACTITIONER MUST KNOW:
THE KNOWLEDGE BASE OF OCCUPATIONAL THERAPY

5. AYRES, AJ: *Development of the body scheme in children.* American Journal of Occupational Therapy, 15:99, 1961, p 4.

6. AYRES, AJ: *The development of perceptual motor abilities: A theoretical basis for treatment of dysfunction.* American Journal of Occupational therapy, 17:221, 1963.

7. AYRES, AJ: *Occupational therapy directed toward neuromuscular integration.* In WILLARD, HS AND SPACKMAN, CS (EDS) Occupational Therapy, ed 3, JB Lippincott, Philadelphia, 1963.

8. AYRES, AJ: *Sensory integration and learning disorders.* Western Psychological Services, Los Angeles, 1972, 266.

9. AYRES, AJ: *The development of sensory integrative theory and practice.* Kendal & Hunt, Dubuque, Iowa, 1974.

10. AZIMA, H and AZIMA, F: *Outline of a dynamic theory of occupational therapy.* American Journal of Occupational Therapy, 13:215, 1959, p 216.

11. AZIMA, H AND WITTKOWER, E: *Apartial field survey of psychiatric occupational therapy.* American Journal of Occupational Therapy, 11:1, 1957.

12. BALDWIN, BT: *Occupational therapy applied to restoration of function of disabled joints.* Walter Reed Monograph, 1919.

13. BANUS, B, et al: The Developmental Therapist (ed 2). Charles B. Slack, Thorofare, NJ, 1979.

14. BARTON, G: *Teaching the sick: a manual of occupational therapy and re-education.* WB Saunders, Philadelphia, 1919.

15. BENNETT, R AND DRIVER, M: *The aims and methods of occupational therapy in the treatment of the after-effects of poliomyelitis.* American Journal of Occupational Therapy, 11:145, 1957.

16. BERGER, P AND LUCKMANN, T: *The social construction of reality.* Anchor Books, New York, 1967.

17. VON BERTALANFFY, L: *General systems theory.* George Braziller, New York, 1968, p 193.

18. VON BERTALANFFY, L: *General systems theory and psychiatry.* In ARIETI, S (ed) *American handbook of psychiatry (Vol. 3).* Basic Books, New York, 1966.

19. BING, R: *Occupational therapy revisited: A paraphrastic journey.* American Journal of Occupational Therapy, 35:499, 1981, p 502, 504.

20. BLANTON, L: *Exercise to develop range of motion of the forearm.* American Journal of Occupational Therapy, 8:263, 1954.

21. BOBATH, B: *The importance of the reduction of muscle tone and the control of mass reflex action in the treatment of spasticity.* Occupational Therapy and Rehabilitation, 27:371, 1948.

22. BOBATH, K AND BOBATH, B: *The facilitation of normal postural reactions and movements in the treatment of cerebral palsy.* Physiotherapy, 50:246, 1964.

23. BOBATH, K AND BOBATH, B: *Cerebral palsy.* In PEARSON, P AND WILLIAMS, C (EDS), *Physical therapy services in the developmental disabilities.* Charles C Thomas, Springfield, Ill, 1972.

24. BOCKOVEN, JS: *Moral treatment in community mental health.* Springer Publishing, New York, 1972.

25. BOULDING, K: *General systems theory — the skeleton of science.* In BUCKELEY, W (ED) *Modern systems research for the behavioral scientist.* Aldine, Chicago, 1968.

26. BOYCE, M: *Plastic splints.* American Journal of Occupational Therapy 6:203, 1952.

27. BRANDT, H: *Research — a guidepost for growth.* American Journal of Occupational Therapy 7:60, 80, 1953.

28. BRONOWSKI, J: *The character of science.* In C. HUGHES (ED) *Custom made* (ed 2). Rand McNally, Chicago, 1976.

29. BROWN, M: *Daily activity inventory and progress record for those with atypical movement.* American Journal of Occupational Therapy, 5:23, 38, 1951.

30. BRUNNSTROM, S: *Motor behavior of adult hemiplegic patients.* American Journal of Occupational Therapy 15:6, 47, 1961.

31. BRUNYATE, R: *Occupational therapy for patients with cerebral palsy.* In WILLARD, HS, AND SPACKMAN, CS (EDS), *Principles of occupational therapy.* JB Lippincott, Philadelphia, 1947.

32. BRYAN, W: *Administrative psychiatry.* WW Norton, New York, 1936.

33. BUHLER, C: *Values in psychotherapy.* Free Press, New York 1962.

34. BURKE, J: *A clinical perspective on motivation: Pawn versus origin.* American Journal of Occupational Therapy 31:254, 1977.

35. CAMPBELL, C: *Weaving as a habit training project.* Occupational Therapy and Rehabilitation 23:124, 1944.

36. CAPLAN, R: *Psychiatry and the community in 19th century America.* Basic Books, New York, 1969.

37. CHRISTRUP, H: *The new look in industrial therapy.* American Journal of Occupational Therapy 11:276, 291, 1957.

38. CLARK, P: *Human development through occupation: A philosophy and conceptual model for practice, Part 2.* American Journal of Occupational Therapy 33:577, 1979.

39. CLARK, P: *Human development through occupation: Theoretical frameworks in contemporary occupational therapy practice, Part 1.* American Journal of Occupational Therapy 33:505, 1979.

40. CONTE, W: *The occupational therapist as a therapist.* American Journal of Occupational Therapy 14:1, 12, 1960.

41. CRAIG, H AND HENDIN J: *Toys for children with cerebral palsy.* American Journal of Occupational Therapy 5:50, 1951.

42. CROMWELL, F: *A procedure for pre-vocation evaluation.* American Journal of Occupational Therapy 13:1, 1959.

43. CURRAN, PA: *A study toward a theory of neuromuscular education through occupational therapy.* American Journal of Occupational Therapy 14:80, l960.

44. CYNKIN, S: *Occupational therapy: Toward health through activities.* Little Brown and Co, Boston, 1979.

45. DIASIO, K: *The modern era — 1960-1970.* American Journal of Occupational Therapy 25:237, 1971.

46. DUBOS, R: *Mirage of health.* Harper & Row, New York, 1959.

47. DUNNING, H: *Environmental occupational therapy.* American Journal of Occupational Therapy, 26:292, 1972.

48. DUNTON, WR: *Occupational therapy: A manual for nurses.* WB Saunders, Philadelphia, 1915.

49. DUNTON, WR: *Reconstruction therapy.* WB Saunders, Philadelphia 1919, p 65, 207.

50. DUNTON, WR: *The educational possibilities of occupational therapy in state hospitals.* Archives of Occupational Therapy, 1:403, 1922.

51. ELLIOTT, R: *Orthetics in poliomyelitis,* American Journal of Occupational Therapy, 11:135, 166, 1957.

52. ELTON, F: *Relationship of occupational therapy to rehabilitation.* Archives of Occupational Therapy, 3:101, 1924.

53. EMMETT, R: *Adaptation of homemaking skills for the hemiplegic woman.* American Journal of Occupational Therapy, 11:283, 290, 1957.

54. ESQUIROL, J: *Mental maladies.* Occupational Therapy and Rehabilitation, 26:181, 1947.

55. FELLOWS, R AND MCKILLIP, M: *Industrial therapy.* American Journal of Occupational Therapy, 4:154, 1950.

56. FIDLER, G: *The role of occupational therapy in a multi-discipline approach to psychiatric illness.* American Journal of Occupational Therapy, 11:8, 35, 1957.

57. FIDLER, G: *Some unique contributions of occupational therapy in treatment of the schizophrenic.* American Journal of Occupational Therapy, 12:9, 36, 1958.

58. FIDLER, G: *A second look at work as a primary force in rehabilitation and treatment.* American Journal of Occupational Therapy, 20:72, 1966.

59. FIDLER, G: *The task-oriented group as a context for treatment.* American Journal of Occupational Therapy. 23:43, 1969.

60. FIDLER, G: *From crafts to competence.* American Journal of Occupational Therapy, 35:567, 1981.

61. FIDLER, G AND FIDLER, J: *Introduction to psychiatric occupational therapy.* Macmillan, New York, 1958.

62. FIDLER, G AND FIDLER, J: *Occupational therapy: A communication process in psychiatry.* Macmillan, New York, 1963.

63. FILSTEAD, W: *Qualitative methods: A needed perspective in evaluation research.* In COOK, T AND REICHARDT, C (EDS): *Qualitative and quantitative methods in evaluation research.* Sage, Beverly Hills, 1979.

64. FIORENTINO, M: *Occupational therapy: Realization to activation.* American Journal of Occupational Therapy, 29:15, 1975.

65. FLOREY, L: *Intrinsic motivation: The dynamics of occupational therapy theory.* American Journal of Occupational Therapy, 23:319, 1969.

66. FORBES, E: *Two devices for use in treating hemiplegics.* American Journal of Occupational Therapy, 5:49, 1951.

67. FRANK, J: *The therapeutic use of self.* American Journal of Occupational Therapy, 12, 215, 1958.

68. FREIDSON, E: *Profession of medicine.* Harper & Row, New York, 1970.

69. FULLER, D: *The need of instruction for nurses in occupations for the sick.* In TRACY, S: *Studies in invalid occupation.* Whitcomb and Barrows, Boston, 1912, p 2, 7.

70. GARDNER, J, AND MORGAN N: *Industrial therapy.* American Journal of Occupational Therapy, 7:250, 1953.

71. GILLETTE, N: *Changing methods in the treatment of psychosocial dysfunction*. American Journal of Occupational Therapy, 21:230, 1967.

72. GILLETTE, N AND KIELHOFNER, G: *The impact of specialization on the professionalization and survival of occupational therapy*. American Journal of Occupational Therapy, 33:20, 1979.

73. GOTTSCHALK, L: *Understanding history: A primer of historical method* (ed. 2). Knopf, New York, 1969.

74. GRAY, M: *Effects of hospitalization on work-play behavior*. American Journal of Occupational Therapy, 26:180, 1972.

75. HASS, L: *Practical occupational therapy*. Bruce Publishing, Milwaukee, 1944.

76. HALL, H: *O.T.: A new profession*. Rumford Press, Concord, 1923, p 1, 57, 48.

77. HALLIBURTON, J: *A note on the resolution of agressive impulses through creative-destructive activity*. Occupational Therapy and Rehabilitation, 23:284, 1944.

78. HEARD, C: *Occupational role acquisition: A perspective on the chronically disabled*. American Journal of Occupational Therapy, 31:243, 1977.

79. HUDSON, B: *What is research?* American Journal of Occupational Therapy, 8:140, 150, 1954.

80. HULTKRANS, R AND SANDEEN, A: *Application of progressive resistive exercise to occupational therapy*. American Journal of Occupational Therapy, 11:238, 1957.

81. HURT, S: *Occupational therapy with orthopedic and surgical conditions*. Occupational Therapy and Rehabilitation, 20:149, 1941.

82. HURT, S: *Occupational therapy in the rehabilitation of the poliomyelitis patient*. American Journal of Occupational Therapy, 2:83, 1948.

83. HUSS, AJ: *Touch with care or a caring touch?* American Journal of Occupational Therapy, 31:11, 1977.

84. ILLICH, I: *Medical nemesis: The expropriation of health*. Pantheon Books, New York, 1976.

85. IRELAND, K: *Tool holding device for a guadriplegic patient*. American Journal of Occupational Therapy, 8:266, 1954.

86. JACKSON, F: *A device to supply a more comprehensive kinetic therapy in occupational therapy*. American Journal of Occupational Therapy, 8:158, 185, 1954.

87. JANTZEN, AC: *Some strengths of occupational therapy*. American Journal of Occupational Therapy, 16:124, 1962.

88. JOHNSON, J: *Occupational therapy: A model for the future*. American Journal of Occupational Therapy, 27:1, 1973.

89. JOHNSON, J: *Old values — new directions: Competence, adaptation, integration*. American Journal of Occupational Therapy, 35:589. 1981.

90. KABAT, H AND ROSENBERG, D: *Concepts and techniques of occupational therapy for neuromuscular disorders*. American Journal of Occupational Therapy, 4:6, 1950.

91. KIDNER, TB: *Work for the tuberculous during and after the cure*. Archives of Occupational Therapy, 1:363, 1922.

92. KIDNER, TB: *Occupational therapy The science of prescribed work for invalids*. W Kohlhammer, Stuttgart, Germany, 1930, p 28, 26, 19.

93. KIELHOFNER, G: *Temporal adaptation: A conceptual framework for occupational therapy*. American Journal of Occupational Therapy, 31:235, 1977.

94. KIELHOFNER, G: *General systems theory: Implications for theory and action in occupational therapy.* American Journal of Occupational Therapy, 32:637, 1978.

95. KING, LJ: *Toward a science of adaptive responses.* American Journal of Occupational Therapy, 32:429, 1978.

96. KOESTLER, A. Beyond atomism and holism—the concept of the holon. In A. KOESTER AND JR SMYTHIES (EDS), *Beyond reductionism.* Boston: Beacon Press, 1969.

97. KUHN, T: *The structure of scientific revolutions* (ED. 2). University of Chicago Press, Chicago, 1970.

98. KUHN, T: *The essential tension.* University of Chicago Press, Chicago, 1977.

99. LASLO, E: *The relevance of general systems theory.* George Braziller, New York, 1972, p 5.

100. LEIFER, R: *In the name of mental health.* Science House, New York, 1969.

101. LEURET, F: *On the moral treatment of insanity.* Occupational Therapy and Rehabilitation, 27:27, 1948.

102. LICHT, S: *Kinetic analysis of crafts and occupations.* Occupational Therapy and Rehabilitation, 26:75, 1947.

103. LICHT, S: *Modern trends in occupational therapy.* Occupational Therapy and Rehabilitation, 26:455, 1947.

104. LICHT, S: *Modifications of tools and activities in kinetic occupational therapy.* Occupational Therapy and Rehabilitation, 26:240, 1947.

105. LICHT, S: *Occupational therapy sourcebook.* Williams & Wilkins, Baltimore, 1948.

106. LLORENS, LA: *Facilitating growth and development: The promise of occupational therapy.* American Journal of Occupational Therapy, 24:93, 1970.

107. LLORENS, LA AND YOUNG, GG: *Fingerpainting for the hostile child.* American Journal of Occupational Therapy, 14:306, 1960.

108. LUCCI, J: *Daily living achievements of the adult traumatic quadriplegic.* American Journal of Occupational Therapy, 12:144, 160, 1958.

109. MAGARO, P, GRIPP, R AND McDOWELL, D: *The mental health industry: A cultural phenomenon.* John Wiley and Sons, New York, 1978.

110. MARSH, C: *Borzoi: Suggestions for a new rallying of occupational therapy.* Archives of Occupational Therapy, 11:169, 1932.

111. MATSUTSUYU, J: *Occupational behavior—a perspective on work and play.* American Journal of Occupational Therapy, 25:291, 1971.

112. McNARY, H: *The scope of occupational therapy.* In WILLARD, HS, AND SPACKMAN, CS, (EDS), *Principles of occupational therapy.* JB Lippincott, Philadelphia, 1947.

113. McNARY, H: *A look at occupational therapy.* American Journal of Occupational Therapy, 12:203, 1958, p 203.

114. MEYER, A: *The philosophy of occupational therapy.* Archives of Occupational Therapy, 1:1, 1922, p 5.

115. MEYERSON, L: *Some observations on the psychological roles of the occupational therapist.* American Journal of Occupational Therapy, 11:131, 1957, p 131.

116. MICHELMAN, S: The importance of creative play. American Journal of Occupational Therapy, 25:285, 1971.

117. MOORE, J: Individual differences and the art of therapy. American Journal of Occupational Therapy, 31:663, 1977.

118. MOSEY, A: *Recapitulation of ontogenesis: A theory for practice of occupational therapy.* American Journal of Occupational Therapy, 22:426, 1968.

119. MOSEY, A: *The concept and use of developmental groups.* American Journal of Occupational Therapy, 24:272, 1970.

120. MOSEY, A: *Involvement in the rehabilitation movement—1942-1960.* American Journal of Occupational Therapy, 25:234, 1971, p 235.

121. MYSAK, ED AND FIORENTINO, MR: *Neurophysiological considerations in occupational therapy for the cerebral palsied.* American Journal of Occupational Therapy, 15:112, 1961.

122. NAVARRO, V: *The industrialization of fetishism or the fetishism of industrialization: A critique of Ivan Illich.* Social Science and Medicine, 9:351, 1975.

123. PECK, JB: *Development and management of transference.* American Journal of Occupational Therapy, 26:78, 1962.

124. PESSIN, J AND FRIEDMAN, I: *The value of art in the treatment of the mentally ill.* Occupational Therapy and Rehabilitation, 28:1, 1949.

125. PETERS, H: *Training for research.* American Journal of Occupational Therapy, 8:177-187, 1954.

126. PRICE, A: *Laterality of upper extremity function in physically handicapped children.* American Journal of Occupational Therapy, 8:241, 276, 1954.

127. PRICE H AND CORCORAN, L: *Work therapy in a private neuro-psychiatric hospital.* Occupational Therapy and Rehabilitation, 24:155, 1945.

128. REESE, M: *Music as occupational therapy for psychiatric patients.* American Journal of Occupational Therapy, 6:14, 49, 1952.

129. REIL, J: *Rhapsodies on the psychic treatment of the insane.* Occupational Therapy and Rehabilitation, 26:342, 1947.

130. REILLY, M: *An occupational therapy curriculum for 1965.* American Journal of Occupational Therapy, 12:293, 1958.

131. REILLY, M: *Research potentiality of occupational therapy.* American Journal of Occupational Therapy, 14:206, 1960.

132. REILLY, M: *Occupational therapy can be one of the great ideas of 20th century medicine.* American Journal of Occupational Therapy, 16:1, 1962.

133. REILLY, M: *A psychiatric occupational therapy program as a teaching model.* American Journal of Occupational Therapy, 20:61, 1966.

134. REILLY, M: *The modernization of occupational therapy.* American Journal of Occupational Therapy, 25:243, 1971.

135. REILLY, M (ED): *Play as exploratory learning.* Sage, Beverly Hills, 1974.

136. REREK, M: *The depression years—1929 to 1941.* American Journal of Occupational Therapy, 25:231, 1971.

137. RILEY, JN: *Western medicine's attempt to become more scientific: Examples from the United States and Thailand.* Social Science and Medicine, 11:549, 1977.

138. RITZER, G: *Sociology: A multiple paradigm science.* The American Sociologist, 10:156, 1975.

139. ROBINSON, A: *Play: The arena for acquisition of rules for competent behavior.* American Journal of Occupational Therapy, 31:248, 1977.

140. ROHRER, J: *Training for research.* American Journal of Occupational Therapy, 8:179, 191, 1954.

141. ROOD, M: *Every one counts.* American Journal of Occupational Therapy, 12:326, 1958.

142. RUSH, B: *Medical inquiries and observation upon the diseases of the mind.* Occupational Therapy and Rehabilitation, 26:177, 1947.

143. SAFILIOS-ROTHSCHILD, C: *The sociology and social psychology of disability and rehabilitation.* Random House, New York, 1970.

144. SCHOLTEN, W: *Occupational therapy as a preliminary to industrial therapy.* Occupational Therapy and Rehabilitation, 21:86, 1942.

145. SHANNON, P: *Work-play theory and the occupational therapy process.* American Journal of Occupational Therapy, 26:169, 1972.

146. SHANNON, P: *The derailment of occupational therapy.* American Journal of Occupational Therapy, 31:229, 1977.

147. SLAGLE, EC: *Training aides for mental patients.* Archives of Occupational Therapy, 1:11, 1922, p 14, 16.

148. SLAGLE, EC: *Occupational therapy: Recent methods and advances in the United States.* Archives of Occupational Therapy, 13:289, 1934.

149. SLAGLE, EC AND ROBESON, H: *Syllabus for training of nurses in occupational therapy* (ED 2). State Hospitals Press, Utica, NY, 1941, p 41, 53, 42, 53, 19, 29.

150. SMITH, HD: *Scientific and medical bases.* In HOPKINS, HL, AND SMITH, HD, (EDS), *Willard and Spackman's occupational therapy* (ed 5). JB Lippincott, Philadelphia, 1978.

151. SOLOMON, A: *Occupational therapy, a psychiatric treatment.* American Journal of Occupational Therapy, 1:1, 1947.

152. SOLOMON, A AND FENTRESS, T: *A critical study of analytically oriented group psychotherapy utilizing the technique of dramatization of the psychodynamics.* Occupational Therapy and Rehabilitation, 26:23, 1947.

153. SPACKMAN, C: *Treatment for limitation of motion of joints, flaccid paralysis and industrial injuries.* In WILLARD, HS, AND SPACKMAN, CS, (EDS), *Principles of occupational therapy,* JB Lippincott, Philadelphia, 1947.

154. SPACKMAN, C: *A history of the practice of occupational therapy for restoration of physical function: 1917-1967.* American Journal of Occupational Therapy, 22:67, 1968.

155. SPENCER, EA: *Functional restoration.* In HOPKINS, HL, AND SMITH, HD, (EDS), *Willard and Spackman's occupational therapy* (ed 5). JB Lippincott, Philadelphia, 1978, p 355.

156. STANLEY, J: *Habit-training.* Occupational Therapy and Rehabilitation, 21:82, 1942.

157. STOCKMEYER, SA: *A sensorimotor approach to treatment.* In PEARSON, P AND WILLIAMS, C. (EDS), *Physical therapy services in the developmental disabilities.* Charles C. Thomas, Springfield, Ill, 1972.

158. SVENSSON, V AND BRENNAN, M: *The opponens splint.* American Journal of Occupational Therapy, 7:98, 1953.

159. *Task force on target populations.* American Journal of Occupational Therapy, 28:158, 1974, p 159.

160. TAKATA, N: *The play history*. American Journal of Occupational Therapy, 23:314, 1969.

161. TOFFLER, A: *The third wave*. Wm Morrow & Co, New York, 1981.

162. TRACY, S: *Studies in invalid occupation*. Whitcomb & Barrows, Boston, 1912, p 171, 15.

163. *Training of teachers for occupational therapy for the rehabilitation of disabled soldiers and sailors*. Government Printing Office, Washington, DC, 1918, p 135, 35, 50.

164. WADE, B: *Occupational therapy for patients with mental disease*. In WILLARD, HS AND SPACKMAN, CS, (EDS), *Principles of occupational therapy*. JB Lippincott, Philadelphia, 1947.

165. WATANABE, S: *Four concepts basic to the occupational therapy process*. American Journal of Occupational Therapy, 22:439, 1968.

166. WEGG, L: *The role of the occupational therapist in vocational rehabilitation*. American Journal of Occupational Therapy, 11:252, 1957.

167. WIEMER, R: *Traditional and nontraditional practice arenas*. In *Occupational therapy: 2001*. American Occupational Therapy Association, Rockville, Md, 1979, p 43.

168. WEISS, P: *Living nature and the knowledge gap*. Saturday Review, 19, 56, November 29, 1969.

169. WEST, W: *Synthesis*. American Journal of Occupational Therapy, 12:225, 1958, p 229.

170. WEST, W (ED): *Psychiatric occupational therapy*. American Occupational Therapy Association, New York, 1959.

171. WEST, W: *The occupational therapist's changing responsibility to the community*. American Journal of Occupational Therapy, 21:312, 1967.

172. WEST, W: *Professional responsibility in times of change*. American Journal of Occupational Therapy, 22:9, 1968.

173. WHITE, L: *Science is "sciencing"*. In HUGHES, C, (ED), *Custom made*. Rand McNally, Chicago, 1976.

174. WOODSIDE, H: *Dimensions of the occupational behaviour model*. Canadian Journal of Occupational Therapy, 43:11, 1976.

175. YERXA, E: *Authentic occupational therapy*. American Journal of Occupational Therapy, 21:1, 1967.

CHAPTER 2

A PARADIGM FOR PRACTICE: THE HIERARCHICAL ORGANIZATION OF OCCUPATIONAL THERAPY KNOWLEDGE

Gary Kielhofner

EDITOR'S INTRODUCTION

All occupational therapists will confirm that they possess considerable knowledge—though the knowledge might be difficult to describe. The premise of this chapter is that the greatest problem in occupational therapy today is not lack of information, but unity of information. An appropriate methaphor for occupational therapy knowledge and practice is endless yards of various threads—threads which this chapter attempts to weave into a coherent fabric. Like the work of weaving, the task of the chapter requires precision, and aesthetic appeal and practicality of the final product will result from matching and fitting appropriate threads.

The clinician is likely to find most useful the section labeled "clinical puzzles," toward which the chapter's initial (and admittedly more technical and labored) discussion is aimed. The clinical implications of the material should make the section which lays out the basic framework of systems worth the reader's effort. Educators are likely to find the middle section of the chapter which examines current knowledge and its gaps to be most relevant to their concerns. Students may wish to examine their education against the hierarchical schema the chapter presents while questioning whether and to what extent they have been educated along the continuum of phenomena that concern occupational therapists. Such a process of self-discovery may become a basis both for appreciating the range of concepts already learned and for selecting future courses of self-study.

Because the logical argument builds and progresses as the chapter proceeds, the reader will find it necessary to become familiar with the full scope of the chapter to benefit from it maximally.

The chapter begins where the previous history of occupational therapy leaves off, articulating possible views of humans, the clinical puzzles, the methods of therapy and the goals of a new unified paradigm of occupational therapy. Readers will find that the chapter attempts to include the current range of knowledge and practice techniques in the new paradigm; it does not suggest, as some might fear, "throwing out the baby with the bathwater." Rather, the chapter aims to give the reader an appreciation of how such vastly different phenomena as joint range of motion and human value systems are quite intimately connected in the human being. To achieve this goal concepts from general system theory will be used as an overall framework. The concept of hierarchy (i.e., the proposition that the world is composed of interlocking levels of phenomena) is the primary basis of the presentation. The reader will find a view of occupational therapy knowledge and practice based on an understanding of different levels of phenomena which are involved in our patients and clients' problems and their processes of adaptation. Since the chapter introduces concepts progressively the reader will find it helpful to refer to the figures which summarize the concepts and their relationships. The concept of hierarchy is used throughout to provide an in depth explanation for the efficacy of occupational therapy and to articulate more fully why purposeful activity is central to the field and why it works as therapy.

GK

If all of human knowledge, everything that's known, is believed to be an enormous hierarchic structure, then the high country of the mind is found at the uppermost reaches of this structure in the most general, the most abstract considerations of all. (Pirsig, Zen and the Art of Motorcycle Maintenance: An Inquiry Into Values)

The occupational therapist in clinical practice faces the singular task of examining a client or patient, arriving at a set of conclusions concerning problems to be addressed, and designing and implementing a course of treatment. In a less obvious fashion, this central business of clinical practice is made possible through the tradition of knowledge and technique. The field's choices concerning how it will generate, organize, and impart abstract knowledge to its practitioners have very real consequences for patients and clients. Ultimately, the field is not less responsible for the knowledge it generates than for what its practitioners do; the two are inextricably interwoven.

This chapter examines a number of critical issues involved in organizing and generating knowledge for practice. It proceeds on the assumption that a new paradigm is required for occupational therapy. This assumption is derived from the conclusion in Chapter 1 that the field must undergo a fundamental reorganization of its knowledge to achieve coherence of current theory and continuity with traditional principles. The pages that follow may be viewed as an attempt to illuminate the range and nature of what will be required to reach that goal.

The concept of paradigm is a more recent and less familiar way of describing knowledge in a field than such abstractions as frame of reference, theory, conceptual model, and the like. The idea of a paradigm does not debunk these older concepts. Rather, it offers a broader, deeper, and more dynamic view of the scientific enterprise. Theories, frames of reference, and models are—if you will—limited "insider" versions of a field's organized knowledge. The concept of paradigm, in contrast, represents an outsider version of the entire enterprise of knowledge generation. As Ritzer[63] notes, theories, frames of reference, and models are only components of far broader paradigms. Kuhn's [42] concept of paradigm also provides a more critical and complete description of the knowledge-related processes and activities of a field, especially those related to recasting information under changing rubrics.

Since this chapter proposes an outline for a *new* paradigm for occupational therapy, some mention of what is involved in a transformation from one paradigm to another is necessary. In writing about differences between a paradigm and its successor Kuhn notes:

> Since new paradigms are born from old ones, they ordinarily incorporate much of the vocabulary and apparatus, both conceptual and manipulative, that the traditional paradigm had previously employed. But they seldom employ these borrowed elements in quite the traditional way. Within the new paradigm, old terms, concepts, and experiments fall into what we must call, though the term is not quite right, a misunderstanding between the two competing schools.[42]

This incommensurability reflects the fact that the shift in paradigms results in an entirely new vision of the world. A new paradigm does not merely add new information about empirical objects and events. It redefines fundamental phenomena of concern. When such central dogma of a field is transformed, all particulars are shifted by fiat. In a very real sense all that was known under the old paradigm is now seen in a new light.

It is this aspect of any new paradigm, its incommensurability with old fundamental ideas, which creates problems in communication. In discussing these ideas with professional colleagues, I have been struck with the need to achieve a stance which appreciates the essential differences in how we perceive aspects of the world. The same clinical example which a disagreeing discussant sees as a challenge to my position, appears to me to be just more evidence of its correctness. In a deep sense the empirical world is presented differently to those who employ differing paradigmatic lenses. Thus, the task of this chapter is not only to present new information; it must also illustrate new ways of seeing.

The fundamental problem in occupational therapy today is not as much a lack of information as it is a lack of coherence about knowledge that has been accumulated. The theory which the field has begun to incorporate from other disciplines and the concepts it has generated now constitute an unwieldy body of knowledge. This accretion creates a dilemma for the practitioner, student, and educator, since there are no priorities or criteria for determining which theories are most relevant to practice, and no general schema for integrating diverse facts into a practical framework.

To reduce perplexity over the discrepancies in current knowledge and to prevent an excess of new information in occupational therapy, a structure to support future theorizing is required. The new paradigm will require a single frame which can accomodate diverse knowledge. The structure must be able to specify properties of areas of knowledge, their interrelationships, and their operational significance to the practice of occupational therapy.

This chapter proposes an approach to the knowledge of the field which corresponds to these requirements. Further, since the field's central business is the art of influencing health with occupation, it will be argued that priorities of knowledge must always be in terms of the ability of concepts to define and explain why and how occupation possesses a reservoir of healing potential. With these goals as a beacon, this chapter examines the utility of organizing occupational therapy knowledge into a hierarchical structure, an idea proposed long ago by Meyer[49] which appears ever more timely today.

To reiterate, the framework will be a blueprint for future theorizing in occupational therapy. It should therefore identify categories of knowledge which explain occupation and specify their relationship, while also facilitating the process of establishing priorities of knowledge in the field. Not by chance, the hierarchical schema also reveals a number of important themes concerning clinical puzzles, methods and rationales of treatment, and goals for the practice of occupational therapy.

THE HIERARCHICAL META-STRUCTURE FOR OCCUPATIONAL THERAPY KNOWLEDGE

Most persons are unaware of the ultimate structure of their rational thinking. Rather, people operate conceptually from a matrix of implicit ideas about the world which seem natural or evident to them. To ask how thinking is structured calls attention to basic categories of knowledge and the ways in which they are interrelated. Even more rare are attempts to accomplish fundamental reordering of conceptual processes. Yet, this is exactly what is involved in paradigm change. Commenting on the requirements to restructure thinking, Weiss notes:

> Instead of enlarging and adapting our tools of expression to the demands of new insights into nature, we often, unwittingly, try to make nature, or rather our thoughts about it, fit into the narrow box of our traditional ways of representing it. . . . For scientific knowledge to process unhampered by such arbitrary constraint, its practitioners must concern themselves not only with the factual content of science, but with the adequacy of the intellectual and verbal tools used for communicating that content and for making it intelligible.[84]

Since the abstract tools employed for ordering knowledge are working features of one's natural ways of thinking, they do not ordinarily require awareness. Rather, as one makes unconscious use of the body as an instrument of routine activities, patterns of conceptualization are subliminal implements of thinking. However, just as learning a new type of physical performance calls attention to one's body and its movements, reorganization of knowledge requires consideration of cognitive manipulations which are otherwise automatically performed.

A reanalysis of the foundations of scientific thinking has begun in this century and it promises to restructure fundamental knowledge in many fields. In their search for generic laws of nature, systems theorists have effected a restatement of the problems of modern scholarship, especially in the biologic and social sciences. Whereas science has progressed to date largely through the examination of cause and effect relationships between the most elementary constituents of phenonema, general system theorists are now proposing that major advances in science will require the study of problems more complex than causation. They have introduced network dynamics, gestalt functions, autoregulation, and a plethora of other extra-causal processes as puzzles for modern science. In so doing, systems theorists have also vetoed the longstanding dogma that explanation is ultimately reducible to elementary cause and effect laws. Science is literally becoming topsy-turvy; now, the scholarly way of "getting to the bottom of things" is a pathway of inquiry leading to the higher regions at which phenomena manifest their essential nature. The concept of hierarchy with its ramifications of a multifarious and pluralistically regulated continuum of phenomena has become part of a fundamental and emerging scientific vision. And it reshapes the very nature of science.

Von Bertalanffy describes it as, "a change in *basic categories* of knowledge . . . to deal with complexities, wholes, systems, organizations . . . a shift or re-orientation in scientific thinking."[7] Earlier science is described as reductionist—a term which refers to its mode of scientific explanation. Consequently, reductionist science begins with cause and effect empiricism and culminates in linear causal explanations. Classical reductionism was based on the assumption that all the parts and their relationships can ultimately be reconstituted into an understanding of the whole.[83] However, as Weiss notes, the reductionist strategy of "*putting the pieces together again . . . can yield no complete explanation of the behavior of even the most elementary living system*".[83] The ultimate goal of reductionism—to reduce explanations to least common denominators of constituent parts and relationships—is now clearly untenable.

In this new perspective, systems are conceptualized as irreducible organized patterns or configurations, rather than collections of parts. The ordering of the whole is thought to be governed by laws other than the cause and effect relationships among parts. Laws governing the organization of the whole cannot be further reduced to laws that describe the relationship of the parts.[7].

Weiss provided the following example to illustrate the irreducibility of phenomena to constituent parts and their relationships. If one were to note all the constituent chemical compounds of a living cell and then, using cause and effect laws of chemistry to specify the series of chemical reactions which would result, it would be found that these reactions are quite different from what actually happens inside the cell. This problem, Weiss points out, leaves us no other conclusion but that there must be *laws of a higher order* that operate in the cell as a living system and not in its chemical constituents and that, importantly, have the power to *organize* and *determine* which of the lower level chemical laws will be called upon in the service of the living system.[83] This process can be likened to the conductor of an orchestra. Each component has its own laws in the notation of the symphony, but the conductor organizes these parts into a whole by specifying superordinate instructions. The cell has its own built-in conductor which orchestrates gestalt functions dependent upon, yet not limited to, chemical chain reactions. This is the basic concept of *hierarchy*—the idea that phenomena are organized into different levels and that higher levels oversee and determine how the potentials of lower levels will unfold.

A HIERARCHICAL SCHEMA FOR ORDERING OCCUPATIONAL THERAPY KNOWLEDGE

The recognition that there were hierarchies of phenomena naturally led scientists to consider how phenomena could be classified in this manner and to search for universal levels of complexity. The schema of hierarchical levels that I find most relevant to occupational therapy is one formulated by Boulding,[9,10] and I have modified and elaborated this schema to achieve more clarity and relevance. In this hierarchy there are differing levels of complexity and recognizable systems in nature which belong to each level. A property of each higher level of complexity is that systems belonging to that level incorporate the features of lower levels into their makeup. At the level to which a system belongs there are emergent qualities and laws which govern how the lower incorporated levels will function. Thus, while the hierarchy serves as a taxonomy to differentiate types of phenomena, it also serves as a schema for revealing the relationship between different levels. I will first describe the levels and their features and then propose laws which govern the interrelationships of levels. The laws of levels and the laws by which levels interrelate form an abstract structure upon which to begin ordering occupational therapy knowledge. Having described the hierarchial schema I will next examine the process of using it to organize the field's knowledge.

FRAMEWORKS. The first and simplest level of Boulding's taxonomy is frameworks. Systems at this level are those which maintain a static pattern. The crystal is an example of such a framework system. Frameworks are also incorporated into the structures of higher phenomena, such as the arrangement of bones, muscles, and nerves in a body. All higher systems incorporate some kind of framework that is reflected in the basic arrangement of their parts.

CLOCKWORKS. The second level is clockworks, and the emergent quality is kinetics. Here systems exhibit motion, but only within the limits of the system's patterned arrangement—its basic structure. At this level the structure of the system absolutely predetermines the motion of its parts. Levers are simple clockwork systems; the solar system is a giant clockwork and the pattern of electrons spinning around the atomic nucleus is a submicroscopic one. Systems belonging to this level transfer movement along a pathway of the structure and its pivotal junctures (i.e., movement about the fulcrum of a lever, around the center of revolution, and so forth).

Features of this level are also incorporated into all higher systems. For instance, the musculo-skeletal system functions as a clockwork system, and economic trade between social groups within a nation or culture reveals clockwork-like processes. When such patterns are manifest in higher systems they are subordinated within layers of higher ruling phenomena.

CYBERNETICS. The third level is that of cybernetics. Here the emergent quality is the ability of systems to regulate some aspect of their own performance according to information received about the consequences of past behavior. Cybernetic systems can only "read" feedback for which they have been programmed and adjust behavior in order to approximate a predetermined ideal since these functions are built into the structure of the system. For example, a thermostat's interaction with external conditions is always in terms of the ideal temperature for which it is rigidly programmed.

Obviously, cybernetic functions are extremely important features of higher level systems. The temperature regulation of mammals is a cybernetic process. In human behavior social feedback is a cybernetic function which is essential to permit persons to recognize the consequences of their action and to adjust behavior accordingly. Behaviorism is a theory that begins with the recognition of cybernetic processes in humans, although it has been rightly criticized for its attempt to reduce all human behavior to a purely cybernetic level of explanation.[18,23]

OPEN SYSTEMS. The fourth level is that of open systems. At this level there is a radical departure from the characteristics of other levels. As Von Bertalanffy [6] notes, all three previous systems belong to a general category of physical or closed systems in which structure is paramount and determines any function of the system. When one reaches the open system level—the level where life is differentiated from inanimate existence—an enormous difference is encountered. Part of the distinction is reflected in the new relationship of structure and function; the latter now fashions the former. Von Bertalanffy offers the following explanation:

> There is a simple reason for the primacy, in the organism of dynamical as against structural order. In contrast to a machine which consists of lasting parts, all organic structures are maintained in a continuous process, in perpetual breaking down and regeneration. The only thing which is really permanent in the organism is the order of processes. Therefore, the ultimate reason of the pattern and order in the living system can be sought only in the laws of the process itself, not in pre-established and enduring structures.[5]

Open systems' structures are more properly considered patterns, or arrangements, that are created and maintained by processes. In the open system the arrangement of parts is not nearly so consequential as the regulative processes that constitute recognizable patterns. Open systems, by virtue of their process-dominated nature, are dynamic orders that are maintained and transformed through their own action. The action of open systems is described as the input and output of information and energy from and to the environment. Their self-ordering and the patterns of internal arrangement they achieve is termed throughput. The cycle of input, throughput, and output is the basic dynamic order of all open systems. This cycle mediates between the internal requirements and potentials of the system and the demands and supports of the environment. Open systems can thereby effect internal rearrangement of parts and processes to maximize the fit between the system's goals and environmental circumstances. This property is called equifinality.[6]

The most important feature of the open system is the dynamic self-regulatory capacity that imposes requirements for gestalt or network conditions on the function of components. Within the open system, processes are not mediated across time and space by means of the linear cause and effect chains which predominate in lower systems. Rather, optimal conditions of the whole are maintained by subordinating lower processes. For example, within the cell—the prototypic open system—chemical reactions are regulated by overall requirements for the dynamic order of the living cell.

Open systems also exibit the quality of spontaneity. Unlike the closed systems of lower levels, these systems act of their own accord and require no external agency to initiate function. The open system incorporates features of frameworks, dynamics, and cybernetics, into its overall makeup. But at this level these features are made possible by the new quality of self-regulation or self-organization. Their existence is thus more fragile and transient as they are incorporated into higher levels. Moreover, they are not rigid patterns and processes, but operate according to the requirements of the overall system. In open systems patterns, dynamics and cybernetic functions can be adjusted when the system as a whole requires it.

The structure of the open system is reflected in its throughput, where the internal patterning of order is maintained. Clockwork processes are reflected in the input and output cycle, and cybernetic functions are incorporated into the system's use of feedback. While these features from lower levels are part of the patterning of the open system, it is the organization of the open system and its properties of spontaneity, self-organization, and equifinality that make it so different from lower level systems.

DIFFERIENTIATED SYSTEMS. Boulding[9] identifies the genetic-societal level as the next stage of complexity. I prefer the term differentiated as more descriptive of systems belonging to this level of complexity which exhibit a differentiation of parts, division of labor, and integration under a leading part.

The plant is a typical system that belongs to this level of complexity. Here the predominance of process over structure becomes even more cogent. Diversification of parts in systems of this type are ontogenic processes. Such systems begin in an undifferentiated or amorphous state and, in the course of growth and development, achieve an individuation of parts and their arrangement into a working matrix, with various constituents contributing different functions to the system's overall operation. Thus, the recognition of a differentiated system results from observation of the system's state along a process of continual self-transformation. While differentiated systems incorporate features of frameworks, dynamics, and cybernetics (i.e., patterned arrangement of parts, dynamic interface and feedback regulation), all contribute to this unfolding process of self-complication. However, it is the open system feature of differentiated systems that directly supports this higher emergent quality. The processes of input, throughput, and output which comprise the basic dynamic of an open system are prerequisites to self-differentiation. An example is the ability of a plant to import nutrients and energy and use them in its throughput process to produce its own differentiated structures (i.e., the transition from undifferentiated seed to adult plant with leaves, branches, etc.).

Differentiation is also incorporated into higher level systems; specialization and division of labor is basic to human social systems and to the function of the central nervous system. By specialization in the various subunits of a larger system, the overall potentialities of the system are broadened and its behavior is more complex.

ICONIC SYSTEMS. Several emergent qualities make up the increased complexity of the next level. Here systems have sensory receptors, motor effectors, and a complex nervous system which links them and allows sophisticated processing of information and production of behavior. Further, their behavior exhibits properties of teleology or purpose. These collective qualities are organized under a ruling phenomenon which Boulding[9] calls the image. This is an internal representation of external features of the environment and rudimentary awareness of self generated by experience. Boulding labels this level the animal level, after its members; I have chosen the term iconic to describe the emergent property of systems at this level, the ability to form an internal representation of external reality. Boulding comments on this emergent quality as follows:

> Here we have the development of specialized information receptors (eyes, ears, etc.) leading to an enormous increase in the intake of information; we have also a great development of the nervous systems, leading ultimately to the brain, as an organizer of the information intake into a knowledge structure or "image." Increasingly as we ascend the scale of animal life, behavior is response not to a specific stimulus but to an "image" or knowledge structure

or view of the environment as a whole. This image is of course determined ultimately by information received into the organism; the relation between the receipt of information and the building up of an image however is exceedingly complex. It is not a simple piling up or accumulation of information received, although this frequently happens, but a structuring of information into something essentially different from the information itself.[9]

One of the most important features of the image capacity is that it allows the individual to learn new behavior from experience. The plant's store of information is "learned" at the species level through evolutionary experience; the "knowledge" of the plant belongs to the species as a whole and is genetically inherited. The animal inherits some species knowledge, but its most important endowment is the integration of specialized sensory receptors and motor effectors with the complex nervous system which allows the emergent image. While the sensory receptors and brain are the basis for this iconic ability, the latter is a recognizable entity in its own right. Incoming physiochemical signals are translated through the image into significant messages. The image is a network of information that allows interpretion and recognition of incoming signals and that allows the system to choose action. As Boulding notes, the image greatly enhances the complexity of behavior. Because of the image the relationship of stimulus to output is much more than a simple clockwork function. A stimuli may or may not lead to a given output, depending on its significance to the image. Further, intensity or type of stimulus is not always correlated with the character of response, since its significance depends on the image. For instance, thunder may produce no flight in a wild animal, though the slightest sound of human footsteps will.

The image makes possible the observable quality of purpose or teleology in the behavior of animals. Boulding's view on the emergence of an image from the nervous system and his postulate that the image is itself an entity, dependent on, but separate from and not reducible to brain function, is supported by the writings of other authors such as Sperry,[71] Hayek[29] and Hofstadter[32].

There is a trend toward even more fluid structures and the primacy of function over structure with each higher level of this hierarchy of complexity. The image represents yet another degree of primacy of process over structure. It is almost completely experience-determined. Since it governs lower level components of the iconic system (i.e., the brain, sensory receptors, and motor effectors) the role of function or experience in such systems is crucial.

As Boulding notes, this phenomenon is extremely complex and very little is known about it. Despite its complexity it is a topic of immediate and extensive relevance to occupational therapy. The field's interest in the relationship of brain function and pathology to adaptation leads it directly to concern with the image and its governing role in higher processes that involve the nervous system.

SYMBOLIC SYSTEMS. The paramount characteristic of human beings is their ability to function symbolically, and it represents an enormous expansion of the functions of the image:

> Man is not differentiated from the lower animals by any increased capacity for intake of information. Human eyes and ears are not much better than those of other mammals, and

the human nose is almost certainly much worse. It is the capacity for organizing information into large and complex images which is the chief glory of our species.[10]

Understanding the image function at the level of humans may be aided by reflecting for a moment on what happens to lower level functions when incorporated into higher systems. Clockwork and cybernetic processes become more fluid and open-ended when incorporated into higher systems, as incorporation of lower level functions and structures into higher systems always results in their becoming more fluid. For instance, a thermostat is a rigid feedback system belonging to the level of cybernetics. Such purely cybernetic systems cannot change their own ideal standard or create new outputs beyond those for which they are programmed. By contrast, cybernetic functions, such as feedback on performance, when incorporated into human systems, are extremely open-ended. The cybernetic functions in human behavior are part of a system which has these abilities. Feedback on failure to achieve a goal in human systems can result in formulation of an entirely new objective or the creation of new *modus operandi* to replace means which failed to attain the goal.

This trend toward fluidity of lower processes parallels what happens to the image at the human level. Lower animals' neurologic hardware is designed through evolution to accommodate only a certain genre of image. An example of such evolutionary programming of mammalian brains for specialized images is the superior ability of a squirrel (whose brain is simpler) over a dog to circumnavigate a post around which a leash is tangled in order to get access to food. This is attributed to the fact that:

> Dogs live in a two-dimensional world: If they want something, they go and get it. Squirrels, on the other hand, live in trees. In their three-dimensional world, a squirrel wanting to go from tree to tree has a choice: it can descend the trunk; go along the ground and then climb the tree; or it can remain in the treetops, seeking a place where the branches of two adjacent trees are in contact. The former strategy would expose the squirrel to its ground-dwelling predators; the latter would therefore be safer, but it would often require the ability to go initially away from the goal so as to achieve it eventually. In other words, the ancestors of present-day squirrels were good at solving detour problems. Rephrasing this more accurately in the language of evolutionary biology: ancestral squirrels that were relatively more adept at solving such problems left more offspring than did those were less well endowed.[2]

The difference of the human brain is that it is programmed through evolution for the ability to acquire almost any image and to generate and share images. As Boulding[10] points out, human symbolism has such freedom that individuals can acquire idiosyncratic images, as in cases of schizophrenic thinking. Since human beings have fewer biologic constraints on the genre of their images, they must rely on the information pool of the social group to structure acquisition of the image. In lower species collective information is shared and maintained primarily through genetic processes. Thus the animal brain arrives at birth preprogrammed for much of the behavior necessary for survival. Humans, on the other hand, maintain more species knowledge in the social tradition and have, as part of the deal, more flexible, but more "ignorant" brains at birth. Species knowledge has been shifted from the biologic to the cultural realm. Indeed, human evolution is characterized by the emergence of social-technical change as part of the succession of factors selecting for adaptive advantage. Thus, the organism best suited for a species which has collective adaptation savvy is one which efficiently acquires (learns) that pool of information. As Boulding points out, the increased complexity of the human brain is not in the service of more sophisticated sensory receptors, or even motor effectors, but in order to support the emergence of a vastly complicated image, whose eventual patterns are largely dependent on what is learned in the cultural milieu.

Symbolization is the term given by Boulding to the emergent ability of the human being which builds on the simpler image of lower species. In Bateson's[3] and Hofstadter's[32] terms the symbol is complex metainformation. The most abstract human symbols are images about images. They are reflexive images which account for acute self-awareness and awareness of highly diffuse environmental variables.

Despite its expansive nature, the symbolic system of human beings has several basic properties which immediately concern occupational therapy. Because of the reflexive character of symbolization, the human being has the ability and, consequently, the need to maintain a *positive* self-awareness.[26] Interrelated with this aspect of the symbolic system is the human consciousness of time and the accompanying grasp of such complex relations as causation.[16,18] Temporal awareness allows one to connect events in time, observe and anticipate consequences, and expect and plan future events. Because of temporal awareness the self-image includes both what one has done in the past and what one hopes to do in the future. This sense of future time allows human purpose to become vastly more complex than the teleological behavior of animals. In humans there is the possibility of purposes which are undertaken for more distant goals which subserve more abstract objectives or ideals.

As in other systems, there must be a superordinate ruling level in the human symbolic system. This is the level of values.[10,77] The human experience of values ultimately determines which purposes will be chosen and pursued, even governing the range of new images that will be formed. The apex of emergent qualities at the human level is the ruling power of value.

It is the human image which accounts for the experience of meaning. According to Boulding[9] the meaning of information is the way in which it impacts or changes what already exists in the individual's collective image. Thus, meaning is always a match between information which is encountered or recalled and how it registers against what is in the present system of images. Meaning can occur at any level of the image hierarchy. For instance, the words on this page have meaning determined by the image of the English language the reader possesses. Concepts conveyed by the words have meaning that depends on the reader's previous understanding of the topics discussed. And, finally, this entire thesis on the paradigm of occupational therapy will have a particular meaning that will depend on the values the reader holds in reference to occupational therapy. Several levels of meaning operate at once, characterizing how the words, concepts, and thesis of this chapter interact with the image system of the reader.

Concepts of meaning and purpose have traditionally been used to describe how the activities used in occupational therapy influence patients and clients. Despite the field's ostensible commitment to the ideal of purposeful and meaningful activity as therapy, there have been only limited attempts to penetrate and understand human symbolic processes and, as a consequence, occupational therapists know very little about meaning and purpose. There exists within the context of hierarchy an inviting, if not crucial, opportunity to understand how meaningful activity impacts the entire human system. As the highest ruling level of the human system, symbolic processes influence the continuum of lower phenomena which make up the organism.

SOCIAL SYSTEMS. Processes which incorporate the human symbolic capacity and involve the collective and interactive behavior of individuals constitute another level of phenomena: social relations. Boulding[9] notes that culture and social relations constitute an emergent level with properties not reducible to the symbols and behaviors of members. Watzlawic, Beavin and Jackson[79] conceptualize social interaction as an identifiable system demonstrating the same coherence as lower level systems. Such analyses illustrate the value of conceptualizing social organizations as a level of phenomena in their own right.

Boulding offers a partial list of emergent qualities at the level of social organizations:

> At this level we must concern ourselves with the content and meaning of messages, the nature and dimensions of value systems, the transcription of images into a historical record, the subtle symbolizations of art, music and poetry, and the complex gamut of human emotion. The empirical universe here is human life and society in all its complexity and richness.[9]

The social organization is built upon the collective and interacting symbols and behaviors of individuals. It necessarily includes the sum of their individual actions, while exhibiting its own coherence and order independent of the contributions of particular persons. Part of this process is historical (i.e., the tradition of meaning, values, artifacts, and practices which characterize the collective culture of a group). Another aspect is the dynamics set in motion by the interaction of groups within the larger group (e.g., economic behavior between various organizations, businesses, etc.).

Another important feature of social organizations is their function in carrying, maintaining, and elaborating knowledge and technology. For instance, the abilities that an occupational therapist possesses are a result of the collective tradition of information which the field generates, stores, and imparts to new members. Similarly, within a family, daily living skills are learned by children as parents and other kin pass on traditions of knowledge. Thus, the social group and its collective meanings complete the human being by providing a pool of information which he or she acquires and uses throughout life.

Boulding[9] includes a transcendental level that I agree exists, but being unable to speculate on its implications for occupation, I have omitted a discussion of it. The hierarchical schema is thus completed and I will turn attention to laws which relate levels of hierarchy.

LAWS OF HIERARCHY

The next step in making the hierarchy useful for organizing occupational therapy knowledge is to identify laws that describe the relations between levels of phenomena. Systems theorists have proposed a number of such laws. These laws of hierarchy are rules which

WHAT THE PRACTITIONER MUST KNOW:
THE KNOWLEDGE BASE OF OCCUPATIONAL THERAPY

govern how complex phenomena interrelate. Considered with the emergent qualities of systems at each level, they constitute a matrix of laws that describe the operations of a continuum of phenomena. The following list of such laws is derived from the writing of Feibleman[19], Koestler[41], and Ozbekhan[55]:

(1) Complexity of levels is cumulative upward. That is, ascending any hierarchy there are increasingly complex systems whose organization includes features of each of the lower levels they incorporate. This means that to theorize about systems at higher levels, explanations must be more complex. One can be misled, by not recognizing a historical feature of emerging science, to believe that current theories represent the complexity of their topics. For instance, by appearing more intricate than biology, physics may incorrectly lead to the conclusion that physical phenomena are more complex than biologic phenomena. Similarly, the state of neuroscience versus psychology may misrepresent the brain as more complicated than the mind. It must be recognized that the complexity of theories today is a sign of the maturity of a science rather than a reflection of the nature of its subject matter. Complexity is a feature of position in the hierarchy of phenomena. Indeed, part of the complexity of higher systems is that they incorporate all the complexity of lower systems and then add some. The brain is no less a collection of atoms than is a stone. And the mind includes as part of its processes all the neurons that constitute the brain. To reiterate, complexity is cumulative upward.

(2) A system which incorporates lower levels into its organization operates with the highest level ruling one just below it, and that level ruling the next below, and so forth. In this way all levels of the system are governed (directly or indirectly) by the highest level. This governing influence always changes how lower levels would operate if they were not integrated into a higher level—a view of agency control across levels of a system that complicates the old picture of linear causation. The influence of the parts of a system on each other is not mediated along chains of relations among the most elementary constituents. Rather, control is by means of triggers that set off gestalt functions, that in turn govern a collection of subunits. The control of complex systems is thus something like an inverted tree, with the trunk as highest level, branching into differentiated lower units (major limbs) which in turn divide into yet smaller units (twigs and leaves). Agency across such a system (i.e., from highest to lowest level) is mediated through layers of hierarchy and may be translated at each juncture of the hierarchy. For instance, a thought in the mind may translate within the brain to chemical impulses which are transformed to yet other impulses at the neuromuscular synapse, and into physical movement at the musculoskeletal level. In such a case, thought controls the motor act through several mediating levels.

(3) The division of systems into levels of hierarchy does not suggest that aspects of any system ever function in isolation. Rather, systems always function as wholes with all subsystems constantly integrated into the overall function. It has been a longstanding error of reductionism to isolate functional parts of systems with the idea that they actually are isolated systems. To continue the example above, even the function of a motor unit is continuously and in critical ways influenced and organized by the image of the organism. It is known that levels of emotional excitement have corresponding effects in the nervous system that in turn influence thresholds at lower nervous system levels. Thus while lower components act, to some degree, as functional gestalts, they are never—in any strict sense—functionally separate.

(4) A disturbance at any level of the hierarchy reverberates with effects at all other levels. If lower levels are disturbed, they tend to constrain the higher level (i.e., joint stiffness constrains nervous system commands for movement). Higher level disturbances tend to result in disorganization (e.g., the abnormal motor movements in athetoid cerebral palsy or in schizophrenia).

(5) The system's capacity for self-repair increases upward in the hierarchy. Since higher level systems possess more potential for variation than lower systems do, they can create new functions to compensate for constraints that lower levels impose. An example is the way in which the image of a congenital bilateral upper extremity amputee is organized to translate hand functions to the lower extremity. This occurs even though the frameworks, neurologic circuitry, and the anatomy of the foot are poorly suited.

(6) Any system functions both as a whole and a part. That is, gestalt systems at any level are parts of a system at a higher level. The cardiovascular system is a recognizable gestalt system within the body. While human beings are gestalt systems, they are also parts of social systems. The balance between being a part and whole reflects the dynamics that maintain a system's organization. For instance, in order to successfully adapt, a human being must exhibit both a degree of autonomy and a willingness to belong to and serve a social group. Thus, it is incorrect to view any system merely as a collection of its parts, or solely as an autonomous gestalt, or only as a part of a higher system. Collectively, all three dimensions represent the reality of how any system operates.

SUMMARY

The preceding discussion has described a hierarchical schema of levels of empirical phenomena and a set of hierarchical laws. With each new level, emergent characteristics were identified which governed lower levels that had been incorporated into the system belonging to that level. Figure 1 portrays the levels, prototypic members of levels, and the qualitative features (laws) of each level, as well as the laws governing the relations between levels. This schema can serve as a framework for organizing occupational therapy knowledge.

HIERARCHY AND THE PARADIGMATIC VIEW OF HUMANS.

A paradigm is a window for looking out on the world. The reigning aspect of paradigm is the unique view of phenomena that it makes possible. Since occupational therapy deals with human problems, its paradigm provides a special view of human beings. In occupational therapy literature several writers have espoused the perspective that any view of human beings must be based on biologic, psychologic and social dimensions.[53,60,65] While these three categories are useful for compartmentalization of occupational therapy knowledge, more exact delineation of knowledge content and organization is necessary and can be achieved by identifying the hierarchical levels represented in each of these three domains. I am proposing a matrix of knowledge (Figure 2) to delineate topics that constitute the occupational therapy view of human beings and set the stage for discussing

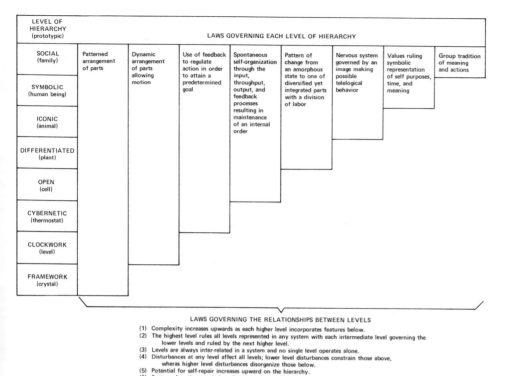

FIGURE 1. Levels of hierarchy and the laws of relationships.

relationships between areas of knowledge content. This map of occupational therapy knowledge has several uses, as demonstrated below.

BIOLOGIC PHENOMENA. In occupational therapy the biologic phenomenon that explains the human capacity for occupation is the neuromuscular system. At the lowest level of the hierarchy—frameworks—occupational therapy knowledge includes the traditional areas of functional anatomy and neuroanatomy that explain the structure of the neuromuscular system. Kinesiology, a highly developed body of knowledge, belongs to the clockwork level and explains the potential of the latter system for motion. Many neurologic phenomena, such as simple reflexes, also operate as clockwork systems. The field's knowledge of these mechanisms is substantial. At the cybernetic level, knowledge of neurologic feedback processes has been recognized and studied (e.g., concepts of inhibition and facilitation of nervous impulses, Golgi tendon organs, and muscle spindles). At the level of open systems neurologic principles of the relationship of sensory input to motor output have been identified. However, other open systems properties such as the holistic, self-maintaining, and spontaneous properties of the brain are little understood.[82] The process of differentiation and integration of sensory receptors and motor effectors has received a great deal of attention in recent neurologically based occupational therapy. Finally, at the iconic level it will eventually be necessary to develop

Levels	Biologic Domain	Psychologic Domain	Social Domain
Social			Tradition of values, meanings, and technology which impact occupation
Symbolic		Values, goals, temporality, interests and personal causation	Impact of culture on personality such as definitions of time, cultural interests, values, and so forth
Iconic	Brain as coordinator of sensory and motor information and as infrastructure of images	Complex network of images that constitute an inner model of the external world	Skilled actions and performances maintained in the group tradition
Differentiated	Differentiation and specialization of nervous and musculoskeletal systems	Differentiation of occupational behaviors and their underlying symbols and images over the lifespan	Divisions of labor and integration of individuals in group
Open	Spontaneous, holistic, and self-maintaining process of sensory input and motor output	Spontaneous urge for activity as organizing principle. Occupational behavior as self-maintaining output	Organizations as self-maintaining systems with input, output, and throughput
Cybernetic	Feedback loops in the nervous system	Feedback regulation of skilled action and social feedback modifying self-concept	Social feedback processes regulating performance of group members
Clockwork	Kinetics of movement simple relexes	Balance of work and play, dynamics of life space	Dyadic interaction and group dynamics
Framework	Anatomy of the musculoskeletal and nervous systems	Pattern of motives and symbols which energize and organize behavior	Social roles and status within group structure

FIGURE 2. Hierarchical knowledge in biopsychosocial domains.

knowledge of the brain's role in organizing information and the brain as the infrastructure for formation, maintenance, and changing of images. Knowledge at this level is largely nonexistent today.

PSYCHOLOGIC PHENOMENA. For purposes of this discussion psychologic phenomena are conceived as the individual's motivational and symbolic processes. In concert with the theme that occupational therapy should focus its knowledge on occupation, this category will include that knowledge which defines the psychologic aspects of human occupation. Thus, knowledge of human sexuality and the bulk of related psychodynamic theory, behaviorism, and other psychologic concepts which are not aimed at explaining occupation is purposely omitted.

Very little is known in occupational therapy about the motives and symbolic processes of occupation. Maslow's[44] hierarchy of needs is an example of such a framework of generic motivational propensities; a comparable framework of needs pertaining to occupation would be a major addition to occupational therapy's understanding of human beings. A preliminary hierarchy of exploration, competence, and achievement was proposed by Reilly[61] and it begins work toward a structure of occupational motives. Similarly, little is known about the framework or arrangement of symbolic structures and processes. Reilly's[61] proposal that values are the ruling symbolic structures in occupation,

Kielhofner and Burke's[37] delineation of symbolic subsystems and their internal structures and deRenne-Stephen's[62] proposals concerning the internal and external structure for imitation represent beginning theories of symbolic processes incorporating framework level phenomena. Also, stage theories of development such as Takata's[74] epochs of play incorporate framework approaches to human occupation.

At the level of clockworks, there is concern with the dynamics of occupation. Shannon's[67] concept of balance of work-play phenomena, Reilly's[60] and Watanabe's[78] concept of life spaces and their dynamic relationship are examples of theories which incorporate this level. At the cybernetic level the regulatory action of feedback is the phenomena of concern. The idea of feedback regulation of skilled action[30,37,57,61] and of habit processes[36] are concepts from this level of complexity. The impact of feedback on the self-image is another concept at this level that enhances understanding of occupation.[12,69]

The level of open systems requires understanding of the basic spontaneous tendency underlying occupation, the processes of input, output, throughput, and feedback that contribute to the self-maintaining properties of the system. Both Boulding[9] and Allport[1] note that only limited knowledge exists at or beyond this level in the life sciences and behavioral sciences. A number of occupational therapists have incorporated open systems concepts into their theoretical frameworks, beginning the generation of knowledge at this level.

Florey's[22] concept of intrinsic motivation as the dynamics of occupation and Kielhofner and Burke's[37] urge to explore and master the world have outlined the basic spontaneous principle underlying the open system's nature of occupation. Reilly[61], Webster[80], Kielhofner and Burke[37], and Paulson[57] have all incorporated open systems concepts of the importation of energy and information to maintain system integrity in their explanations of work, play, and occupational choice. Fidler and Fidler's[21] concept of doing and becoming reflects the principles of self-organization of open systems.

At the level of differentiated systems we recognize the process of progressive diversification and integration of phenomena. Here one confronts such difficult topics as how the ambiguous awareness of the human neonate translates into the highly complex system of symbolic representation of the world and self which guides occupation. The differentiation of symbols in play,[50,61,64] the differentiation of interests,[45] and the process of making an occupational choice[57,80] are part and parcel of phenomena at this level.

At the iconic level the emergent phenomena is the image. Only rudimentary explanations of its nature and dynamics have been offered.[9] The image is an internal model of the external world. Many authors agree that it is a network of rules which govern organization of information.[15,29,32] Thus the image is a rule-bound system of awareness of experience. At the level of the image beginning work has been done by Robinson[64] and Reilly[61] who have examined the formation of rules of competent behavior that make skill possible. Similarly, Kielhofner, Barris and Watts[36] have proposed habits as rule-governed processes which organize occupational behavior; that work also reflects this level of complexity.

The symbolic capacity of human beings is the apex of occupational ability. At this level the image is freed from time and space, and human beings can reflect on their own behavior, imagine past and future events, create purposes and the like. In occupational therapy literature the concepts of temporal awareness,[34,54] awareness of self-worth and agenthood,[12] valued goals,[37] interests,[45] and personal meaning,[85] have begun to advance our understanding of symbolic properties of human occupation.

SOCIAL PHENOMENA. The importance of the social dimension in occupation has always been recognized in the field. Moral treatment, the predecessor of occupational therapy, was a process of creating a social environment in which mentally ill individuals could recover. Social expectation, support, and recognition have always been understood as important dimensions of occupational therapy. More recently, it has been proposed that occupation is both a means of entry into the social world and a means of contributing to the social system.[37,46,64,67] The influences of the social system on the individual's occupational life have also been recognized.[40] Thus, social phenomena are clearly important topics for occupational therapy.

At the level of frameworks we recognize social phenomena such as the various role positions and standard patterns of interaction which make up the structure of any social system. The concept of occupational role and the opportunities and expectations it brings to the individual has been proposed as a major factor in occupational behavior.[30,46] At the level of clockworks we recognize such dynamic social patterns as dyadic interaction[51] and group dynamics,[20,52] and the implication of these processes for competent occupational performance. Feedback processes and their regulatory functions have been identified in social systems, as patterns of regulation in organizations always incorporate important feedback functions.[33,81] Such principles of group feedback processes are used in occupational therapy groups. However, much remains to be understood at this level.

Social processes have been recognized and conceptualized as open systems processes,[33,79,81] but the implication of these processes for occupational therapy practice remains largely unexplored. Understanding how the dynamics of group exchanges of information and self-maintaining and self-transforming processes of groups impact the growth and progressive organization of members eventually will be important for occupational therapy's use of therapeutic groups. At the level of differentiation we recognize the familiar patterns of division of labor and integration of activities in groups. The performance of individuals within groups is guided by this process; as groups evolve into differentiated and integrated systems, the function of individuals becomes more specialized and interrelated with those of other group members. This process places greater demands on individual members as the organization becomes more complex. Once again, the implications of such processes have gone largely unexplored in occupational therapy.

At the level of iconics are the image-determined underlying patterns of social groups and the way they structure behavior. Below the level of human awareness a plethora of images guides how persons interact physically and temporally and maintain the technical way of life the group has developed[27]. These patterns form a deep fabric of social life and are learned by new members largely through imitation. At the symbolic level cultural tradition and its definitions of meaning, purpose, and value, which impact the individual's occupational behavior, are phenomena of concern to occupational therapy. Finally, at the social system level one must recognize the social group as a functional whole whose requirements influence the thoughts and behavior of individuals. As Koestler[41] points out, human beings must be understood as both autonomous wholes and as parts of a larger social system. Allport[1] notes that while we tend to think of the individual personality as residing "within the skin," the reality is that human beings are both a function of internal makeup and of external relations and interactions. It is both impossible and incorrect to attempt understanding of individuals without incorporating a view of their interrelatedness with an external social world. The balance of internal and external processes are the fundamental dynamic of the human system.

SUMMARY

This discussion has outlined the relationship of biopsychosocial knowledge and phenomena to the levels of hierarchy, revealing broad areas of information relevant to the practice of occupational therapy. It should be apparent that the current status of knowledge in the field is not equal across all dimensions. The most well developed and nearly complete information is at the lower levels of the hierarchy and in the domain of biologic phenomena. Ascending the hierarchy toward more complex phenomena, or moving from biologic to psychologic or social domains of knowledge, there are less well developed bodies of information. In short, the least knowledge is available in areas where the most knowledge is needed. Since higher levels of the hierarchy in any system exert an all-important governing influence over the lower levels, knowledge of the higher levels is essential. Occupational behavior encompasses the biologic, psychologic and social domains across many levels of complexity, and understanding requires knowledge in all of these areas. Even the simplest everyday occupation reveals itself as part of a complex and integrated system of relationships between domains and levels of phenomena. For example, dressing oneself reflects cultural mores governing dressing style and its symbolization of the person's position in the social group. Further, the behavior involves a personal view of self, an image which guides skillful action needed to perform the act, the nervous system and musculoskeletal system hardware used, and so forth. All of these and other domains of reality intermesh as one performs a deceptively simple daily routine. Ultimately, the view of human beings the field generates must acknowledge the breadth and scope of occupational phenomena. It behooves occupational therapy to examine closely priorities of knowledge development as well as the requirements of knowledge for practice. Current approaches to identifying the knowledge underlying occupational therapy practice, while eclectic, involve no systematic identification of the domains or levels of knowledge dealt with. A more rigorous approach to identifying the knowledge of the field (both that which is currently available and that which is required but undeveloped) could guide the field's decisions for education, research, and theory development. Such a systematic approach to the genesis and dissemination of knowledge would enhance the development of a coherent paradigm.

In addition to identifying gaps in knowledge, the discussion implies a further problem in occupational therapy theory.

Knowledge accumulated about biologic lower level phenomena is not integrated with that of psychologic higher level phenomena. Similarly, knowledge of the individual in the psychologic domain is not well integrated with knowledge of how persons function as part of the social system. Thus, the field operates with artifical divisions across domains of knowledge and between levels of knowledge. The two most important dichotomies of knowledge are the mind-body dualism and the person-environment dualism of current thinking. Our view of human beings in the new paradigm must ultimately be based on a resolution of these two important gaps in occupational therapy knowledge.

MIND-BRAIN UNITY

In his Slagle lecture, Bing[8] identified mind-body unity as a central proposition of early occupational therapy, a finding consistent with the preceding historical analysis. Current thinking in the field neglects this original concept.

The neurosciences have a predisposition to reduce behavior that has mental aspects to neurophysiologic explanations.[70] Neurophysiology has traditionally showed disinterest toward mental phenomena and does not recognize the causative influence of mental processes on brain physiology, though the reverse *is* assumed.[70] Similarly, in occupational therapy the impact of brain function and dysfunction on mental processes is assumed without due consideration of the reverse. According to the hierarchical principles just reviewed, symbolic processes should govern neurophysiology at the same time the brain serves as the foundation of these conscious processes. Sperry[71] offers a compelling theory of mind-brain phenomenon that reflects hierarchical principles. He considers mental processes to be an integral part of the brain process itself. Sperry[71] posits conscious mental processes as emergent properties of the brain which are interdependent with the brain but which are also "distinct and special in their own right." He proposes further, in line with hierarchical thinking, that conscious processes exert a ruling influence over aspects of brain physiology:

> The conscious properties of cerebral activity are conceived to have analogous causal effects in brain function that control subset events in the flow pattern of neural excitation. In this holistic sense the present proposal may be said to place mind over matter, but not as any disembodied or supernatural agent.[70]

Sperry points out that in his view conscious processes do not interfere with nervous system physiology but that they do "supervene" and rule at the molar level. He offers a basis for a resolution of mind-brain dichotomy that may enhance the potential for a long overdue connection between purposeful activity and its influence on brain physiology and coordinated and adaptive sensory-motor patterns. Such a perspective on mind-brain phenomenon requires that the basic relation of sensory input to motor output be reconceptualized. Rather than sensory impulses being "routed through a central network system into a motor response,"[70] one must conceive of sensory information entering and impinging on the dynamics of an integrated system.[3,9] It is the state of that system (including the status of symbolic processes), which determines how sensory information will be read and interpreted and what, if any, output will be enacted. The meaning of sensory input depends not only on the properties of the sensory message, but also on the interaction of its properties with the readiness of the system to decode and attribute significance to those properties. Sperry and other writers such as Hayek[29] and Hofstadter[32] seek an alternative to Cartesian dualism that achieves a view of the mind as an entity in its own right at the expense of its being disembodied or disconnected from the brain. They also eschew those propositions which reduce mental events to epiphenomenal aspects of neurophysiologic processes. In their view mind or mental events are continuous with the material phenomenon of the brain. Yet neither can be transposed into the other without an inevitable distortion of what is meant at a particular level. Neurophysiologic events cannot be explained as mental events, and vice versa, although they are continuous and interrelated.

Moreover, this does not imply an absolute isomorphism between neurologic events and the symbols which emerge from them. Bateson[3] and Smythies[68] both make the point that mechanical production of "thoughts" by neurophysiologic processes is not what is meant by the mind emerging from brain function. It is not presently known what the physiologic correlates of symbolic processes are. Hofstadter[32] proposes that symbols may be rooted in the relations between processes, so that a single brain cell might participate in production of many symbols. Neurophysiologic events which contribute to symbols may be layered, overlapping, and concurrent in both space and time. Hayek[29] postulates that the symbolic process is seated in the overall organization of neurologic processes. In his view symbolic processes are synonomous with the rules governing operation of the brain at the highest level. These rules (like the rules governing the living cell) are not located in any particular time or space in the system, but rather throughout the brain or the cell, and as the fundamental principles of their ongoing order. This view is consistent with Collier's[15] notion that elementary consciousness emerges from the organizational properties of protoplasmic processes. Sperry[70] adds another dimension to the relatedness of symbolic and neurophysiologic processes by noting that although each has an influence on the other (brain making possible mental events and the latter having effects in the brain), no temporal sequence is implied. Rather, he suggests that symbolic processes and their neurophysiologic events are simultaneous, and that this does not preclude the ruling influence of symbols over physiology.

The symbolic level is the highest level on a continuum of organization of information which begins with sensory receptors and culminates with the arrival of impulses in a vast information processing system which operates on them to make decisions about action. Symbolic processes are thus intimately linked to the primary function of organizing information for action. As Collier[15] points out, the fact that not all symbolic processes result in action does not preclude their being primarily in the service of action. Such diverse writers as Piaget[58] and Sudnow[72] share the conviction that symbolic processes (thought and conscious experience) arise fundamentally out of the creation of action by the organism and remain linked in essential ways to action. If this is the case, mental processes are closely interrelated with occupation. Indeed, they require occupation for their existence.

Theorists suggest that play is a fundamental process in the emergence of symbolic capacity.[11,61] This writer's view is that play serves as the process for co-developing and co-differentiating symbolic and neurophysiologic processes. A recent paper by Parhman, Lindquist and Gonzales[56] linking play and sensory integration, offers a preliminary but cogent schema consistent with this proposition.

The viewpoint that symbolic processes remain linked in essential ways to action is supported by Berger and Luckman.[4] They propose that consciousness is always intentional; thus it operates as a system which considers and wills courses of action. It is a fundamental postulate in areas of sociology that symbolic processes are maintained, constructed, and reconstituted in ongoing action.[4,13,47,48,66] This holds tremendous implications for occupational therapy, since occupation is important as a dynamic medium of symbolic processes. Purposeful activity is thus at the very crux of both symbolic and neurophysiologic events. This is not surprising. Rather, it is a predictable characteristic of the open systems nature of the mind-brain system; as an open system it maintains itself through its own action.

The ideas offered here are intended primarily to stimulate interest and action in the complex area of mind-brain unity. I would like to close the discussion by enumerating briefly how a unified view might reorganize some present knowledge in the field. Occupational therapy is concerned with several kinds of phenomena which have clear neurophysiologic bases: perception, sensory integration, and motor competence. However, most of the theory development concerning these phenomena has ignored or paid only passing attention to the role of symbolic processes which ultimately rule in this realm. Further, the current view of neurophysiologic dysfunction preceding and preventing symbolic operation is only partly true. The intimate connection of these two processes means that we are dealing with a unified system that has to be addressed as a gestalt. In specific terms, it would mean that perceptual, sensory integrative, and motor processes will need to be understood in terms of the imagery processes of imaginative and fantasy play, purposeful intention, meaningful features of the environment, and so forth. Perception cannot occur without an image. Sensory integration must be processed in concert with symbolic processes in play. Coordinated motor movement is always intentional or purposeful. The challenge of theorizing in the future will be to specify how such interconnected processes operate.

PERSON-SOCIAL SYSTEM UNITY

Occupational therapy shares with other disciplines a perspective which falsely dichotomizes persons and their social systems. As Allport[1] notes, psychology has tended toward constructing a version of human beings as isolated entities, ignoring the importance of interaction with the external social environment. Von Bertalannfy[7] faults the predominant isolationist views of human beings and the mechanistic metaphors which have been used to explain human behavior. If humans are thought to be like machines, then there is little need to be concerned with the nature of their environments and the interactions and influences between the human system and the environment. However, as the open systems character of the human being is recognized, one is increasingly aware of the importance of the environment in the shaping and maintaining of the system's integrity. Unity of the human system with the social environment is not a platitude, but is an essential part of the human condition which must be recognized if the organization of the human system is to be understood in any meaningful way.

In the same way that the mind emerges from the brain as a new ruling level, the social system emerges from, but also governs, the collectivity of individuals as they interact. Similarly, the social system exerts an important ruling influence on the individual thought and action of its members. The interface between person and social group is best appreciated from the perspective of evolution. In the course of the species' emergence, social evolution became both a moving force in selection and a buffer between the individual and the selective press of the environment. The individual adapted *both through and to* the cultural tradition.

Social systems are created from patterns of events (i.e., interactions of persons) and thus they have no structure apart from the dynamics of members participation.[1] Thus, just as the mind is dependent on the brain for its existence, social systems depend on the collective participation of individuals. The social system, like the mind, also exerts a governing effect on its infrastructure. As the mind rules the brain, so the social system rules throughts and the actions of its members.

Katz and Kahn[33] identify three ways in which social systems govern human behavior: (a) environmental pressures, (b) shared values and expectations, and (c) rule enforcement. As groups encounter various environmental pressures (e.g., availability of food, information, and other resources) the group requires a division of labor and specific contributions by members. Thus, the social group mediates the demands of physical and social ecology for survival, goal attainment, and so forth. By definition, groups have values and expectations; these collective feelings and convictions place demands on members to pursue certain courses of action and avoid others. Finally, to maintain their integrity, groups, consisting only of events which members produce, must place limits on the types of events which members can engage in. Members are thus governed by implicit and explicit rules.

Sociologists further propose that the group provides each member with a basic world view.[4] Social groups not only require certain behavior of their members, but by virtue of the traditions of knowledge in groups, provide ways of interpreting and understanding the external world. This fundamental world view (which includes such basic perceptions as time and space) is learned in a long period of enculturation during which the personality is formed.[27] Such enculturation results in a mature individual who, for the most part, sees the world as his cultural peers do, and who is predisposed to interpret events and respond to them in socially typical ways.

The social world continues throughout life to serve as a source of reaffirmation and elaboration of the world view which its members have come to inherit. Some sociologists stress how reality, as the individual experiences it, is constructed in an ongoing way by the active and collective efforts of social members.[4,13,25,48] Thus the internal reality which an individual experiences is first constructed and maintained by the social order.

Sutton-Smith[73] proposes that the child's enculturation begins in earliest infant play where the basis of the child's perspective on self and on the external world is constructed. Play serves as a metaphor for the child's reflexivity or self-awareness—that trait which separates the symbolic from the iconic level. Thus, while humans have the capacity for symbolization, the cultural milieu is the arena in which it is constructed. The deep interdependence of the human mind and the social world which shapes, informs, and elaborates mental capacity is a complex subject about which we have only beginning knowledge, yet it promises to reveal more about humanity than any other line of inquiry in the social and behavioral sciences.

The social system not only provides a generalized matrix of information, values, mores, norms, and other prohibitive and prescriptive elements, but also provides a guiding structure for individualized participation in the form of social roles. Each individual acts out social life in terms of a number of roles that define position in the group and which, in turn, prescribe what they may and may not do.[33,75] As Cicourel[14] points out, this is a dynamic process in which individuals literally negotiate their way through social roles by balancing personal propensities and abilities against implicit and explicit expectations for their role.

The social role is a most useful concept for understanding the relationship between the individual and the social group. At the level of the social system the role is the unit of participation. Within organizations individuals may come and go, but the role and its function remain relatively constant if the social system is to survive. The role is a functional aspect of any organization which is to some degree vital for its continuation. The function of an individual within the role matters primarily in terms of how well that person fills the function. Thus the system requires a rather constant set of role expectations despite changes in role occupants. Without such constancy the social system's integrity could not be assured. The need of the system to thus govern its components is apparent.

Without the set of role prescriptions individuals could not readily act in a manner which would allow the continuation of the social system; their collective enterprise would be chaotic and unstable. Further, without their perspectives inherited from cultural traditions, the basis for interaction would be eliminated. Human life would be like the biblical Tower of Babel in which individuals could not coordinate their efforts or understand each other. Thus the social system provides both the means by which individuals can participate in collective action, and in doing so, it governs the mental processes and behavior of each individual.

CONCLUSION: THE VIEW OF HUMAN BEINGS IN THE EMERGING PARADIGM

In the preceding pages I have attempted to construct a preliminary framework for organizing the knowledge of occupational therapy and to examine its implications for the field's view of human beings. We now recognize that knowledge in the field encompasses biologic, psychologic and social domains, and crosses several levels of complexity. Plotting the biopsychosocial dimensions against the levels of hierarchy, we have a map of the basic territory of information that will make up the field's body of knowledge defining human beings. According to this framework, human beings are viewed in hierarchical terms. Lower level processes involving primarily the nervous and musculoskeletal systems are seen in terms of higher level functions into which they are integrated. In turn, humans are recognized as members of social systems into which their thoughts and actions must be integrated. In addition to our need to see lower level phenomena in terms of their integration into higher levels, we also require a more unified perspective of the major domains of knowledge. Current dichotomies between the mind and the brain and between the individual and the social system contribute to the fragmentation of occupational therapy knowledge.

The emerging paradigm of occupational therapy will thus be a multi-level perspective that recognizes the interrelatedness of phenomena. The continuum from motor movement to cultural tradition constitutes the phenomena of human occupation. While incorporating this range of knowledge, the field must achieve a coherent perspective that views human beings as integrated systems of biologic and psychologic processes that function within larger social processes. The structure of hierarchical levels and the rules which govern relations between levels should serve to cement concepts together into a unified gestalt.

OCCUPATIONAL THERAPY PUZZLES

In paradigmatic change the new view of the phenomena inevitably leads to a redefinition of the puzzles which practitioners will solve.[42] As shown in Chapter 1, a change in the clinical puzzles of occupational therapy accompanied paradigm change. The discussion above proposes a new view of humans which similarly has inherent in it a proposal for changing the clinical problems the field would address. It is part of the shift in focus from underlying components of occupation, which belong to lower levels of the hierarchy, to occupational behavior at the symbolic and social levels.

In her paper outlining the differences between occupational therapy and medicine, Rogers[65] called for a movement beyond the current diagnoses of medicine to a new taxonomy of occupational dysfunction. The idea flows naturally from the theme of centering theory and practice on occupation and turning from component structures to overall gestalt patterns. Diagnostic systems in medicine describe disorder in component structures, whereas concepts of occupational dysfunction would describe patterns of disorganization in the human system's interaction with the environment.[65] Problems faced in occupational therapy may often emanate from underlying pathology, but they are manifest in the disorganization of daily living patterns, the loss of skills for a chosen lifestyle, the interference of disability with the attainment of valued goals, and so forth. The list of symbolic dysfunctions which populate occupational therapy clinics includes: idleness, boredom, hopelessness, passiveness, and dependence. The processes with which therapists hope to replace these disabilities include courage, hope, commitment, and confidence. These are the processes which occur at the highest level of organization in the human system—the level of symbol and value.

A taxonomy of occupational dysfunction would necessarily go beyond the level of dysfunction of bodily or intrapsychic functions to describe the occupational dysfunctions of daily life performance in productive life roles, daily living tasks, and ludic occupations and their concomitant disruptions of time and purpose. The diagnostic system of medicine does not give this information. For instance, the occupational dysfunction of a university professor become paraplegic is not the same as the occupational dysfunction of the paraplegic truck driver. The hand injury to the accountant is not the same as the hand injury to the clock maker. The ways in which dysfunction of lower levels will reverberate through the higher levels cannot be predicted from the bottom up. In this case the university professor and the accountant have in common that they must adjust to their work roles. The truck driver and clock maker must relinquish theirs. Thus, the differential diagnosis of productive life role loss and productive life role adjustment might well be a more relevant diagnosis for occupational therapy. In similar vein, one might recognize in the schizophrenic and the cord injured football player the dysfunction of occupational choice, since neither has viable options in current self-identity for work. The person with degenerative arthritis and the person with multiple sclerosis have in common the problem of maintaining competence for daily living tasks in the context of decreasing functional capacity. The unique contribution of occupational therapy in the overall understanding of health problems thus would be in the area of identifying how occupational life is affected by disease, trauma, and social conditions, and how disruptions of occupational life have further implications for the health and competence of persons.

This writer's clinical practice has confirmed a belief that such a perspective on occupational dysfunction is both viable and effective for patient care. For example, in working with adolescents and adults, the identification of disruption or suppression of normal play was a meaningful clinical category. Individuals whose life circumstances and neuromuscular or emotional deficits had contributed to their being poor players or nonplayers were encountered many times. Since play is an important behavior for development,[76] the extent to which the lack of normal play was disabling to the individual beyond other internal deficits could be specified. By concentrating effort on the restoration or elicitation of normal play, therapy not only improved normal occupational behavior, but also influenced development in other areas.[38]

Development of a taxonomy of occupational dysfunction to serve as our system of clinical puzzles will be a major conceptual task for the formulation of a new paradigm. The payoffs of such effort would be the identification of a unique set of puzzles for occupational therapy clinical practice, the organization of clinical thinking in occupational therapy around a central core of identified dysfunctions, and the enhancement of the process of developing systematic puzzle-solving or treatment techniques.

As Rogers[65] notes, classification is not enough. Any designation of occupational therapy problems must also include a means of conceptualizing disorder in the system. It will also have to include a conceptualization of the many levels of phenomena which are affected by injury, disease process, or circumstances which threaten the integrity of occupational behavior in an individual. Our present schema of levels of complexity can be used to illuminate the multilevel or hierarchical nature of dysfunction.

A common occupational therapy problem, spinal cord injury, will illustrate the hierarchical nature of some of the disturbances affecting an individual's occupational behavior. (Table 1). Severing of the human spinal cord creates a disturbance primarily at the clockwork level. Without proper innervation the dynamic function of motor movement is disrupted. At the framework level we find subsequent disorganization: muscles atrophy, and eventually the skeletal framework may undergo some loss of integrity. Severe constraints are imposed throughout the system. Nervous impulses from deinnervated areas cannot reach the central nervous system; thus, sensory loss ensues. Without this feedback regulatory systems which assure relief of pressure and blood supply or those which protect the lower extemities by signaling pain cannot function. At the open system level the output of the system in the biologic, psychologic and social domains is disrupted. Motor output, output for goal attainment, and output of social role performance are constrained. Along with this disruption of output there is also a threat to the integrity of self-maintaining nature of the system. Physical, psychologic, and social disorganization can easily follow. At the level of differentiation, there is a disruption of bodily division of labor: the arms may become primary tools for mobility; sight must replace tactile sense for feedback concerning position and other states of the lower extremities. Thus, organization of the diversified and integrated functions of the body is disturbed and a new division of labor and integration of parts is required. Similar disorganization and requirements for reorganization occur in the psychologic and social domains. At the

TABLE 1. Levels of Dysfunction in Spinal Cord Injury

LEVELS OF COMPLEXITY	DYSFUNCTIONS
Social	Disengagement from social roles, stigma
Symbolic	Disruption of purposes, goals, meaning in life, and sense of causation
Iconic	Images governing skilled action are no longer viable
Differentiated	Division of labor and integration of functions in biologic, psychologic and social areas disrupted
Open	Output blocked with consequent threat to self-maintenance
Cybernetic	Sensory feedback disrupted
Clockwork	Movement disrupted
Framework	Structure of musculoskeletal system threatened

iconic level old images governing skilled action are no longer useful since the motor apparatus they formerly called upon cannot respond; many basic skills must then be relearned. At the symbolic level the sense of self as a cause, values, purposes, and meaning in life are disrupted. Finally, the individual may become disengaged from the social network in several ways. Social roles may be lost, stigma may serve to alter the nature of all social relations, and new roles of patient and invalid may begin to take over. Dysfunction reverberates throughout the system.

The case of mental illness serves to illustrate dysfunction emanating from the other end of the hierarchy (Table 2). More and more, psychiatric problems are recognized to be functions of the social system of the individual.[31,43,79] For instance, developing children exposed to chaotic and emotionally turbulent families may develop inconsistent values, distortions of the temporal order, and a sense of ineffectiveness and helplessness. These symbolic disturbances create poor conditions for the learning of images for competent action, resulting in problems ranging from social ineffectiveness to poor motor skills. Thought processes do not become sufficiently differentiated and integrated; the individual may not even fully differentiate self from others. Open system functions are disrupted and the system as a whole continues disorganization, with the result that feedback from the environment is absent, negative, or improperly interpreted. Finally, disturbances in the neuromuscular system may be manifest with distortions of movement and posture.

Too often there is failure to recognize the multiple levels of disorganization which occur in patients of all types. The dynamics of a disorganized system are more complex than the discrete problems therapists are accustomed to dealing with. Moreover, because these dysfunctions reverberate throughout an integrated system, not only are some aspects of the dysfunction undetected, but the most important dysfunction—the disturbance of the whole—is missed.

PUZZLE-SOLVING: THE NATURE OF CLINICAL PRACTICE UNDER A NEW PARADIGM

A shift in the clinical puzzles of occupational therapy will, of necessity, require re-examination of clinical practice, the field's puzzle-solving techniques. Occupational ther-

TABLE 2. Levels of Dysfunction in Mental Illness

LEVELS OF COMPLEXITY	DYSFUNCTIONS
Social	Chaotic and emotionally turbulent family
Symbolic	Distortion of temporal order, sense of ineffectiveness
Iconic	Failure to learn images to guide skilled action
Differientated	Thought processes and sense of self not differentiated and integrated
Open	Inconsistent output, poor environmental interaction
Cybernetic	Feedback absent, negative or improperly interpreted
Clockwork	Movement patterns distorted
Framework	Postural mechanisms abnormal

apy puzzle-solving must focus on the use of occupations that naturally reorganize and remediate dysfunction throughout the hierarchy, and on the adaptation of tools and environments to permit those with intractable limitations at lower levels to engage in occupational behavior.

The use of occupations as therapy is the oldest and most central theme in occupational therapy. The employment of play, games, arts and crafts, creative music, productive pursuits, and so forth comprise the art and science of the field. Unfortunately, this therapeutic use of occupation has increasingly been eschewed by occupational therapists.

Some of the most basic knowledge in occupational therapy spells out how the musculoskeletal system and its dynamics make possible the performance of everyday activities. A growing body of neurologically-based theories defines ways in which the nervous system underlies similar performance. Therapists readily recognize how disease or trauma which affects these systems can undermine the health and occupational performance of individuals. No small part of present practice is oriented to techniques that attempt restoration of these anatomic and neurologic subsystems.

Traditional belief has held that occupation has a unique capacity to restore behavior and maintain the organization of systems affected by disease and trauma. However, as suggested in Chapter 1, much of the explanation of the healing power of occupation has been reduced to the direct influence of activity on the nervous system or motor system. In the hierarchical schema, the relationship between meaningful or purposeful activity and lower level functions is exceedingly complex, involving the interaction of effects through several levels of complexity. It is apparent that much of the richness of occupation's health-maintaining and health-restoring character has been oversimplified and underestimated. Activation of the human symbolic capacity through occupation reverberates throughout the image, the nervous system, and its musculoskeletal and sensory hardware. According to laws of hierarchy the human system operates as a dynamic whole with the higher levels in unique position to govern the lower. Yerxa[85] provides an example of this symbolic impact on the neuromuscular system in the incident of a woman unable to move her arm, and who when presented with a glass of water, suddenly was able to reach out and grasp it. The following examples should further illuminate the hierarchical principles involved in occupation and its influence on dysfunction. Norman Cousins in his book, *Anatomy of an Illness*, relates the following story about Pablo Casals, the renowned cellist:

> I met him for the first time at his home in Puerto Rico just a few weeks before his ninetieth birthday. I was fascinated by his daily routine. About 8 A.M. his lovely young wife Marta would help him start the day. His various infirmities made it difficult for him to dress himself. Judging from his difficulty in walking and from the way he held his arms, I guessed he was suffering from rheumatoid arthritis. His emphysema was evident in his labored breathing. He came into the living room on Marta's arm. He was badly stooped. His head was pitched forward, and he walked with a shuffle. His hands were swollen and his fingers were clenched. Even before going to the breakfast table, Don Pablo went to the piano—which, I learned, was a daily ritual. He arranged himself with some difficulty on the piano bench, then with discernible effort, raised his swollen and clenched fingers above the keyboard. I was not prepared for the miracle that was about to happen. The fingers slowly unlocked and reached toward the keys like buds of a plant toward the sunlight. His back straightened. He seemed to breathe more freely. Now his fingers settled on the keys. Then came the opening bars of Bach's *Wohltemperierte Klavier,* played with great sensitivity and control. . . . Then he plunged into a Brahms concerto and his fingers, now agile and powerful, raced across the keyboard with dazzling speed. His entire body seemed fused with the music; it was no longer stiff and shrunken but supple and graceful and completely freed of its arthritic coils. Having finished the piece, he stood up by himself, far straighter and taller than when he had come into the room. He walked to the breakfast table with no trace of a shuffle, ate heartily, talked animatedly, finished the meal, then went for a walk on the beach.[17]

A few years ago in a research project at the University of California at Los Angeles, I was studying the daily life adaptation of developmentally disabled persons in the community. In one of our study sites, a residential facility, I met a most remarkable middle-aged man who was afflicted with athetoid cerebral palsy. Despite this man's extreme motor impairment which made every movement and every effort to speak a monumental task, he lived an astonishingly full occupational life. Each day he dressed himself in suit and tie, literally spending hours on his grooming. He pursued hobbies of electronics and carpentry and rode a three-wheeled bicycle throughout West Los Angeles. The man was constantly busy, constantly planning new projects, constantly involved in the commerce of everyday life. My research interest led me to take detailed field notes on the simplest of his everyday activities. I was repeatedly amazed that he managed to do anything at all. Then one day, as I watched him drink a cup of coffee the secret of his competency unfolded for me. Soon thereafter I wrote the following note on the incident:

> I found Paul in the kitchen eating. I sat with him for a while as he ate and said a few things to him from time to time. It is amazing to watch Paul eat. I have the feeling that if I were given his body at this moment, I would be absolutely unable to do anything useful with it. Despite all its writhings and distortions, Paul's body does all the things it has to and the care with which he organizes and executes each movement is striking. Paul is a truly *graceful* cerebral palsied person. It is near mystery to watch him wind his unruly hands around a cup of tea which is purposefully not too hot so as not to burn him should a sudden involuntary movement dump it into his mouth or over his face. He slowly places one hand toward the cup, nudging it with the other to focus the movement. When his hand is in place, he makes a grasping movement which sends off a whole parade of involuntary contractions throughout his arm. The second hand is still steadying things during all this. Then, the second hand

moves just as carefully to embrace the other one. Now, with this two-handed grasp in which his fingers literally encircle and hide the cup, he brings his face and hands to meet halfway and sips the tea with lips and throat that move uncontrollably. The tea spills, he makes gurgling and loud sipping noises and chokes a bit on the tea. In the midst of all this, Paul remains impeccably calm and dignified. A great spirit of inner calm and strength emanates through a withered, contorted and unruly body.

In pouring over other notes on this man, I found over and over again a very simple fact. Each of the things that this man did mattered; they were meaningful to him in the context of how he carried out his daily life. Each aspect of his functional performance, however difficult and trying to execute, was nonetheless worth doing. His nervous system remained dysfunctional. But the meaning he found in the activities of daily living organized his every movement. Like Casals, he was made *graceful* by the occupations that meant so much to him and that he performed as daily rituals. His gracefulness was not a conventional or easily observable feature of his performance, but a deep seated phenomenon involving the creation of internal images which allowed him to master his own unruly movements. His life tasks were permeated with his acquired ability to effectively use what others might find an unmanageable body.

These examples illustrate ways in which phenomena at higher levels of the hierarchy can rule or govern the operation of lower levels. This is the most fundamental characteristic of any hierarchy, as each emerging level builds on the levels below, while also governing them. Moreover, because the degree of freedom of higher levels is wide, they can adapt to limitations or disruptions of lower levels to maintain the integrity of the whole.

In each of these cases there was a dysfunction at the level of movement. In one case there was an anatomical disruption producing pain, stiffness, and deformity, and in the other a dysfunction in the neurologic hardware that coordinates motor movement. For each person the problem was overcome or adjusted at a higher level.

Casals' deep personal involvement in classical music resonated through his nervous and motor subsystems. Here the sheer governing force of a healthy set of higher images reverberate downward through levels of the system to evoke motor performance.

The second case is perhaps the more interesting one. One problem which an individual with athetoid cerbral palsy faces is that the intention to move evokes extraneous movements. What apparently allowed this man to gracefully execute athetoid movement was the formation of images about his movements and the extraneous movements they evoked. These higher level images could then incorporate plans to achieve purposes which compensated for the problems that arose when intentions were being executed. Thus, by knowing what his body would do when he intended an act, Paul could command another act to counter or compensate for the error of the first one. His problem probably was complicated by the fact that the second act would itself have some degree of error that needed to be compensated for at yet another level of image. Whatever their nature, a hierarchy of images allowed him to act *gracefully* even though his neurologic hardware for effecting action was faulty.

These examples provide an insight into the complex yet very real way in which occupation plays a central role in life adaptation. The purposeful nature of occupations includes a vast store of potential effects for maintaining and restoring the system throughout its many levels. Occupations have an organizational ability far beyond the direct effects of movement on muscle physiology, and even the latter may have a much more complicated connection than previously supposed.

Understanding this hierachical schema and its function greatly enhances the ways in which occupational therapy can conceptualize the role of occupation in healing and health. It provides a new structure for thinking about relations between human beings' levels of organization, their complexity, and their interrelatedness that promises to explain more cogently why occupation can be therapy.

But demands of using occupation therapeutically are substantial and will require a great deal of development in the field. It is surprising, for instance, that the science of achieving purposefulness in the occupational therapy clinic remains undeveloped. Therapists in clinical practice have no recourse to a body of knowledge to develop purposeful activities for patients; rather they must make do with common sense. However, the therapeutic use of occupations should always begin with a careful approach to the highest levels of the hierarchy. Just as engaging a patient in an activity that incorporates neurologic principles is poor therapy, to engage a patients in a craft which is culturally insignificant or which ignores their self-image is also counter-therapeutic. Because activity analysis requires careful attention throughout the hierarchy, the impact of occupations on higher levels should be thoroughly planned.

Remediation at the lower levels does not assure remediation at the higher levels; however, remediation at the higher levels has tremendous payoff for the lower levels. Nothing ends depression like a new goal. Nothing overcomes perceptual difficulty like fun. Nothing erases pain like interest. This is why the higher levels demand careful study and application in clinical practice. For example, therapeutic approaches for achieving changes in the nervous system will have to take into consideration the role of the symbolic level in organizing and influencing neurologic processes. Thus, techniques whose major aim is modification of neurophysiology still require a focus on the higher levels. The early maturation of the nervous system is guided by the imagery process that occurs in childhood play; this is the natural medium for achieving neurologic changes. Moreover, since neurophysiologic and symbolic processes are continuous, their organization must be in concert.

This hierarchical schema should be fundamental to all uses of occupation for remediation in occupational therapy. Here are several principles derived from rules of hierarchy which should guide therapy: (a) Changes in lower levels are always mediated through the organizing agency of higher levels, thus higher levels are the prime focus in therapy; (b) maintenance of any positive changes will depend on the integrity of higher levels, thus failure to attend to the organization of higher levels could eventually undermine lower level gains; (c) when permanent disorganization occurs at lower levels, the higher levels are also affected, but they can be changed to compensate for lower level dysfunctions.

The earlier example of achieving sensory integration through play is an instance of the first principle. A further example would be the long-standing principle that purposeful activity better elicits coordinated movement than does pure exercise. The dynamics of this process are to be found in the hierarchical arrangement of symbolic processes over neurophysiologic components of coordinated movement. Examples of the second principle are the decubiti and rejected splints which result from the patient's experience of purposelessness in facing daily life. The example of Pablo Casals at the piano is a fine illustration of how further disability can be prevented through the operation of higher levels. Finally, the man with athetoid cerebral palsy is a reminder of the ability of higher levels to achieve a state of organization despite limitations at lower levels.

When such hierarchical principles are recognized and implemented in occupational therapy practice, the importance of the modality becomes more apparent. The purpose and value of activities become their most important organizing features.

A new form of activity analysis is required that includes a consideration of the clinical atmosphere, the mode of presenting an activity, the cultural values and symbols embodied in the activity, and the reigning spirit of the setting. Esprit de corps, craftsmanship, sportsmanship, the challenge of standards of performance, security to fail in the process of learning are all essential ingredients in occupations which effectively organize the behavior of individuals. Effective use of occupation demands that the therapist know how to orchestrate such circumstances.

Occupational therapy clinics should not inspire awe with impressive contraptions, but should evoke curiosity and a willingness to experiment. They should provide challenges and opportunities, and above all, they should offer *occupations of value*. Clinics should offer a broad spectrum of occupations including those which are currently popular and valued in society.

The greatest threat to the efficacy of occupational therapy today is not lack of technical knowledge, but the loss of an appreciation of the cultural nature of occupations and the impact of their value and purpose on human beings. Despite its lack of theoretical acumen and scientific grounding, the early paradigm of occupational therapy offered an efficacious service because it was firmly grounded in a vision of how occupation organized human volition and a recognition that reorganization of the system had to begin with the symbolic process. There are real limits to what technology and knowledge aimed at lower levels can do. Limits are fewer at higher levels because of their greater degree of freedom. History is replete with accounts of individuals who overcame devastating trauma to body and mind because of their attachment to values found in the occupations they pursued. As Frankl[23] acknowledges, one of the major ways in which humans achieve meaning in their lives (the others being love and suffering) is through purposeful action. The domain of occupational therapy is in this symbolic sphere of the human being, the ability to regenerate body and mind through the application of effort in occupations which have personal and cultural significance.

GOALS OF THE PARADIGM

Paradigms ultimately bind their users to a set of goals for knowledge development and puzzle solution. The goals specified by the proposed view of humans are straightforward. Within this proposed paradigm, occupational therapy would be committed to quality of life that can be had in the achievement of values through occupation. Next, occupational therapy would pursue the goals of reducing human incapacity through the organizing effects of occupation on body and mind. Lastly, therapy would address itself to the objective of creating in the culture, in social groups, in neighborhoods, and in families the resources and opportunities for individuals to occupy themselves in the business of caring for self, of contributing to the world's commodities and knowledge, and of celebrating existence in play.

These goals are so fundamental to human nature and so complex that the field will be committed to a noble and demanding enterprise. Such goals will occupy the best efforts of generations of dedicated persons. Occupational therapy once before set its vision toward such lofty goals and gained the commitment of great scholars, humanitarians, and practical persons. The field's goals should be based on a recognition of this inherent greatness—in Reilly's[59] words, not just the greatness of an idea which served a generation or even a century, but the greatness of an idea which advances civilization. Nothing less should be the goal of occupational therapy.

REFERENCES

1. ALLPORT, GW: *The open system in personality theory.* In BUCKLEY, W (ED): *Modern system's research for the behavioral scientist.* Aldine, Chicago, 1968.

2. BARASH, DP: *Sociobiology and behavior.* Elsevier, New York, 1977, p 4.

3. BATESON, G: *Mind and nature: A necessary unity.* Bantam Books, New York, 1980.

4. BERGER, PL AND LUCKMAN, T: *The social construction of reality: A treatise in the sociology of knowledge.* Anchor Books, New York, 1967.

5. VON BERTALANFFY, L: *General system theory: A new approach to unity of science.* Human Biology, 23:347, 1951, p 360.

6. VON BERTALANFFY, L: *General system theory—A critical review.* In BUCKLEY, W (ED): *Modern systems research for the behavioral scientist.* Aldine, Chicago, 1968.

7. VON BERTALANFFY, L: *Chance or Law.* In KOESTLER, A AND SMYTHIES, JR (EDS): *Beyond reductionism.* Beacon Press, Boston, 1969.

8. BING, RK: *Occupational therapy revisited: A paraphrastic journey.* American Journal of Occupational Therapy, 35:499, 1981.

9. BOULDING, K: *General systems theory—The skeleton of science.* In BUCKLEY, W (ED): *Modern systems research for the behavioral scientist.* Aldine, Chicago, 1968, p 7, 8.

10. BOULDING, K: *The image.* University of Michigan Press, Ann Arbor, Mich. 1973, p 24.

11. BRUNER, J, JOLLY, A AND SYLVA, K (EDS): *Play: Its role in development and evolution.* Basic Books, New York, 1976.

12. BURKE, JP: *A clinical perspective on motivation: Pawn versus origin.* American Journal of Occupational Therapy, 31:254, 1977.

13. CICOUREL, AV: *Method and measurement in sociology.* The Free Press, New York, 1964.

14. CICOUREL, AV: *Basic and normative rules in the negotiation of status and role.* In SUDNOW, D (ED), *Studies in social interaction.* The Free Press, New York, 1972.

15. COLLIER, RM: *A dynamic regulatory theory of consciousness.* In COLEMAN, J (ED): *Psychology and effective behavior.* Scott, Foresman & Company, Glenview, Ill, 1969.

16. COTTLE, TJ: *Time's Children.* Little, Brown & Company, Boston, 1971.

17. COUSINS, N: *Anatomy of an illness as perceived by the patient.* Bantam Books, New York, 1981, p 72.

18. DE CHARMS, R: *Personal causation*. Academic Press, New York, 1968.

19. FEIBLEMAN, JK: *Theory of integrative levels*. In COLEMAN, J. (ED): *Psychology and effective behavior*. Scott, Foresman & Co., Glenview, Ill 1969.

20. FIDLER, GS: *The task-oriented group as a context for treatment*. American Journal of Occupational Therapy, 23:43, 1969.

21. FIDLER, GS: AND FIDLER, JW: *Doing and becoming: Purposeful action and self-actualization*. American Journal of Occupational Therapy, 32, 305, 1978.

22. FLOREY, LL: *Intrinsic motivation: The dynamics of occupational therapy theory*. American Journal of Occupational Therapy, 23, 319-322, 1969.

23. FRANKL, VE: *Reductionism and nihilism*. In KOESTLER, A AND SMYTHIES, JR (EDS): *Beyond Reductionism*. Beacon Press, Boston, 1969.

24. FREUD, S: *The ego and the id* (Riviere, J, trans). WW Norton, New York, 1960. (Originally published 1937)

25. GARFINKEL, H: *Studies in ethnomethodology*. Prentice Hall, New York, 1967.

26. GOLDSCHMIDT, W: *Ethology, ecology, and ethnological realities*. In COELHO, GV, HAMBURG, DA & ADAMS, JE (EDS), *Coping and adaptation*. New York: Basic Books, 1974.

27. HALL, ET: *The silent language*. Anchor Press, Garden City, New York, 1973.

28. HAYEK, FA: *The primacy of the abstract*. In KOESTLER, A AND SMYTHIES, RJ (EDS), *Beyond Reductionism*. Beacon Press, Boston, 1969.

29. HAYEK, FA: *The sensory order*. University of Chicago Press, Chicago, 1976.

30. HEARD, C: *Occupational role acquisition: A perspective on the chronically disabled*. American Journal of Occupational Therapy, 31:243, 1977.

31. HENRY, J: *Pathways to madness*. Vintage Books, New York, 1971.

32. HOFSTADTER, DR: *Godel, Escher, Bach: An internal golden braid*. Basic Books, New York, 1979.

33. KATZ, D AND KAHN, RL: *The social psychology of organizations*. John Wiley & Sons, New York, 1966.

34. KIELHOFNER, G: *Temporal adaptation: A conceptual framework for occupational therapy*. American Journal of Occupational Therapy, 31:235, 1977.

35. KIELHOFNER, G: *Occupation*. In HOPKINS, H AND SMITH, N (EDS): *Willard and Spackman's Occupational Therapy, Ed 6*. JB Lippincott, Philadelphia. In press.

36. KIELHOFNER, G, BARRIS, R AND WATTS, JH: *Habits and habit dysfunction: A clinical perspective for psychosocial occupational therapy*. Occupational Therapy and Mental Health. In press, 1982.

37. KIELHOFNER, G AND BURKE, J: *A model of human occupation, Part one. Conceptual framework and content*. American Journal of Occupational Therapy, 34:572, 1980.

38. KIELHOFNER, G AND MIYAKE, S: *The therapeutic use of games with mentally retarded adults*. American Journal of Occupational Therapy, 35:375, 1981.

39. KING, LJ: *A sensory-integrative approach to schizophrenia*. American Journal of Occupational Therapy, 28:529, 1974.

40. KLAVINS, R: *Work-play behavior: Cultural influences*. American Journal of Occupational Therapy, 26:176, 1972.

41. KOESTLER, A: *Beyond atomism and holism—the concept of the holon.* In KOESTLER, A. AND SMITHIES JR (EDS), *Beyond reductionism.* Beacon Press, Boston, 1969.

42. KUHN, TS: *The structure of scientific revolutions* (ED 2). University of Chicago Press, Chicago, 1974, p 149.

43. LAING, RD AND ESTERSON, A: *Sanity, madness, and the family.* Penguin Books, Baltimore, 1976.

44. MASLOW, A: *Towards a psychology of being.* Van Nostrand, Princeton, 1962.

45. MATSUTSUYU, JS: *The interest check list.* American Journal of Occupational Therapy, 23:323, 1969.

46. MATSUTSUYU, JS: *Occupational behavior: A perspective on work and play.* American Journal of Occupational Therapy, 25:291, 1971.

47. MEAD, GH: *Mind, self and society.* University of Chicago Press, Chicago, 1962.

48. MEHAN, H AND WOOD, H: *The reality of ethnomethodology.* John Wiley & Sons, New York, 1975.

49. MEYER, A: *The philosophy of occupation therapy.* Archives of Occupational Therapy, 1:1, 1922.

50. MICHELMAN, SS: *Play and the deficit child.* In Reilly, M. (ED): *Play as exploratory learning.* Sage Publications, Beverly Hills, 1974.

51. MOSEY, AC: *Recapitulation of ontogenesis: A theory for practice of occupational therapy.* American Journal of Occupational Therapy, 22:426, 1968.

52. MOSEY, AC: *The concept and use of developmental groups.* American Journal of Occupational Therapy, 23:272, 1970.

53. MOSEY, AC: *An alternative: The biopsychosocial model.* American Journal of Occupational Therapy, 28:137, 1974.

54. NEVILLE, A: *Temporal adaptation: Application with short-term psychiatric patients.* American Journal of Occupational Therapy, 34:328, 1980.

55. OZBEKHAN, H: *Planning and human action.* In Weiss, PA (ED): *Hierarchically organized systems in theory and practice.* Hafner Publishing, New York, 1971.

56. LINDQUIST, JE, MACK, W AND PARHAM, D: *A synthesis of occupational behavior and sensory integration concepts in theory and practice, Part 1. Theoretical foundations.* American Journal of Occupational Therapy, 36:365, 1982.

57. PAULSON, CP: *Juvenile delinquency and occupational choice.* American Journal of Occupational Therapy, 34:565, 1980.

58. PIAGET, J: *Play, dreams and imitation in childhood* (GATTEGNO, C, AND HODGSON, FM, trans.). Norton, New York, 1951.

59. REILLY, M: *Occupational therapy can be one of the great ideas of 20th century medicine.* American Journal of Occupational Therapy, 16:1, 1962.

60. REILLY, M: *A psychiatric occupational therapy program as a teaching model.* American Journal of Occupational Therapy, 20:61, 1966.

61. REILLY, M: *Play as exploratory learning.* Sage Publications, Beverly Hills, 1974.

62. deRENNE-STEPHAN, C: *Imitation: A mechanism of play behavior.* American Journal of Occupational Therapy, 34, 95, 1980.

63. RITZER, G: *Sociology: A multiple paradigm science.* The American Sociologist, 10:156, 1975.

64. ROBINSON, AL: *Play: The arena for acquisition of rules for competent behavior.* American Journal of Occupational Therapy, 31:248, 1977.

65. ROGERS, JC: *Order and disorder in medicine and occupational therapy.* American Journal of Occupational Therapy, 36:29, 1982.

66. SCHUTZ, A: *The phenomenology of the social world* (WALSH, G, LEHNERT F, AND WALSH, G, trans). Northwestern University Press, 1967 (Originally published 1952)

67. SHANNON, PD: *Work-play theory and the occupational therapy process.* American Journal of Occupational Therapy, 26:169, 1972.

68. SMYTHIES, JR: *Aspects of consciousness.* In KOESTLER, A AND SMYTHIES, JR (EDS): *Beyond reductionism.* Beacon Press, Boston, 1969.

69. SMITH, MB: *Competence and adaptation: A perspective on therapeutic ends and means.* American Journal of Occupational Therapy, 28:11, 1974.

70. SPERRY, RW: *A modified concept of consciousness.* Psychological Review, 76:532, 1969, p 533.

71. SPERRY, RW: *An objective approach to subjective experience.* Psychological Review 77:585, 1970.

72. SUDNOW, D: *Ways of the hand: The organization of improvised conduct.* Bantam Books, New York, 1978.

73. SUTTON-SMITH, B: *A "sportive" theory of play.* In SCHWARTZMAN, HB, (ED): *Play and culture.* Leisure Press, West Point, NY, 1980.

74. TAKATA, N: *Play as a prescription.* In Reilly, M (ED), *Play as exploratory learning.* Sage Publications, Beverly Hills, 1974.

75. TURNER, R: *Role-taking: Process versus conformity.* In M. Rose (ED): *Human behavior and social processes.* Houghton Mifflin, Boston, 1962.

76. VANDENBERG, B AND KIELHOFNER, G: *Play in evolution, culture, and individual adaptation: Implications for therapy.* American Journal of Occupational Therapy, 36:20, 1982.

77. VICKERS, G: *Value systems and social processes.* Basic Books, New York, 1968.

78. WATANABE, S: *Four concepts basic to the occupational therapy process.* American Journal of Occupational Therapy, 22:439, 1968.

79. WATZLAWICK, P, BEAVIN, J, AND JACKSON, D: *Pragmatics of human communication.* WW NORTON, New York, 1967.

80. WEBSTER, PS: *Occupational role development in the young adult with mild mental retardation.* American Journal of Occupational Therapy, 34:13, 1980.

81. WEICK, KE: *The social psychology of organizing.* Addison-Wesley, Reading, Mass, 1969.

82. WEISS, PA: *One plus one does not equal two.* In QUARTON, G, MELNECHUK, T, AND SCHMITT, F, (EDS): *The neurosciences: A study program.* Rockefeller University Press, New York, 1967.

83. WEISS, PA: *The living system: Determinism stratified.* In KOESTLER, A, AND SMYTHIES, JR, (EDS): *Beyond reductionism.* Beacon Press, Boston, 1969

84. WEISS, PA: *Hierarchically organized systems in theory and practice.* Hafner Publishing, New York, 1971, p 1.

85. YERXA, EJ: *Authentic occupational therapy.* American Journal of Occupational Therapy, 21:1, 1967.

Chapter 3

THE STUDY OF HUMAN OCCUPATION

Joan C. Rogers

EDITOR'S INTRODUCTION

The preceding chapters offer two ways of viewing current knowledge in occupational therapy. Chapter 1 traces its historical development and Chapter 2 provides a synthesis under the rubric of general systems theory. The reader will recall that occupational behavior was proposed as an appropriate body of knowledge to compose the field's paradigm since it was closely aligned with the early principles of practice and offered a broad but coherent approach to patient problems. Chapter 2 demonstrated that the concepts represented in the occupational behavior school are not exclusive of other viewpoints and theories and offered some means of integrating these bodies of knowledge. Chapter 3 accomplishes the important task of providing a systematic view of the occupational behavior tradition and its major features. The chapter presents a broad and accurate account of the structure, content, and themes of occupational behavior. Since two of these themes are general systems theory and the history of practice, the chapter also puts earlier chapters into perspective as arguments which arise from the occupational behavior tradition.

The term occupational behavior was originally designed to be descriptive of the everyday activities of human beings. It has also come to signify the ideas represented by the work of Reilly and associated writers and clinicians. Occupational therapists' knowledge of its connotations ranges from faint awareness to intimate familiarity. Readers at any point on this continuum should find this chapter a valuable resource. It clearly identifies the concepts of occupational behavior, their sources in interdisciplinary literature, and their integration into a coherent perspective. Such an articulation is offered for the first time and should serve to demystify much that has heretofore been obscure. The author clearly identifies and explains the major themes of occupational behavior, and also suggests resources for further study.

The chapter contains periodic tables which summarize the subconcepts associated with each major concept discussed. These tables also offer the reader ready references for further study. Finally, the chapter provides a comprehensive listing of clinical instruments designed from the occupational behavior perspective.

GK

Because our profession is focused on influencing the health of people there will always be a need to include in our body of knowledge the fundamental material of anatomy, neurophysiology, personality theory, social processes and the pathological states to which these functional areas are subject. However, I do not feel that this is our unique content. We should have as a special contribution a profound understanding of the nature of work. (Reilly, Occupational Therapy Can Be One of the Great Ideas of Twentieth Century Medicine)

"Why do I need to learn this?" "How am I going to use it?" "I simply work with the concrete problems of patients, why do I need abstract theory?" Questions concerning the knowledge needed to practice occupational therapy are frequently posed by clinicians and students alike. Such questions challenge those concerned with the development, organization, transmission, and use of knowledge in occupational therapy. This chapter is designed to provide one way of answering questions concerning the relevance of knowledge for practice.

A justification is offered for the knowledge requirements for occupational therapy practice in the pages that follow. The rationale is based on the conviction that *human occupation is the appropriate focus of occupational therapy science*. The critical concepts for study will be identified as well as the key processes. The ideas presented are summarized in outline form at the end of each major section. Since the discussion only introduces complex topics that require further study, a list of readings supporting the ideas examined is also given. These readings may collectively be regarded as a basic "textbook" in human occupation. The chapter concludes with a discussion of the implications of the study of human occupation for education and research.

Thus, on completing this chapter, the reader will appreciate the range of knowledge needed by occupational therapists and why this knowledge must be mastered if occupational therapy is to be based on an understanding of human occupation. In addition, the reader will have a guide to additional information pertinent to the concepts and processes presented.

ORIENTATION FOR LEARNING

In Chapter 1 occupational behavior was identified as a philosophical school of thought along with the kinesiologic and developmental schools. Occupational behavior was presented as furnishing the elements for a new paradigm of practice based on the occupational nature of humans and the dynamics of occupation for facilitating health and well-being. Since the occupational behavior frame of reference seeks to integrate knowledge of occupation[84], it may be used as a guide for selecting the core concepts for the study of human occupation. Hence, at the outset, the student of human occupation should be aware of several essential features of the occupational behavior perspective.

First, the occupational behavior perspective is based on scientific knowledge.[79,81,82,83] Such knowledge has as its primary purpose *the disciplining of the student's mind* in the powers of observation and critical judgment relevant to the field of practice.[79] Second, the course of study is *interdisciplinary* in nature.[80,86,87] This implies that occupational behavior is a multidimensional concept that requires knowledge from many sciences to be understood and explained. Thus, the occupational behavior frame of reference acknowledges the need to delve into disciplines such as psychology, anthropology, social psychology, sociology, and social ecology as well as biomedicine, psychiatry, anatomy, physiology, neurology, and kinesiology. Occupational behavior theorists have concentrated on developing occupational therapy science by bringing in knowledge from the behavioral and biologic sciences relevant to human occupation. This has resulted in the specification of concepts that complement reductionist concepts already available in the field.

The third feature is that the occupational behavior perspective is a *generic frame of reference*. This means that it applies to all areas of occupational therapy practice. It may be used with children as well as adults and is appropriate for both physical and psychosocial dysfunctions. Because of its broad applicability, the occupational behavior perspective is well suited to serve as the organizing paradigm for occupational therapy.[85] Lastly, knowledge of occupational behavior is organized in developmental and systems terms.[87] The developmental vocabulary allows one to look at changes in occupational behavior from infancy through senescence, while the systems vocabulary facilitates a view of the multiple factors influencing occupational behavior at one point in time.

The orientation for learning about human occupation is thus conceptual rather than technical. When conceptual understandings support practice, the therapist is better prepared to develop and use the skills of practice.[79] This focus on organized scientific knowledge, as opposed to techniques for practice, characterizes professions and distinguishes professional occupational therapy from technical occupational therapy.

A summary of orientation for professional education is presented in Table 1.

CONCEPTS AND PROCESSES FOR STUDY

The study of human occupation requires an exploration of several concepts and processes. The concepts define the structure of the subject matter of human occupation, while the processes delineate the operations through which this knowledge is created and put to functional use. The essential concepts are: (a) history of practice, (b) occupation as a health determinant, (c) the occupational nature of humans, (d) the ontogeny of work, (e) the phylogeny of work, (f) the occupational environment, (g) occupational role dysfunction, and (h) occupation as a change strategy. The processes vital to the framework are (a) criticism, (b) general systems thinking, (c) qualitative research, (d) the case method, and (e) consultation. The discussion that follows provides a rationale for the inclusion of these concepts and processes in the course of study. The discussion emphasizes aspects of human occupation brought to occupational therapy by occupational

TABLE 1. Orientation for Professional Education

Subconcepts	Purpose	References
Human occupation Intellectual discipline Interdisciplinary orientation Generic application Developmental and systems characteristics	To provide a focus for occupational therapy science To call attention to the theory and theoretical assumptions that direct the use of professional skills	Reilly[79] Reilly[81] Reilly[80] Reilly[82] Reilly[83] Reilly[84] Reilly[85] Reilly[86] Reilly[87] Reilly[88] Chapters 2, 8

behavior theorists. Relationships between the tenets of the occupational behavior perspective and the inner mechanism paradigm (see Chapter 1)—the kinesiologic, neurologic, and intrapsychic approaches—will be delineated.

HISTORY OF PRACTICE

Professions emerge in response to societal needs or desires for specialized services. The first stage in the evolution of a profession is reached when a group of individuals begins to fill a need. These individuals develop a sense of shared values and identity and band together, first informally, then formally, to define their services, develop knowledge and skills, and recruit and educate new practitioners.

By studying the advent of a profession, its mandate or raison d'etre is clarified. Through historical analysis, continuity and discontinuity in the ways in which the mandate has been expressed over time are probed. Explanations for varying directions of development or for lack of development are sought in events internal and external to the profession. The insight on the past gained from historical study allows one to develop a sense of professional identity and to extrapolate future trends.

Studying the history of occupational therapy is thus intended to provide answers to questions such as: What vital client needs were we born to serve? In what manner were we to serve these needs? What changes have taken place in our technology? What has been the source of motivation for change? How adequately have we responded to societal change? Have we achieved status as a full profession as opposed to a semi-profession? Have we deviated from the purposes for which we were founded? Historical study thus provides an opportunity to re-examine our legacy, our parameters of practice, and our methodologies. It encourages us to confront ourselves as a professional entity, and to reflect on critical questions about our developmental processes and our state of health.

Knowledge of the origins and historical development of occupational therapy provides the foundation for appreciating the importance of the study of occupation. The focus on human occupation is based on the finding that our mandate is to develop, maintain, or improve the capacity of the severely and chronically disabled to cope with daily living tasks to achieve satisfying occupation. In other words, history reveals that we

WHAT THE PRACTITIONER MUST KNOW:
THE KNOWLEDGE BASE OF OCCUPATIONAL THERAPY

need to study occupation to understand the occupational needs we serve. Historical analysis, conducted within[3,23,72,89,99] and outside[27] occupational therapy, reveals the impact of the philosophy of reductionism on the direction of occupational therapy practice. Reductionism seeks to explain and understand a complex phenomenon by breaking it down into its elementary parts. Within medicine, reductionism took hold as the medical model, viewing health as an absence of disease and emphasizing pathology and symptom reduction. Within occupational therapy, reductionism gained momentum in the 1950s. It deflected us from our focus on the occupational nature of humans to the inner mechanisms associated with kinesiologic, neurologic, and intrapsychic function. Imitating medicine, occupational therapy developed techniques to reduce pathology. Our strategies for alleviating the disabling effects of pathology on daily life were increasingly laid aside, despite the recognition that symptom reduction technology was inadequate for helping the disabled to become functioning members of society.

History reveals that the roots of occupational therapy can be traced to moral treatment that prevailed in American psychiatry in the early nineteenth century. This was based on a humanistic philosophy that viewed the mentally ill as innocent sufferers who succumbed to external stress. Treatment consisted of normal activities carried out in an environment supportive of daily living occupations to promote meaningful involvement. Moral treatment was abandoned with the advent of scientific medicine, which regarded mental illness as a relatively incurable, organic disease. Social commitment to compassionate care was also impaired by overcrowded facilities and prejudiced attitudes toward patients.

The first decades of the twentieth century saw a revival of moral treatment in the form of occupational therapy. Forces contributing to the emergence of occupational therapy were a psychologic and environmental perception of mental illness and public recognition of the negligent conditions existing in mental hospitals. Meyer,[68] a neuropathologist, articulated the first paradigm of human occupation. He viewed mental illness as a deterioration of habits caused by reactions to environmental stresses. Activity and the environment were organized, graded, and adapted to promote a healthy lifestyle. Major ideological contributions to occupational therapy philosophy were made by early leaders. Slagle[100] devised a habit training program which began on the ward with simple, familiar tasks requiring minimal attention, progressed to a workshop setting, and terminated in a pre-work situation incorporating complex, novel tasks requiring monitoring. Hass[37] introduced concepts of craftsmanship, orderly work environments, and high quality instruction as means of organizing disordered behaviors. Bryan[17] proposed matching patients' aptitudes and interests to hospital jobs to promote reality orientation, mental organization, and work habits. From its inception on the back wards of mental hospitals, occupational therapy was extended to tuberculosis sanitoriums, supporting the utility of graded occupation for both the mentally and physically disabled.[43]

The occupational behavior perspective represents a recommitment to the ideas put forth in the early paradigm of occupation. The major conceptual building blocks for the occupational behavior perspective are drawn from the early paradigm. First, there is an emphasis on the *health* of persons in terms of their productive participation in society. Second, health is seen as correlated with *daily experience,* which consists of *work, play, rest,* and *sleep.* Third, daily experience takes place in a complex *physical, temporal,* and *social* environment, which is a critical factor in shaping behavior. Fourth, occupational dysfunction that may be recognized by symptoms such as boredom, futility, indifference, lack of self-respect, immobility, and disorientation, disrupts daily life. Fifth, daily life may be reorganized through engagement in occupations, such as work, play, crafts, and sports. Sixth, the occupational therapist assists the process of organizing behavior by habit training and socialization of patients to the expectations of the culture. The learning of habits and internalization of social norms requires role models, practice with activities graded from playful to productive, and an environment supportive of high quality productivity.

These are the beliefs and values that the occupational behavior perspective seeks to revive from early practice to meet the needs that occupational therapy was born to serve: the occupational problems of the severely and chronically disabled. Through an understanding of the history of occupational therapy the student develops an appreciation of the potential and goals of practice based on human occupation.

A summary of the history of practice is presented in Table 2.

OCCUPATION AS A HEALTH DETERMINANT

The essential premise of the occupational behavior perspective is "that man, through the use of his hands as they are energized by his mind and will, can influence the state of his own health."[80] Support for this premise may be gleaned through study of the positive effects of occupation and the negative effects of inactivity on humans.

Research investigating the relationship between activity and well-being may be gleaned from many sources: psychology, behavioral genetics, gerontology, psychiatry, orthopedics and aerospace to name a few. This interdisciplinary literature supports the notion that activity is preferable to inactivity and also indicates that for each individual there is an optimal level of activity that is health-promoting. Purposeful activity in one sphere of human functioning, such as social or motoric, has been shown to cause alterations in other spheres. Participation in activity has been observed to enhance one's self concept and feelings of self control, improve mental alertness and acuity, promote physical robustness and agility, foster social competence, reduce stress, and contribute to overall life satisfaction. Knowledge of the attributes and effects of various activities, and of the personal circumstances under which various activities influence well-being, assists the therapist to provide activities conducive to health in the treatment milieu.

The second approach to assessing activity as a health determinant allows one to judge the value of activity by considering what happens in its absence. Generally, occupational therapists are more familiar with the effects of prolonged inactivity on physical movement than on other body processes. The interdisciplinary focus of the occupational behavior perspective considers a broader biologic view and also adds the psychologic and social effects of inactivity. The collection of biologic and psychosocial complications resulting from inactivity is referred to as *hypokinetic disease* or the *disuse syndrome*.

In studying the disuse syndrome, attention is directed toward changes in the digestive, urinary, cardiovascular, respiratory and metabolic systems as well as the more familiar neuromuscular, skeletal, and integumentary systems. Hence, the deleterious conditions of urinary renal stones, cardiovascular deconditioning, venous stasis, thrombus formation, orthostatic hypotension, pulmonary stasis, respiratory acidosis, and pulmonary emboli are scrutinized, as well as those of decubitus ulcers, backache, disuse

TABLE 2. History of Practice

Subconcepts	Purpose	References
Overview	To indicate historical trends in the models of occupational therapy practice	Bing[3] Diasio[23] Erickson[27] Kielhofner & Burke[48] Mosey[72] Rerek[89] Shannon[99]
Moral treatment and the early paradigm of occupation	To clarify the reasons for the inception of occupational therapy To outline the societal needs served by the founders of occupational therapy; the population that was the recipient of occupational therapy services; and the early technology To place the focus of occupational therapy science on human occupation in historical perspective	Bockoven[6] Bockoven[7] Bryan[17] Engelhardt[26] Gillette & Kielhofner[31] Haas[37] Kidner[43] Marsh[64,65] Meyer[68] Slagle[100] Chapter 1

osteoporosis, and contractures. Knowledge of the disuse syndrome is completed through an investigation of psychosocial functions. Hence, the characteristics of dependency, disorientation, decreased motivation, and lethargy are added to the symptomatology of inactivity. In studying the effects of inactivity one is challenged to learn not only what happens, but also why it happens; whether the condition is preventable, reversible, or irreversible; and the best way of achieving prevention or reversion. Thus, study of the introduction and withdrawal of activity in relation to human functioning provides support for occupational therapy's philosophy, furnishes constructs and theories for its knowledge base, and suggests principles and techniques for intervention.

A summary of occupation as a health determinant is presented in Table 3.

THE OCCUPATIONAL NATURE OF HUMANS

A profession's unique service is derived from the assumptions about the nature of humans that underlie its intervention strategies. Different professions serve different needs, and hence operate on different assumptions about human nature. For example, a physician serves human biomedical needs, sees humans as composites of anatomic and physiologic variables, and uses medications and surgery to cure disease. A pastor serves spiritual needs through prayer and counseling.

Historical analysis reveals that occupational therapy assumes responsibility for the human need for occupation. The precise way in which this need will be met depends upon an understanding of the occupational nature of humans. A clearly articulated view of human occupation provides the therapist with guidelines for clinical decisions concerning the population to be treated, the types of problems to be treated, and the methods and technologies for intervention. The occupational behavior frame of reference looks at humans as achievers in occupation. The focus lies "in the non-sexual area of human

TABLE 3. Occupation as a Health Determinant

Subconcepts	Purpose	References
Introduction of activity	To outline the positive effects of participation in occupation	Snow[103]
	To infer principles of intervention	
Withdrawal of activity	To support the value of activity for health and well being by considering the deleterious effects of inactivity	Brinker[13] Burt[20] Parent[75] Suedfeld[105]
	To infer principles of intervention	U.S. Department of Health[118] Chapters 2, 5, 10, 13

productivity and creativity."[80] Human productivity and creativity require action. This action is expressed in self-care, work, and leisure occupations. Further, these occupations have developmental aspects. The life span manifestations of self-care, work, and play are referred to as occupational behavior. This incorporates an occupational component, involving time management as demanded by age-appropriate daily living functions, and a behavioral component concerned with the level of competent performance required for adaptation.

Occupational behavior theory and research is still in its infancy. Because of the critical significance of the view of humans in defining and specifying services, much of the research undertaken to date has concentrated on formulating a clearer picture of the occupational nature of humans. Kielhofner and Burke[49] recently synthesized this research into a cohesive systems model. The components of the model may be used to identify concepts for in depth study.

Humans are viewed as open systems comprised of three hierarchically arranged subsystems: performance, habituation, and volition. Humans exist in and interact with a macrosystem — the environment — which contains people, events, and objects. It is this constant interaction that defines humans as open, as opposed to closed, systems. The interaction consists largely of an input of information about people, events, and objects in the environment that enables the individual to produce an action that meets environmental demands. Underlying the systems model is the premise that individuals are intrinsically motivated to explore and master the environment and that such mastery yields a sense of achievement.

The *performance* subsystem is responsible for *producing action.* The unit of focus is *skill,* which requires *perception, problem solving, decision-making,* and *movement.* Skills are flexible strategies that allow goal accomplishment under varying environmental conditions. To perform skillfully one requires knowledge of the task, technical ability to complete the task, and a feedback mechanism to determine the degree of success of task accomplishment. Skill gives one a sense of being a *cause* or *origin* of action to achieve ends.

Skills are organized into *habits* and *roles.* The *habituation* subsystem maintains behavior in routines and hence allows occupations to be conducted efficiently. Role refers to a position in a social group and the requirements of the position. When organized according to social norms, habits and role behavior enable one to act in socially approved ways.

While the performance subsystem allows action and the habituation subsystem efficiently and flexibly organizes action, it is the *volition* subsystem that provides the motivation to act. Hence, the volition subsystem determines action. Its motivational components are *personal causation, valued goals,* and *interests.* Personal causation refers to a self-image of competence or incompetence. This is derived from a pattern of success or failure in managing environmental interactions. The expectation of success or failure influences a decision to act or not to act. Valued goals refers to a preference for certain actions to achieve productive ends. They organize *time* by relating past, present, and future actions to achievements. Valued goals are able to sustain actions that are unpleasant or involve delayed gratification. Like valued goals, interests are also preferences for action. However, interests are primarily oriented toward pleasurable engagement in activity. Interests lead to active participation in satisfying occupational activities and also serve to maintain self-initiated activity. Interests attract and hold attention and determine how an individual will spend free time.

The three motivational components, personal causation, valued goals, and interests are differentiated out of the innate global urge to explore and master the environment. There is a movement from curious exploration that energizes *skill development,* to *competency* that energizes *habit formation,* to *achievement motivation* that supports *role socialization.*

The enactment of occupational behavior is thus a complex process requiring an understanding of the multiple variables influencing achievement. The conceptual building blocks needed by the student for understanding humans as occupational achievers are: roles, habits, skills, perception, problem-solving, decision-making, personal causation, goals, interests, time, exploration, competence, achievement, and environment. These concepts traverse the biologic, psychologic, and social sciences. This bio-psycho-social synthesis is in contrast to the kinesiologic and neurologic approaches which use biologic concepts and the intrapsychic approach which borrows from psychology and psychiatry.

A summary of the occupational nature of humans is presented in Table 4.

THE ONTOGENY OF WORK

Occupational behavior is developmentally acquired. Development entails the translation of skills to habits for a sequence of life roles beginning with preschooler, progressing to student and worker, and culminating in the retiree role. Knowledge of work ontogeny provides an understanding of normal developmental milestones and processes. This knowledge is used to plan developmentally based treatment. In the occupational behavior perspective, developmentally based treatment implies treatment goals directed toward facilitating age-appropriate occupations through methods which enhance normal developmental processes.

The study of work ontogeny begins in childhood play. Through play, children become acquainted with the world in which they live and with their capacities for managing it. Play supports the emerging worker role through the development of motor,

TABLE 4. The Occupational Nature of Humans

Subconcepts	Purpose	References
Overview	To demonstrate the role of perceptions of human nature in defining professional services To describe the view of human nature that provides direction for intervention based on the occupational behavior perspective	Boulding[11] Kielhofner & Burke[49] Kielhofner[46,47] Koestler[57] Woodside[119] Chapter 4
Motivation	To highlight the intrinsic quality of the human need for occupation	Burke[19] Florey[30] McClelland[63] Reilly[86] Rotter[93] Smith[101] Smith[102] White[116] White[117] Chapters 4, 13

cognitive, and social skills. In the process of exploring and testing the environment, the child learns rules or expectancies for competent behavior. Occupational choices are made and tried out in make-believe play. Mastery of personal self-care skills is also begun during the preschool years.

Movement from the preschool to the student role necessitates a restructuring of time. School work and chores compete with play for time. As time is divided to accommodate work, a sense of obligation and basic attitudes toward work and leisure are developed.

During adolescence, values emerge to guide the life plan. Interests narrow and stabilize. Participation in hobbies allows the adolescent to acquire dexterity and to develop attitudes of workmanship. Games and social events provide practice in competitive and cooperative interaction. The occupational choice process continues with the reduction of childhood fantasy choices to a number of alternatives which take personal assets into account. Part-time employment allows further reality testing. The selection of an occupation is also influenced by societal needs. Once a selection is made, competence in the occupational role is developed and economic self-care is secured.

Adulthood is characterized by achievement in family (procreative) and community (productive) roles. Work is a major factor in self-identity and time organization. The role of play changes from skill preparation for work to a "re-creation" for work. When occupational change is anticipated, the occupational choice process may be repeated. The retiree moves through a similar process of exploration and decision-making when planning retirement activities. In retirement, temporal adaptation and occupational satisfaction is generally sought in leisure pursuits and volunteer work. With increasing age, personal self-care may again become difficult to perform.

Knowledge of work ontogenesis provides one with concepts concerning developmental change in occupational behavior. Such change relates the transition from one occupational role to another, for example, change from the pre-school to the student role. Change is both quantitative and qualitative. New skills are acquired and previous skills are reorganized and transformed. The change from one state to another is brought about by action—by choosing to act and by acting. Man has three levels of orientation for action: biologic, psychologic, and sociocultural. Learning proceeds from rules to skills to habits to roles. This process is repeated over and over again each time the person encounters novelty in the environment. Novelty may embody new roles or new role requirements. Each role in the developmental sequence embodies skills and habits that must be acquired for successful progression to future roles.

Thus, it is apparent that the individual and the environment each contribute to behavior. Adaptation is the process through which the individual makes a sufficient response to meet the demands of the environment. At any point in time, the individual and the environment maintain a level of adaptation that aids the survival, functioning, and maintenance of the individual. The relationship between the individual and the environment is constantly changing, and adaptation is limited by personal capacities and environmental opportunities. The change process operates with reference to the present and past status of the individual and the environment.

The yield from the study of work ontogenesis is an understanding of the developmental nature of human occupation. Achievement behavior is related to humans as players and workers. Play with objects, motion, companions, symbols, and rules is analyzed from various theoretical perspectives and interpreted in terms of its meaning for adult occupations. Theories of occupational choice and vocational development facilitate an understanding of how one prepares for, maintains, and exits from occupational roles. Factors contributing to occupational satisfaction, dissatisfaction, and stress are also critical to examine. The interplay between ludic (play/leisure) and productive (work) occupations is traced over the life span and contributes to an appreciation of the value of play, arts and crafts, games, sports and work to health.

A summary of the ontogeny of work is presented in Table 5.

TABLE 5. The Ontogeny of Work

Subconcepts	Purpose	References
Overview	To describe occupational behavior over the life span	Kielhofner[46] Matsutsuyu[67] Shannon[97] Sundstrom[106] Woodside[119]
Play/Leisure	To identify the role of ludic occupations in human development	Bruner[15,16] Berlyne[2] Florey[30] Michelman[69] Reilly[87] Robinson[90] Takata[108]
Work	To identify the role of productive occupations in human development	Black[5] Ginzberg[32] Roe[91] Schein[95] Sundstrom[106]

THE PHYLOGENY OF WORK

A long evolutionary process has contributed to the human capacity to work. The history of the human species in regard to work is termed the phylogeny of work. At first glance, work phylogenesis may seem to be quite removed from the occupational therapy process. However, knowledge of the evolution of culture furthers one's understanding of how behavior is organized. Parallels between the history of the human species and individual ontogeny lend meaning to the treatment principle that ontogeny recapitulates phylogeny.

An evolutionary view of human occupations evidences changes in the use of time and nature of occupation. Primitive man was hard pressed to obtain food through hunting, fishing and searching for edible berries and roots. Daily life was spent in meeting survival needs. Leisure came about when hunting and agriculture became more efficient as a result of the use and development of tools and social structures. Over the centuries, humans have developed complex technologies and social institutions to ease adaptation. Work has become more sedentary and mechanistic. Less time is required to fulfill basic food, clothing, and shelter requirements. The productive use of increased leisure time has become problematic in modern society.

The development of coordination between the eye, the hand, and the brain is particularly important to occupational therapists, because of its significance for purposeful activity. Evolutionary evidence supports the thesis that biologic adaptation followed, rather than preceded, the making of tools. In other words, humans adapt to tasks. Biologic structures are a result of environmental forces, including culture. Furthermore, adaptation proceeds as a bio-psycho-social whole with various capacities evolving simultaneously. Evolutionary milestones related to the human capacity to interact with the environment are cephalo-caudal development, accommodative vision, bipedal locomotion, manipulation, and vocal communication. Collectively, these gave humans a new perception of the environment and a new way of controlling it.[104]

The evolution of eye-hand-brain coordination reflects a complex, interdependent sequence of events. Bipedal locomotion freed the hands for manipulation, while upright posture also enabled visual control of the hands. Simultaneously, the brain was stimulated to direct skilled movement. Thus, evolutionary data illustrate a synchronous development of eye, hand, and brain. The occupational behavior perspective gleans the principle of mutual causation from the knowledge of the co-adaptation of the eye, hand, and brain. This principle is in contrast to the one-way causation inherent in reductionism. In the latter scheme, a single cause introduces a single effect, and science seeks to describe their relationship.

Evolutionary trends also highlight the fact that humans used tools long before they fabricated them. Tool transitions have proceeded from the use of the body as a tool, to the use of naturally occurring objects, to the adaptation of naturally occurring objects, to the making of tools. Tool making has progressed from hand tools, to power tools and machinery, to digital technology.

The ability to make tools represents a significant event in human history. In contrast to tool use, which can be accomplished with perceptual thinking, tool fabrication requires conceptual thinking. To make a tool, one has to imagine something that does not exist and devise a plan to make something that has not been made before. Since tools and the products made with them express intellectual capacity, they provide useful information about grading activity. Many cultural changes were precipitated by tool development. For instance, tools were shared within a group and instruction in tool use and making was communicated.

The study of human evolution reveals that the development of the tool-maker meant the introduction of a long period of immaturity. Humans do not differ from nonhuman primates in the general sequence of events from conception through birth. However, in humans the period from birth to maturity is prolonged. This extended period is generally believed to have been introduced to provide a relatively pressure-free time to learn the complex skills required for human adaptation.

Knowledge of work phylogeny thus demonstrates the interaction between the environment and the biologic structure, intellectual capacity, and social organization of humans. The response of humans as a whole or as individuals to environmental demands has wide range implications for eliciting adaptive behavior. Adaptation is seen as dependent on the mastery of tools that have become increasingly complex as society has moved from an agrarian to a technological culture. Work phylogeny records the grading of occupations in accordance with manual, cognitive, and social skills.

A summary of the phylogeny of work is presented in Table 6.

ENVIRONMENT AS A DETERMINANT OF OCCUPATION

Occupational behavior takes place in a lifelong series of interactions with the environment. Phylogenesis indicates that human adaptation is a function of environmental pressure. The rules of hierarchy described in Chapter 2, derived from the systems view of humans as occupational beings, also support the environment as a determinant of behavior. The environment in the form of social regulations, organizations, and institutions exerts a regulating force on an individual's actions. The history of occupational therapy documents the fact that occupational therapy's roots lie in providing a normalizing environment for individuals experiencing disruptions in daily occupations as a result of severe and chronic conditions. To act as an environmental manager for eliciting occupational behavior, therapists must understand the environment and how it influences occupation.

TABLE 6. The Phylogeny of Work

Subconcepts	Purpose	References
Evolutionary trends in eye-hand-brain coordination, tool use, tool making, time use, occupation	To discern parallels between work ontogeny and work phylogeny	Campbell[21] Napier[73] Oakley[74] Reilly[87] Spuhler[104] Tobias[110] Washburn[113] Chapter 2
	To illustrate the principle of graded occupation from an evolutionary viewpoint	
	To demonstrate the role of the environment in human adaptation	
	To point out the educational significance of immaturity	

Humans are oriented to the environment principally through culture. Culture refers to learned patterns of behavior. Persons of different ethnic backgrounds are known to have different belief systems concerning such factors as family roles and responsibilities, orientation toward time, work and play values, and health and illness perceptions. Within the broad American culture there are multiple ethnic subcultures, including, among others, the Black American, the Mexican American, the Asian American. Persons in certain geographical regions, such as Appalachia, may also exhibit distinctive traits. The primary method used to transmit culture from generation to generation is child rearing. An understanding of cultural diversity assists therapists to communicate and interact more effectively with persons whose cultural orientation is different from their own, and enables them to plan treatment activities that are culturally relevant.

The environment consists of persons, places, and events. The focal point for each of these elements changes as the individual matures. Developmental tasks such as those outlined by Havinghurst,[39] provide an organizational scheme for viewing major life events. The specific events leading to task achievement will be uniquely defined. The initial socializing agent is the family. During school years the people environment expands to include teachers, peers, and nonrelated adults in addition to parents, siblings and relatives. In adulthood, one's spouse, confidants, fellow workers, and social acquaintances are especially influential.

During the course of development, the environment expands from the home to the school, the workplace, the church, and various leisure settings. In the case of illness, disability, or social deviance, places such as hospitals, prisons, and halfway houses become significant behavioral determinants. The architectural features of these places are merely one of the determinants of occupation of interest to the therapist. While barrier-free environments facilitate the mobility of persons with physical handicaps, physical space may also be arranged to promote stimulation of a physical, mental, or social nature. A "friendly visitors" program can be established in a long-term care facility for residents who have few social contacts. A spinal cord-injured person on a stryker frame may experience competence and enjoyment in computer games. By analyzing the objects present in an environment, the environment's stimulus capabilities can be gauged.

In each of these environments, people are organized into groups. Group behavior is governed by norms, which are learned through social interaction. These norms define appropriate and inappropriate behavior and may or may not support competence in occupational behavior. For example, parental expectations for a "well-behaved" child may imply a "quiet" child and may curtail the child's exploration of the home.

In summary, knowledge of the influence of enriched and deprived environments on behavior is needed to support the occupational therapist's role as an environmental engineer in developing occupational behavior. The concept of architectural barriers as a deterrent to competent performance is broadened to include attitudinal barriers. Since occupational behavior is a function of the environment, the therapist requires knowledge of many social systems. Home, school, work, leisure, and treatment environments are examined for their potential in terms of people, objects, and events, to support self-care, work and play.

A summary of the environment as a determinant of occupation is presented in Table 7.

TABLE 7. The Environment as a Determinant of Occupation

Subconcepts	Purpose	References
People/Group	To establish culture and social norms as regulators of occupation	Chapple[22] Figone[29] Havighurst[39] Klavins[54] Kluckhohn[55] Shannon[97] Touchstone[111]
Physical Setting	To identify the characteristics of various settings in terms of their capacity to support occupation	Dunning[25] Gray[36] Proshansky[78] Chapters 4, 15

OCCUPATIONAL ROLE DYSFUNCTION

Intervention is directed toward the remediation of a problem. A problem represents something that is wrong and requires correction. Knowledge of the problem is needed so that appropriate intervention may be initiated. Occupational therapy addresses problems in daily living. For problem definition, the occupational behavior frame of reference builds on a social-psychologic definition of illness, rather than a medical one. The social-psychologic perspective regards illness as an impairment of one's capacity to perform social roles, while the medical perspective sees it as an anatomic or physiologic aberration. While medicine prevents and alleviates disease and illness, occupational therapy prevents and alleviates the functional incapacities associated with disease and illness. Hence, the social-psychologic model of illness fits better with occupational therapy philosophy than does the medical model. The problem in the occupational behavior frame of reference is conceptualized as *occupational role dysfunction* and involves insufficiencies in rules, skills, and habits that contribute to role performance.

The concept of role allows the occupational therapist to view medical problems in the context of daily functioning, rather than as disease entities. Clients are seen primarily as having disruptions in preschool, student, worker, or retired roles, and secondarily as persons with diseases such as arthritis or schizophrenia.

Occupational roles demand a set of habits and skills. If these skills are not intact, incompetent behavior and ineffective interaction with the environment ensues. Based on the conviction that blocking the human need to master, alter, or improve the environment results in severe dysfunction and unhappiness, occupational therapy is directed toward habit and skill acquisition to improve role functioning and the quality of life.

Because of the emphasis on role functioning, it is commonly thought that proponents of the occupational behavior framework have completely cast aside the medical model. This is not the case. They recognize that knowledge of medicine is needed to understand the impact of disease and medical treatment on occupational role. However, this recognition is accompanied by the realization that diagnostic categories tell us little about daily function. From a behavioral perspective, many diseases whose medical indicators are diverse yield similar problems in daily living; and many diseases whose medical indicators are similar yield diverse problems in daily living. Occupational behavior advocates recognize this and account for it by conceptualizing the problem to be treated at a higher level of generalization than disease. Role function provides the focal point for treatment, with medical problems as part of the necessary background information. Problems of motor control, sensory integration, and intrapsychic functions are approached in terms of their implications for occupational role dysfunctions. The significance of these problems is evaluated according to their impact on occupational role performance. Thus, the clinical exploration of occupational role is an *addition to* the assessment of medically defined physical and emotional problems.

Use of role theory in occupational therapy science results in an expansion of the definition of functional problems and furnishes new insights into the etiology of functional problems associated with medical conditions. Role disruptions stemming from the retirement process, social deviance, and sensory or cultural deprivation cannot be explained by disease entities. Role theory introduces deficiencies in rule-bound behavior, skills, and social expectations as alternative causal factors. Hence, role theory gives a more comprehensive view of the etiology of occupational role dysfunctions than does the medical model. To understand the nature of many problems in daily living, knowledge of medical pathology must be supplemented with knowledge of aging, social deviance, sensory and environmental deprivation, and other nondisease factors.

A summary of occupational role dysfunction is presented in Table 8.

OCCUPATION AS INTERVENTION

The occupational therapist is trained to assist clients to alter their occupational behavior to increase their competence in their daily occupations. To serve in this capacity, the therapist requires an assessment technology to facilitate a clear statement of the client's problems and strengths, and a strategy for helping clients to acquire skills related to adaptive needs.

The intervention process is initiated with an assessment of the current state of the client and of his or her occupational history. Since occupational behavior is regarded as a function of motivation, skill, and external challenge, it is the adaptive relationship between the client and the environment that is the focal point of assessment. This requires that assessment procedures used in reductionistic practice approaches—the kinesiologic, neurologic, and intrapsychic—be supplemented by assessments designed to evaluate role behaviors.

Some of the assessments of occupational role have been formulated by occupational therapists specifically for use with the occupational behavior perspective (Table 9), while others have been borrowed from other disciplines (Table 10). Tables 9 and 10 provide a listing of commonly used instruments and their purpose. The method of data collection is also given. A review of Tables 9 and 10 indicates that use of the instruments requires skills in testing, interviewing, observing, and history-taking. Observation, interview, and testing all provide information on current functioning. History-taking is the only method allowing discernment of patterns of change and hence an examination of the past to understand the present. Since the occupational behavior perspective relates

TABLE 8. Occupational Role Dysfunction

Subconcepts	Purpose	References
Role	To facilitate the interpretation of medical problems in terms of daily functioning	Black[5] Heard[40] Sarbin[94]
Problem definition (diagnosis)	To stipulate dysfunctions in occupational role as the object of occupational therapy intervention	Kielhofner[47] Rogers[92] Chapter 2

deficits in current roles to skill deficiencies in previous roles, history-taking assumes particular significance as an assessment technique.

The problems identified through assessment are translated to goals that specify the nature of the adaptation needed to maintain or raise daily living performance. The point of entry for occupational therapy intervention is provided by the client's responsiveness to environmental conditions. The "just right" challenge enables clients to transcend their present adaptive capacity. Play, hobbies, games, chores, work, and cultural and educational activities constitute the treatment technology. The occupational therapist raises the client's level of adaptive competence by managing the environment and teaching skills and habits.

Environmental opportunities promote and strengthen skill development, while environmental deprivation hampers and retards this process. Disability may be viewed as a form of environmental deprivation which disrupts skill acquisition. Occupational therapy is the health-related discipline that provides an environment which supports the acquisition and renewal of skills. Treatment is carried out in a milieu supportive of occupation. This requires objects, people, events, and places that support occupation.

Objects enrich the stimulus capabilities of the environment, encouraging exploratory behavior and furnishing the potential for learning tool use and material use. To instill attitudes of craftsmanship, workmanship, and sportsmanship, the proper tools are provided for tasks to be done. These are kept in condition and stored in an orderly manner.

People in the environment exert their influence by establishing expectancies for client performance. The attitude conveyed by the therapist is respect for clients and belief in their own efficacy. Performance expectations are established in conjunction with the client to insure that they are relevant and clearly understood. Role models are made available to prompt learning via imitation and anticipatory socialization. The client's significant others are included in all phases of treatment to provide them with the information, instruction, and practice necessary to facilitate occupational performance.

Events are structured to provide normal developmental opportunities. Failure in one role is hypothesized to be caused by a failure to build the necessary skills and habits at an earlier stage of occupation. Thus, treatment is structured to develop or remediate deficits in occupational behavior through normal developmental activities sequenced according to developmental principles. Events are structured according to the following tenets:

TABLE 9. Instruments Developed for Use With the Occupational Behavior Perspective

Instrument	Reference	Purpose	Data Collection Method
Decision-Making Skills	Westphal[115]	To assess, using craft activities, the decision making process in regard to goal setting, problem recognition, attitude, information seeking, organization of information, solution selection, and outcome	Observation
NPI Interest Checklist	Matsutsuyu[66]	To describe the interest state by intensity in the areas of manual activities, physical sports, social recreation, cultural education, and activities of daily living	Self-administered questionnaire
Occupational History	Morhead[71]	To describe socialization in chilhood roles; exploration and decision-making concerning occupational choice; patterns of achievement and failure; career movement; work satisfaction, and interaction patterns	History-taking
Time Instrument	Larrington[60]	To assess time use in terms of the basic notion of time, temporal guidance and organization as these relate to success or failure in life role tasks	Self-administered questionnaire
An Inventory for the Assessment of Depersonalization and Occupational Skill Loss during Hospitalization	Gray[35]	To assess the conditions or events contributing to depersonalization (loss of security, privacy, self-identity, self-esteem, and contact with the outside world) and loss of occupational skills (loss of personal-care skills; work, home, and school skills, social skills; recreational skills; and decision-making skills)	Participant-observation

Assessment	Reference	Purpose	Method
Environmental Questionnaire	Dunning[24]	To describe the client's environment in terms of space, people, and tasks	Semi-structured interview
The Play History	Takata[107,109]	To diagnose the level of play development concerning materials, actions, people, and setting; 0 to 16 years	History-taking
A Play Scale	Knox[56]	To determine play age and describe play behavior regarding space and material management, imitation, and participation; 0 to 16 years	Observation
A Play Skills Inventory	Hurff,[41]	To describe development and play abilities concerning sensation, motor, perception and intellect; 8 to 12 years	Testing
A Play Agenda	Michelman[70]	To identify environments, experiences, and activities that promote interaction with the environment, foster mastery of symbols in art experiences and play; and develop risk-taking, problem-solving, and decision-making abilities	Observation
Inventory of Occupational Choice Skills	Shannon[98]	To assess frequency of participation in selected play-chore activities as a means of determining the development of self-discovery, decision-making, and work-role experimentation skills	Self-administered questionnaire
Adolescent Role Assessment	Black[4]	To assess performance in a variety of roles related to the occupational choice process—childhood play, family, school, peer socialization, occupational choice and work	Semi-structured interview
The Assessment Process	Chapters 2, 10, 12, 14	To provide perspective on how to assess persons with complex occupational dysfunctions	

TABLE 10. Instruments Commonly Used in the Occupational Behavior Perspective

Instrument	Reference	Purpose	Data Collection Method
Life Goals Inventory	Buhler & Coleman[18]	To find out what people want or expect to get from life, what they want more than anything else, and what they do not care about at all.	Testing
Generalized Expectations for Internal Versus External Control of Reinforcement	Rotter[93]	To measure the extent to which an individual believes his destiny to be internally or externally controlled	Testing
Social Competencies	Phillips[77]	To describe competence in terms of education, occupation, leisure, and marital status	Structured interview
Value Orientations Inventory	Kluckholn & Strodtbeck[55]	To assess value orientations in regard to: relational orientation, man-nature orientation, time orientation, activity orientation and human nature orientation	Structured interview

(a) A client's interests may be used to engage participation

(b) Play, arts and crafts, games, chores, and educational and cultural activities provide opportunities for self-discovery of values, attitudes, aspirations, and abilities

(c) Play, arts and crafts, games, chores, and educational and cultural activities provide opportunities for decision-making

(d) Work and leisure skills may be reprogrammed through play

(e) The teaching of skill begins with a playful phase and proceeds through structured learning and achievement phases

(f) Skills of daily living are learned through repetition

(g) A repetitive environment and skill mastery promotes habit formation

(h) Novel tasks evoke new behaviors

(i) An overall sense of success in task performance is needed to promote skill acquisition

(j) Time management is a skill and must be practiced to provide balance in work, rest, and leisure roles.

The environment incorporates or simulates as closely as possible the conditions under which the skill is to be performed post-discharge. In medical settings, the occupational therapist is an advocate for normalizing the environment to promote role behavior.

The technology for eliciting and guiding change thus resides in knowledge of socialization, of interest development, of skill acquisition, of developmental tasks, and of environmental management. Thus, in addition to providing new perspectives on the causes of dysfunctions in occupational role, use of the social-psychological concept of role furnishes new concepts for intervention. Arts and crafts, for instance, are not used only to exercise muscles or stimulate proprioceptors, but rather as a means of learning how to use tools and materials and to develop future work aptitudes and attitudes. Occupation is graded to directly influence the client's functional living skills.

A summary of occupation as intervention is presented in Table 11.

PROCESSES

A profession requires processes to both develop and apply its knowledge base. Of the five processes selected for study, criticism, general systems thinking, and qualitative research develop and refine the knowledge base underlying practice. Case method is the problem-solving process used in treating clients, while consultation is the indirect service methodology.

CRITICISM

Criticism is the process of appraising, with *knowledge* and *propriety*, the positive and negative features of a product or performance. To appraise with knowledge, the critic should have substantial expertise about the thing under criticism. Such expertise requires intensive study. To appraise with propriety, the critic should maintain an objective attitude. Criticism uses the cognitive skills of analysis, synthesis, and evaluation. These are applied in a systematic manner to the formulation of evidence to substantiate conclusions.

TABLE 11. Occupation as Intervention

Subconcepts	Purpose	References
Assessments of occupational role	To indicate the instruments used to evaluate strengths and weaknesses in occupational role	See Tables 9 and 10
Environmental management and the teaching of skills and habits	To demonstrate the application of the occupational behavior perspective	Bell[1] Borys[9] Brum & Wheeler[12] Goodwin[34] Heard[40] Hurff[41] Kielhofner[45] Kielhofner & Takata[51] Kielhofner, Burke & Igi[50] Kielhofner & Miyake[52] Kiev[53] Lahein[59] Paulson[76] Reilly[82] Webster[114] Chapters 2, 9, 12, 13, 14

Occupational therapists require critical thinking skills to spur progress in their own thinking. The purpose of criticism is to improve or refine the product or performance under scrutiny. For instance, criticism may be used to evaluate the adequacy of the reasoning process applied in evaluating and treating clients with the intent of improving the services delivered. Criticism may also be applied to the outcomes of the treatment process. Criticism is a critical component of professional behavior which aims at quality client care. In striving to become a self-critic, each therapist needs to learn to articulate ideas and to accept and give criticism.

Criticism is also needed to elaborate and revise the complex knowledge of the occupational behavior perspective. Classically, occupational behavior theorists are recognized for their attack on the medical model and the inner mechanism paradigm. There is much less awareness of the fact that criticism represents an overall policy and is also applied to the ideas of the occupational behavior framework. Occupational behavior theorists operate on the premise that an objective assessment of the positive and negative features of a phenomenon contributes to a greater understanding of its nature. Additional insight may be provided by disputes or debates about the interpretation of an item. In his analysis of the progress of a discipline, Kuhn[58] delineated the role of criticism in stimulating theorizing. Deficiencies in the data are brought into focus, trends are discerned, and new relationships are proposed.

New concepts and conceptual revisions are introduced into the occupational behavior framework only after the concepts have been tested for their philosophical and logical coherence with the framework's assumptions and principles. While the process of knowledge development is eclectic, or draws from many sources, it is also highly selective. Knowledge entering the occupational behavior framework is filtered for its direct relevance to human occupation.

In recent decades, the education of a professional has become extremely cumbersome because of the knowledge explosion. The quantity of material to be learned has become prohibitive and selections must be made. As an applied human services field, occupational therapy will always borrow knowledge, to some extent, from other disciplines. In a sense, the occupational therapy knowledge base at the present time suffers not from too little knowledge but rather from too little organization. This was the underlying theme of Chapter 2. To use an analogy, it is as though we have put together a Sunday outfit, item by item, without taking into account the need to coordinate colors and sizes. The result is a suit of clothes whose items are incompatible in color scheme and size, and hence probably cannot be worn by the same person or at the same time. In the case of the knowledge base, the effect of accumulating knowledge without integrating it is fragmentation and incoherence. Occupational behavior theorists seek to manage the knowledge explosion by using human occupation as the core concept for selecting and organizing knowledge, and criticism as the process for selecting and organizing knowledge.

GENERAL SYSTEMS THINKING

Through study of the history of occupational therapy, one gleans an appreciation of practice based on humans as musculoskeletal, perceptual-motor, or intrapsychic beings. These models were derived from a mechanistic philosophy, which seeks to comprend human behavior by studying its parts in isolation. Occupation is a complex bio-psycho-social, developmental phenomenon. Occupation cannot be understood by dealing with humans as disassembled musculo-skeletal, perceptual-motor or intrapsychic functions. To explain the occupational nature of humans requires that persons be viewed as wholes. Occupational behavior requires a thinking method that adequately encompasses the multiple dimensions of human beings. This methodology is provided by general systems theory.

General systems theory is a systematic method of reasoning designed to synthesize and integrate fragmented knowledge within and between disciplines. Synthesis and integration occurs by generalizing and abstracting across bodies of knowledge to uncover commonalities or general rules. These rules may be applied to phenomena as diverse as hospitals, humans, and the amoeba. Through concepts such as system, boundary, input, feedback, and output, general systems theory provides a common frame of reference for looking at phenomena that have traditionally been studied from many different frames of reference. It has the advantage of allowing the student to study the bio-psycho-social components of occupation as a whole and in the same language. The application of generic laws to occupational behavior fosters insight into the essential qualities of occupation.

Since most of us have been taught to think according to the mechanistic method, use of general systems thinking requires a conceptual reorientation. The focus of thought changes from parts to wholes and from elements to the interrelationships and organization between and among elements. This transformation may be facilitated through repeated application of systems rules. Chapters 2 and 14 demonstrate the application of systems thinking to theory and practice.

QUALITATIVE RESEARCH

An additional method for studying phenomena holistically is provided by qualitative research methodologies. In qualitative research, the object of study is not reduced to an isolated variable or a hypothesis about the relationship between two variables. Instead, it is studied as a whole in all its complexity. Qualitative research methodologies rely heavily on participant observations, personal documents, and unstructured interviewing to maintain the quality of the data in the subjects' own words and behaviors. Thus, they are especially beneficial for investigating the daily behaviors of self-care, work, and play.

CASE METHOD

The adoption of a scientific method represents a critical development in a profession and in a professional. This provides the means through which the body of knowledge is applied to service-related problems. The method of problem-solving must be appropriate for the needs addressed by the profession.

The case method was selected as the scientific method for the occupational behavior frame of reference. This is a form of scientific thinking which allows a number of factors to be examined stimultaneously. These factors are often studied intensively and for an extended length of time. The unit of concern, or the case, may be a client, a group, an institution, or a situation.

The steps of the case method are followed in many professions. The method is made specific for each discipline by its guiding frame of reference. Accordingly, the occupational behavior perspective is used to determine the client data to be collected. Data are gathered by a combination of observational, testing, interview, and history-taking techniques as noted above. Data analysis is also directed by the occupational behavior framework and leads to a role function diagnosis. This consists of a description of the client's assets and liabilities in an occupational role. The diagnosis is used to devise a role reconstruction plan. The plan makes use of assets to eliminate, control, or alleviate deficits, and indicates how assets may be protected and deficits remediated. The final step in the case method is an evaluation of the adequacy of the plan for meeting the client's needs.

Application of the case method depends on a thorough understanding of the frame of reference, skilled use of data collection tools, competence in problem definition and treatment planning, and a critique of the action plan. These professional behaviors may best be gained through a sequence of clinical experiences that includes observing a master clinician using the case method, practicing the case method in treating clients, and researching the results achieved through case method application.

CONSULTATION

Occupational behavior takes place in an environment consisting of persons, places, and events. Although these elements are extrinsic to the client, they are largely responsible for maintaining and prompting behavioral change. Personal changes in occupational behavior seen in treatment environments will not necessarily carry over to the environments of daily life. To elicit and sustain personal change, occupational therapy intervention must also be directed toward the client's environments. Consultation is the mode through which environmental intervention is accomplished.

Consultation is an indirect service. It is the process whereby expert knowledge, skills, and attitudes are transmitted to someone other than the client for the purpose of benefiting the client. The therapist, as a consultant, may serve in various change agent roles. The consultant may exert pressure to change, assist others in learning how to change, provide solutions to problems, or suggest resources. Consultation may involve working with individuals, small groups, organizations, and communities.

Consultation requires knowledge of authority, group dynamics, verbal and nonverbal communication, and ethnic values. Through actual field experience, one learns how to establish contact, define a consultative relationship, gather diagnostic data, select and implement a change strategy, evaluate the results of the intervention, and disengage from the helping relationship.

A summary of processes is presented in Table 12.

IMPLICATIONS FOR EDUCATION AND RESEARCH

It has been shown that human occupation requires knowledge that is scientific and interdisciplinary. The readiness to absorb such knowledge is determined by the level of general education achieved prior to *basic* occupational therapy education.[79] The knowledge requirements for practice based on the occupational behavior perspective are broad, complex, and rigorous. A strong liberal education, which introduces the student

TABLE 12. Processes

Process	Purpose	References
Criticism	To appraise one's own clinical thinking and the philosophical and logical coherence of the elements of occupational behavior theory	Kuhn[58] Leininger[61] Reilly[80]
General systems thinking	To integrate and organize interdisciplinary knowledge	Boulding[10] Feibleman[28] Kielhofner[44] Reilly[87] von Bertelanffy[112]
Qualitative research	To study occupational behavior holistically	Bogdan & Taylor[8] Glaser & Strauss[33]
Case method	To direct the occupational therapy process when it involves direct service to patients	Line[62]
Consultation	To direct the occupational therapy process when it involves indirect service to patients	Brown et al[14]

to multiple academic disciplines and their cognitive processes, furnishes the intellectual foundation for studying human occupation. Basic occupational therapy education builds on this background by transmitting the knowledge that has been accumulated, and teaches the skills and techniques needed to apply it.

At the *advanced* professional level, the study of human occupation remains general—applicable to all medical conditions. The emphasis is on developing theory, constructing evaluation instruments, and testing theory in practice. These research activities are centered on self-care, productive and ludic (play/leisure) occupations. Knowledge developed and tested at the advanced professional level is introduced into basic professional education once its clinical usefulness has been ascertained. Thus, advanced clinicians assume a vital role in formulating the entry level curriculum. Client contact is an integral part of advanced professional education and fosters a productive exchange between abstract concepts and clinical data.

Continuing education may serve two functions in regard to the study of human occupation. One function is to interest therapists, whose basic professional education was not oriented around human occupation, to return to school for graduate study in this area. The other is to assist those with a good foundation in human occupation to update knowledge and technology as new developments occur.

At the present time, much of the knowledge filtered from other disciplines for its relevance to human occupation has related to infancy, early childhood, and adolescence. In other words, more attention has been given to intervention through play than through work and leisure. Additions to occupational therapy science in regard to adulthood and aging are needed to expand the developmental base for practice. Another priority for research lies in investigating the scientific properties of existing occupational behavior instruments and in developing new assessment tools.

In conclusion, occupational therapy is immersed in the process of evolving from a procedure-oriented technical field to a theory-based profession. This transition depends on the development of a conceptual framework which links together accumulated

TABLE 13. Implications for Education and Research

Concept	Purpose	References
Liberal education	Provides the readiness for scientific, interdisciplinary study	Chapters 2, 4, 6, 7, 8
Basic occupational therapy education	Provides entry level knowledge and skills for practice based on knowledge of human occupation Provides the foundation for graduate education in occupational therapy	
Advanced occupational therapy education	Provides the knowledge and skills to develop the scientific basis of practice	
Continuing education in occupational therapy	Update knowledge and skills for practice Stimulate interest in advanced study	
Research Priorities	Theory development concerning work and leisure Formulation of assessment tools	

knowledge and technology in such a way as to guide the practitioner in the occupational therapy process. In this chapter, human occupation was delineated as the focus of occupational therapy science. Human occupation enables a unified view of practice and an integration of the facts, principles, skills, and techniques from the kinesiologic, neurologic, and intrapsychic approaches. Thus, human occupation provides a framework for teaching professional occupational therapy students how to base practice on knowledge. The chapter presented a systematic approach to the study of human occupation involving the scientific processes of questioning, conceptualizing, evaluating, and revising.

A summary of implications for education and research is presented in Table 13.

REFERENCES

1. BELL, CH: *Competition as a motivational incentive.* American Journal of Occupational Therapy, 29:277, 1975.

2. BERLYNE, DE: *Curiosity and exploration.* Science. 52:25, 1966.

3. BING, RK: *Occupational therapy revisited: A paraphrastic journey.* American Journal of Occupational Therapy, 35:499, 1981.

4. BLACK, MM: *Adolescent role assessment.* American Journal of Occupational Therapy, 30:73, 1976.

5. BLACK, MM: *The occupational career.* American Journal of Occupational Therapy, 30:225, 1976.

6. BOCKOVEN, JS: *Moral Treatment in American Psychiatry.* Springer Publishing Company, New York, 1963.

7. BOCKOVEN, JS: *Legacy of moral treatment—1800's to 1910.* American Journal of Occupational Therapy, 25:223, 1971.

8. BOGDAN, R AND TAYLOR, SJ: *Introduction to Qualitative Research Methods: A Phenomenological Approach to the Social Sciences.* John Wiley & Sons, New York, 1975.

9. BORYS, SS: *Implications of interest theory.* American Journal of Occupational Therapy, 28:35, 1974.

10. BOULDING, K: *General systems theory: The skeleton of science.* In Buckley, W (ED): *Modern Systems Research for the Behavioral Scientist.* Aldine Publishing Company, Chicago, 1968.

11. BOULDING, K: *The Image.* University of Michigan Press, Ann Arbor, 1975.

12. BRIM, OG AND WHEELER, S: *Socialization After Childhood: Two Essays.* John Wiley & Sons, New York, 1966.

13. BRINKER, MC: *The Effects of Bed Rest and Inactivity on the Cardiovascular, Respiratory, and Urinary Systems.* Unpublished master's thesis, Division of Occupational Therapy, University of North Carolina, Chapel Hill, NC, 1981.

14. BROWN, D, ET AL: *Consultation: Strategy for Improving Education.* Allyn and Bacon, Boston, 1979.

15. BRUNER, JS: *The skill of relevance or the relevance of skills.* Saturday Review, 20:66, 1970.

16. BRUNER, JS: *The nature and uses of immaturity.* American Psychologist, 27:687, 1972.

17. BRYAN, WA: *Administrative Psychiatry.* WW Norton, New York, 1936.

18. BUHLER, C AND COLEMAN, W: *Life Goal Inventory.* Unpublished manuscript, 1965.

19. BURKE, JP: *A clinical perspective on motivation: Pawn versus origin.* American Journal of Occupational Therapy, 31:254, 1977.

20. BURT, CM: *Hypokinetic Disease: The Effects of Inactivity on the Musculoskeletal System, and Related Skin and Nerve Tissue.* Unpublished master's thesis. Division of Occupational Therapy, University of North Carolina, Chapel Hill, 1981.

21. CAMPBELL, B: *The evolution of the human hand.* In Cohen, YI (ED): *Man in Adaptation: The Biosocial Background.* Adline Publishing Company, Chicago, 1968.

22. CHAPPLE, E: *Rehabilitation: The Dynamic Change.* Center for Research in Education, Cornell University, Ithaca, New York, 1970.

23. DIASIO, K: *The modern era — 1960-1970.* American Journal of Occupational Therapy, 25:237, 1971.

24. DUNNING, H: *Environmental Occupational Therapy.* Unpublished master's thesis, Department of Occupational Therapy, University of Southern California, 1972.

25. DUNNING, H: *Environmental occupational therapy.* American Journal of Occupational Therapy, 26:292, 1972.

26. ENGELHARDT, HT: *Defining occupational therapy: The meaning of therapy and the virtues of occupation.* American Journal of Occupational Therapy, 31:666, 1977.

27. ERICKSON, JM: *Activity, Recovery, Growth: The Communal Role of Planned Activities.* WW Norton, New York, 1976.

28. FEIBLEMAN, JK: *Theory of integrative levels.* In Coleman, JC, (ED): *Psychology and Effective Behavior.* Scott Foresman and Company, Glenview, Ill, 1969.

29. FIGONE, J: *A Model for Family Involvement in Pediatric Occupational Therapy.* Unpublished master's thesis. Department of Occupational Therapy, University of Southern California, 1977.

30. FLOREY, LL: *Intrinsic motivation: The dynamics of occupational therapy theory.* American Journal of Occupational Therapy, 23:319, 1969.

31. GILLETTE, N AND KIELHOFNER, G: *The impact of specialization on the professionalization and survival of occupational therapy.* American Journal of Occupational Therapy, 33:20, 1979.

32. GINZBERG, E: *Toward a theory of occupational choice: A restatement.* Vocational Guidance Quarterly, 20:169, 1972.

33. GLASER, BG AND STRAUSS, AL: *The Discovery of Grounded Theory: Strategies for Qualitative Research.* Aldine Publishing Company, Chicago, 1967.

34. GOODWIN, E: *Implementation of the occupational behavior model: A personal account.* Canadian Journal of Occupational Therapy 43:14, 1976.

35. GRAY, M: *An Assessment of Depersonalization and Occupational Skill Loss During Hospitalization.* Unpublished master's thesis, Department of Occupational Therapy, University of Southern California, 1969.

36. GRAY, M *Effects of hospitalization on work-play behavior.* American Journal of Occupational Therapy, 26:180, 1972.

37. HAAS, LJ: *Practical Occupational Therapy.* Bruce Publishing Company, Milwaukee, 1946.

38. HALL, AD AND FAGEN, RE: *Definition of systems.* In Buckley, W, (ED): *Modern Systems Research for the Behavioral Scientist.* Aldine Publishing Company, Chicago, 1968.

39. HAVIGHURST, RJ: *Developmental Tasks and Education*. Longmans, Green, New York, 1952.

40. HEARD, C: *Occupational role acquisition: A perspective on the chronically disabled*. American Journal of Occupational Therapy, 31:243, 1977.

41. HURFF, J: *A play skills inventory*. In Reilly, M (ED): *Play, as Exploratory Learning*. Sage Publications, Beverly Hills, 1974.

42. HURFF, J: *A play skills inventory: A competency monitoring tool for the 10 year old*. American Journal of Occupational Therapy, 34:651, 1980.

43. KIDNER, TB: *Occupational therapy—Its aims and development*. Occupational Therapy and Rehabilitation, 11:233, 1932.

44. KIELHOFNER, G: *General systems theory: Implications for theory and action in occupational therapy*. American Journal of Occupational Therapy, 32:637, 1978.

45. KIELHOFNER, G: *The temporal dimension in the lives of retarded adults: A problem of interaction and intervention*. American Journal of Occupational Therapy, 33:161, 1979.

46. KIELHOFNER, G: *A model of human occupation, Part 2. Ontogenesis from the perspective of temporal adaptation*. American Journal of Occupational Therapy, 34:657, 1980.

47. KIELHOFNER, G: *A model of human occupation, Part 3, Benign and vicious cycles*. American Journal of Occupational Therapy, 34:731, 1980.

48. KIELHOFNER, G AND BURKE, JP: *Occupational therapy after 60 years: An account of changing identity and knowledge*. American Journal of Occupational Therapy, 31:675, 1977.

49. KIELHOFNER, G AND BURKE, JP: *A model of human occupation, Part 1. Conceptual framework and content*. American Journal of Occupational Therapy, 34:572, 1980.

50. KIELHOFNER, G, BURKE, JP AND IGI, CH: *A model of human occupation, Part 4, Assessment and intervention*. American Journal of Occupational Therapy, 34:777, 1980.

51. KIELHOFNER, G AND TAKATA, CH: *A study of mentally retarded persons: Applied research in occupational therapy*. American Journal of Occupational Therapy, 34:252, 1980.

52. KIELHOFNER, G AND MIYAKE, S: *The therapeutic use of games with mentally retarded adults*. American Journal of Occupational Therapy, 35:375, 1981.

53. KIEV, A: *A Strategy for Daily Living*. The Free Press, New York, 1973.

54. KLAVINS, R: *Work-play behavior: cultural variations*. American Journal of Occupational Therapy, 26:176, 1972.

55. KLUCKHOHN, F AND STRODTBECK, F: *Variations in Value Orientations*. Row, Peterson, Evanston, Ill, 1962.

56. KNOX, S: *A play scale*. In Reilly, M (ED): *Play as Exploratory Learning*. Sage Publications, Beverly Hills, 1974.

57. KOESTLER, A: *The Ghost in the Machine*. Henry Regnery, Chicago, 1967.

58. KUHN, T: *The Structure of Scientific Revolutions*. University of Chicago Press, Chicago, 1962.

59. LAKEIN, A: *How To Get Control of Your Time and Your Life*. New American Library, New York, 1973.

60. LARRINGTON, GG: *An Exploratory Study of the Temporal Aspects of Adaptive Functioning*. Unpublished master's thesis. Department of Occupational Therapy, University of Southern California, 1970.

61. LEININGER, MM: *The Research Critique.* Nursing Research, 17:444, 1968.

62. LINE, J: *Case method as a scientific form of clinical thinking.* American Journal of Occupational Therapy, 23:308, 1969.

63. McCLELLAND, DC: *The Achieving Society.* The Free Press, New York, 1961.

64. MARSH, LC: *Shall we apply industrial psychiatry to psychiatry?* Occupational Therapy and Rehabilitation, 12:1, 1932.

65. MARSH, LC: *Borzori: Suggestions for a new rallying of occupational therapy.* Occupational Therapy and Rehabilitation 11:169, 1932.

66. MATSUTSUYU, JS: *The interest check list.* American Journal of Occupational Therapy, 23:323, 1969.

67. MATSUTSUYU, J: *Occupational behavior—a perspective on work and play.* American Journal of Occupational Therapy, 25:291, 1971.

68. MEYER, A: *The philosophy of occupational therapy.* Archives of Occupational Therapy, 1:1, 1922.

69. MICHELMAN, SS: *The importance of creative play.* American Journal of Occupational Therapy, 25:285, 1971.

70. MICHELMAN, SS: *Play and the deficit child.* In Reilly, M (ED): *Play as Exploratory Learning.* Sage Publications, 1974, Beverly Hills.

71. MOORHEAD, L: *The occupational history.* American Journal of Occupational Therapy, 23:329, 1969.

72. MOSEY, A: *Involvement in the rehabilitation movement—1942-1960.* American Journal of Occupational Therapy, 25:234, 1971.

73. NAPIER, J: *Hands.* Pantheon Books, New York, 1980.

74. OAKLEY, KP: *Man the Tool-Maker.* University of Chicago Press, Chicago, 1960.

75. PARENT, LH: *Effects of a low-stimulus environment on behavior.* American Journal of Occupational Therapy, 32:19, 1978.

76. PAULSON, C.P.: *Juvenile delinquency and occupational choice.* American Journal of Occupational Therapy, 34:565, 1980.

77. PHILLIPS, L: *Human Adaptation and Its Failures.* Academic Press, New York, 1968.

78. PROSHANSKY, HM, ITTELSON, WH, AND RIVLIN, LG: (Eds), *Environmental Psychology: Man and His Physical Setting.* Holt Rinehart and Winston, New York, 1970.

79. REILLY, M: *An occupational therapy curriculum for 1965.* American Journal of Occupational Therapy, 12:293, 1958.

80. REILLY, M: *Occupational Therapy can be one of the great ideas of 20th century medicine.* American Journal of Occupational Therapy, 16:1, 1962.

81. REILLY, M: *Research potentiality of occupational therapy.* American Journal of Occupational Therapy, 14:206, 1960.

82. REILLY, M: *A psychiatric occupational program as a teaching model.* American Journal of Occupational Therapy, 20:61, 1966.

83. REILLY, M: *The challenge of the future to an occupational therapist.* American Journal of Occupational Therapy, 20:221, 1966.

84. REILLY, M: *The educational process.* American Journal of Occupational Therapy, 23:299, 1969.

85. REILLY, M: *The modernization of occupational therapy.* The American Journal of Occupational Therapy, 25:243, 1971.

86. REILLY, M: *Competency as a battered concept.* In Ring, BC and Schroder, DR (EDS): *11th Annual Distinguished Lecture Series in Special Education and Rehabilitation.* School of Education, University of Southern California, Los Angeles, 1973.

87. REILLY, M (ED): *Play as Exploratory Learning: Studies of Curiosity Behavior.* Sage Publications, Beverly Hills, 1974.

88. REILLY, M: *A response to: Defining occupational therapy: The meaning of therapy and the virtues of occupation.* American Journal of Occupational Therapy, 31:673, 1977.

89. REREK, M: *The depression years — 1929 to 1941.* The American Journal of Occupational Therapy, 25:231, 1971.

90. ROBINSON, AL: *Play: The arena for acquisition of rules for competent behavior.* American Journal of Occupational Therapy, 31:248, 1977.

91. ROE, A: *Early determinants of vocational choice.* Journal of Counseling Psychology, 4:212, 1957.

92. ROGERS, J: *Order and disorder in medicine and occupational therapy.* American Journal of Occupational Therapy, 36:29, 1982.

93. ROTTER, JB: *Generalized expectancies for internal versus external control of reinforcement.* Psychological Monographs, 80:1, 1966.

94. SARBIN, TR: *Role theory.* In Lindzey, G (ED): *Handbook of Social Psychology.* Addison-Wesley, Menlo Park, Ca, 1968.

95. SCHEIN, EH: *The individual, the organization, and the career — A conceptual scheme.* Journal of Applied Behavior Science, 7:401, 1971.

96. SHANNON, P: *Work-play theory and the occupational therapy process.* American Journal of Occupational Therapy, 26:169, 1972.

97. SHANNON, PD: *The adolescent experience.* American Journal of Occupational Therapy, 26:284, 1972.

98. SHANNON, PD: *Occupational choice: Decision-making play.* In Reilly, M (ED): *Play as Exploratory Learning.* Sage Publications, Beverly Hills, 1974.

99. SHANNON, P: *The derailment of occupational therapy.* American Journal of Occupational Therapy, 31:229, 1977.

100. SLAGLE, EC: *Occupational Therapy: recent methods and advances in the United States.* Occupational Therapy and Rehabilitation 13:289, 1934.

101. SMITH, MB: *Competence and socialization.* In Clausen, J (ED): *Socialization and Society.* Little, Brown & Company, Boston, 1968.

102. SMITH, MB: *Competence and adaptation.* American Journal of Occupational Therapy, 28:11, 1974.

103. SNOW, TL: *Purposeful Activity: A Literature Review.* Unpublished master's thesis, Division of Occupational Therapy, University of North Carolina, Chapel Hill, 1980.

104. SPUHLER, JN: *The Evolution of Man's Capacity for Culture:* Wayne State University Press, Detroit, 1965.

105. SUEDFELD, P: *Restricted Environmental Stimulation: Research and Clinical Application.* John Wiley and Sons, New York, 1980.

106. SUNDSTROM, C: *The physiological aspects of work and play.* American Journal of Occupational Therapy, 26:173, 1972.

107. TAKATA, N: *The play history.* American Journal of Occupational Therapy, 23:314, 1969.

108. TAKATA, N: *The play milieu—A preliminary appraisal.* American Journal of Occupational Therapy, 25:281, 1971.

108. TAKATA, N: *The play milieu—A preliminary appraisal.* American Journal of Occupational Therapy, 25:281, 1971.

109. TAKATA, N: *Play as a prescription.* In Reilly, M (ED): *Play as Exploratory Learning.* Sage Publications, Beverly Hills, 1974.

110. TOBIAS, PV: *The brain behind the hands. Skilled activities in man and his poor relations.* South African Journal of Occupational Therapy, 1:4, 1966.

111. TOUCHSTONE, JM: *The Occupational Therapy Process and the Mexican American.* Unpublished master's thesis, Division of Occupational Therapy, University of North Carolina, Chapel Hill, 1981.

112. VON BERTALANFFY, L: *General systems theory—a critical review.* In Buckley (ED) *Modern Systems Research for the Behavioral Scientist.* Aldine Publishing Company, Chicago, 1968.

113. WASHBURN, SL: *Tools and human evolution.* Scientific American, 203:63, 1960.

114. WEBSTER, PS: *Occupational role development in the young adult with mild retardation.* American Journal of Occupational Therapy, 34:13, 1980.

115. WESTPHAL, MA: *A Study of Decision Making.* Unpublished master's thesis, Department of Occupational Therapy, University of Southern California, 1967.

116. WHITE, R: *Motivation reconsidered: The concept of competence.* Psychological Review, 66:297, 1959.

117. WHITE, RW: *The urge toward competence.* American Journal of Occupational Therapy, 25:271, 1971.

118. US Department of Health, Education, and Welfare, Public Health Service — National Institutes of Health, The National Institute of Child Health and Human Development, *Perspectives on Human Deprivation,* 1968.

119. WOODSIDE, H: *Dimensions of the occupational behavior model.* Canadian Journal of Occupational Therapy, 43:11, 1976.

CHAPTER 4

DEFINING OCCUPATION: IMPORTING AND ORGANIZING INTERDISCIPLINARY KNOWLEDGE

Janice Posatery Burke

EDITOR'S INTRODUCTION

It is commonly accepted that occupational therapists employ knowledge derived from many disciplines. Thus, occupational therapy is an interdisciplinary topic requiring careful scholarship. In this chapter the reader is given an example of interdisciplinary thinking and its underlying processes.

The chapter begins with an acknowledgment that occupational behavior is a complex phenomenon demanding a full range of biologic, psychologic and social concepts. Arguing that the latter two areas are the least well developed of occupational therapy, the chapter demonstrates how to bring such knowledge into the field. Before proceeding to this task the author provides a set of guidelines for importing and organizing interdisciplinary knowledge. These prescriptions serve as a structure for the remaining discussion.

The author builds on the theme that the field needs to focus on occupation as its central area of knowledge. Interdisciplinary knowledge is incorporated into a definition of occupation. The reader will find this chapter instructive not only for understanding some of the rules of scholarship, but for considering the use of ideas in clinical practice. The chapter shows that issues raised about theoretical consistency are consequential for practice.

Occupational therapy is often characterized as a hodge-podge of techniques practiced by a therapeutic jack-of-all-trades. This chapter offers suggestions for a systematic approach to knowledge and practice and its message is important.

In 1916, the word occupation in occupational therapy simply meant work. . . . Early therapists found increasing difficulty in bringing the patient's job tasks into field hospitals and hospitals. In 1918, it was recognized that crafts met all the therapeutic qualifications of occupations. . . . We saw them as simulators of occupation and then began to look more upon the simulation than on the underlying dynamics of the occupational task and lost our initial orientation to occupation itself. (Weimer, Traditional and Nontraditional Practice Arenas: Occupational Therapy:2001)

Occupational therapy originated with a belief that occupation has a unique ability to restore and maintain organization of human systems affected by disease and trauma. This definition of the therapeutic process provided early leaders with the tools to extend the reach of occupational therapy. Their approach to the care and rehabilitation of patients in insane asylums of the day proved equally applicable to victims of future wars and such chronically disabling diseases as tuberculosis and polio. Today, the viability of human occupation as a central theme for the future practice of occupational therapy is dependent upon the field's abiliy to update our understanding of the complex nature of this concept.

Reilly has reminded therapists that this health care field was founded and must support principles embedded in a humanistic philosophy that "implies that its inherited purpose was to protect and improve the quality of hour-by-hour, day-by-day adaptation of the dysfunctional patient".[26] Her orientation contrasts with that of others who have called for theoretical and technical viewpoints that focus on a narrower scientific and medical based concept of practice. Reilly's[26] central theme is that the field should modernize traditional concepts by importing and organizing interdisciplinary knowledge of occupation and its therapeutic potentials. On the 60th anniversary of the field Engelhardt reiterated the unique and traditional commitment of occupational therapy to daily life through the use of occupation as a therapeutic medium:

> Occupational therapy offers a meaning of therapy that accents the process of human adaptation through involvement in recreation and in physical and mental activities generally. Occupational therapy makes a special contribution to our understanding of the importance and the value of human enterprise whereby humans adapt and thrive in their environments by structuring their time in tasks that lead to recreation and pleasure. In viewing humans as engaged in activities, realizing themselves through their occupation, occupational therapy supports a view of the whole person in functional adaptation.[10]

This orientation to the dynamic interaction of the individual and the environment goes beyond a disease or symptom related view of the person who is suffering from an illness or physical trauma. Thus, it demands knowledge beyond the traditional scope of medicine to support therapists' insight into the complexity of factors that are part of each individual's occupational life. A thorough understanding of the components that make up human occupational behavior is thus necessary for successful therapeutic intervention. A more complete understanding of the occupational nature of persons results in a better grasp of the magnitude of disruption that disease causes in daily lives. For example, we can better understand the despair and disinterest in therapy shown by a recent quadraplegic who is a family man and hard worker with highly valued ability as a stone cutter. We can also understand the depression and lack of interest in planning for the future in the sixty-year-old woman with severe deformities and permanent physical limitations resulting from a car accident, who has always prided herself on her independence and her strong interest in traveling. The issues to be confronted in the occupational therapy clinic are no longer just those related to increasing functional abilities, but are more precisely defined according to the goals and objectives that will serve the patient in re-establishing and selecting new methods for continuing their chosen occupational lives.

THE COMPLEXITY OF OCCUPATIONAL BEHAVIOR AND THE INTERDISCIPLINARY KNOWLEDGE BASE

All human behavior is an amalgamation of various genetic, developmental and biologic factors modified by the social, cultural, and psychologic system in which people live and work.[14] An interdisciplinary definition of occupation which acknowledges this complexity must provide an integrated view of the biologic, psychologic and social aspects of daily life that impact all individuals. As noted in Chapter 2, the occupational therapist is well versed in the biologic influences on individuals as evidenced by kinesiologic and neurologic documentation within the field. The areas most in need of expanded knowledge are thus in the psychologic and social domains.

This chapter illustrates some aspects of the process of selecting interdisciplinary knowledge for occupational therapy. It examines a range of concepts drawn from the behavioral and social sciences and considers their relevance for occupational therapy.

THE PROCESS OF SELECTING INTERDISCIPLINARY KNOWLEDGE

Selecting a group of diverse concepts for special use requires systematic processes of interdisciplinary thinking, as noted in earlier chapters. Simply combining parts to form a montage of ideas invariably fails to achieve critical linkages that allow knowledge to cohere as a functional whole. These linkages are in place only when information is selected for its compatibility with the desired objective, as illustrated in the following example.

There has been much interest in childhood play as an important developmental phenomenon. The work of such writers as Piaget[24] and Bruner[4] identifies play as critical for learning motor, cognitive, and social skills. Clearly, the absence of play in a child is of clinical significance. With an eclectic approach to play, one might select principles and knowledge from behaviorism, thereby warranting clinical intervention to increase play through a system of rewards. While this approach is benign in intent and practical in its use of available theory, it is also inconsistent. Piaget[24] and Bruner[4] theorized that the motive for play is intrinsic, asserting that play is done for its own sake and is self-reinforcing. Behaviorist theories are built on the premise of extrinsic motivation: that behavior functions in response to external rewards. Thus the two theories are incompatible in that they do not conform to first principles concerning the fundamental nature of play.

But more than theoretical purity is involved. In a study by Green and Lepper[15] positive reinforcement (social praise) had the paradoxical effect of decreasing free play. From an intrinsic theory perspective this result is understandable; external reinforcement may destroy the motive for play. Another flaw in the behavioral approach is noted by Mogford[23]. In her discussion of play and handicapped children she points out that reinforcement may produce behaviors that only appear to be play. They are not true play since they are pursued for extrinsic rewards and do not reflect the learning process inherent in self-motivated play.

As this example demonstrates, selecting interdisciplinary concepts must begin with a determination of the nature of the concepts and their theoretical compatibility if they are to be integrated into an useful and effective body of knowledge for practice. The following guidelines are proposed for integrating interdisciplinary concepts: (1) Clearly establish the need for selecting the concept by identifying its purpose for the field's knowledge base (i.e., propose the question which the concept is intended to answer); (2) identify the theoretical tradition(s) behind the concept in order to illuminate the premises that support it; (3) select only concepts which spring from compatible premises; (4) illustrate the relationship of the concepts to occupational therapy by organizing them into statements concerning the field's areas of concern.

This chapter illustrates how a few social science concepts can be selected; it is not intended to be exhaustive. The reader may refer to Chapter 2 for a more comprehensive discussion of relevant concepts. Consideration of theoretical traditions behind concepts will be a brief and exposition of the issues and ideas involved. Finally, the definition of occupation offered at the conclusion of the discussion is not a delimiting definition. It is offered as an expansion of the predominant concept of occupation as merely purposeful activity, but it assumes that the definition will continue to be elaborated. This is primarily a discussion of process; it concerns the dynamics of selecting and organizing knowledge for the field. The eventual theoretical structures that undergird practice will only be as sound as the processes from which they are derived.

THE NEED FOR SOCIAL SCIENCE CONCEPTS. The first proposed guideline requires clarification of the need for concepts. It has already been shown that occupational therapy requires a fuller understanding of occupation as the core of its knowledge base. This can be elaborated by several questions concerning occupation: What are the motivational forces that contribute to a person's occupational behavior? What are the dynamics of the interface of the person's behavior with society? What determines the individual content, value and significance of occupation? How do persons acquire occupational behavior?

MOTIVATION FOR OCCUPATION

Early explanations of motivation focused on the physiologic and later the psychologic determinants of behavior.[12] Freud contributed significant constructs regarding the theory of instincts as part of a psychodynamic theory of motivation. Freud saw instincts as the principal drives or motivators of behavior that functioned to satiate a need state in an organism that arose as a result of a somatic process.[3] These powerful and persistent internal stimuli promoted activities that led to a reduction of the drive.[31]

The Freudian view of development saw the need for gratification as the most important feature contributing to emotional well being and formation of the personality. Later revisions of this theory shifted emphasis from instinctual influences to human relations as basic influences on the organism. Again, emphasis on need states dominated the view of human motivation: the need for mother's love, parental approval, peer and sibling acceptance.

Another major tradition, behaviorism, similarly views behavior as a function of drives arising from tissue needs and resulting in consummatory behavior. Behaviorist concepts focus on the environment as a source of drive-reducing resources.[9,32] The organism is presumed to seek elements in the environment which satisfy drives and to learn in the course doing so.

The Freudian and behaviorist traditions portray human behavior as a means of reducing tension caused by tissue states. They see the organism as unconsciously seeking homeostasis, with behavior oriented to this end and learning accruing as a result.

In an attempt to explain motivation or persistence in an activity after drives have been satisfied or when they are absent, White used the concept of competence:

> The competence of an organism means its fitness or ability to carry on those transactions with the environment which result in its maintaining itself, growing and flourishing.[32]

The concept of competence, unlike earlier conceptualizations, does not explain behavior as based solely on tissue deficits or need states. Rather, White postulates an effectance motive which includes urges for manipulation, exploration, and activity of all types. This effectance urge leads the organism to seek out effective interaction with the environment.[33] By continually engaging in and learning about the world around, individuals become better equipped to meet the demands of danger or survival situations they may encounter.[30] Learning is viewed as an ongoing process that occurs regardless of tissue needs at any time.

Berlyne[2] theorized about the role of the central nervous system as it relates to effectance motivation. He explained that the nervous system is programmed so that perceptual and intellectual activities are engaged in for their own sake. According to Berlyne human organisms experience pleasurable states of "conflict and arousal" when they encounter information about the environment. Individuals select the information they will attend to based on their optimal levels of arousal and their individual interest in novel stimuli. The exploratory behaviors that are activated by such stimuli are unique to each individual as he or she engages in environmental interaction.[3]

These competency-based notions of motivation provide an explanation of behavior centered on the need for all individuals to explore and effect change in their environment. Richard DeCharms[9] developed the concept of personal causation in an attempt to further define the internal factors that influence the effectance motive. He rejected traditional theories of motivation as based on mind-body dualism and as too hedonistically focused. DeCharms argued that they were insufficient ways of defining behavior that is not necessarily "driven". He argued that a conceptualization of motivation as an affective state that causes behavior is inadequate since

> it presupposes a para-mechanical interpretation of the relationship between affect and behavior. Basically, affect must precede behavior and cause it, almost in the sense of energizing it or at least directing it.[9]

DeCharms offers an expanded view of motivation which he terms personal causation. This concept proposes that behavior is a function not only of physical events (such as tissue states) but also of personal causes (i.e., the experience of being a cause). Behavior develops in the newborn in a complex interweaving of learning from experience and the urge to have an effect on the environment. Children repeatedly observe themselves causing change in objects in their physical world, gradually developing an understanding of their ability to move physical things, as in pulling a string to bring an object within easy reach. These effects provide information to children regarding their feelings of causation.[9,21] As time passes the child formulates a view of himself or herself as capable of having an effect on a widening variety of areas.

The basic postulate put forth by DeCharms is that "man's primary motivational propensity is to be effective in producing changes in his environment"[9] Two dominant modes of behavior representing extreme ends of the effectance continuum are labeled origin and pawn. Individuals manifesting pawnlike behavior are more likely to feel they have little choice in what they do and are less able to feel in control of their actions. By contrast, origins feel they have control of what happens to them and are more alert to opportunities in their environment.[9] Those who believe they can control their own destiny are more likely to be alert to aspects of the environment that provide useful information for their future behavior, to take steps to improve their situations, place greater value on skills and be concerned with their abilities.[1] At the other extreme are the persons who believe that what happens to them is a result of chance, fate, or powerful others.[16]

CHOOSING CONCEPTS FOR OCCUPATIONAL THERAPY. The relevance of motivational constructs to occupational therapy is their ability to explain why persons engage in occupation. Thus, concepts of motivation that do this best are chosen for occupational therapy.

THEORETICAL TRADITION. The concepts of motivation represent two major theoretical traditions. The first sees the basic motivational tendency of humans arising from tissue needs with the goal of tension reduction. Psychodynamic theories and behaviorist theories share this common framework, locating the biologic determinants of motivation in the disruption of homeostatic states of viscera (e.g., hunger, thirst, sex) and their psychologic manifestation as drives. This tradition sees humans as largely passive organisms who seek tranquillity and satisfaction of desire in order to reach homeostasis. Motivation is covert and tension reducing and behavior is engaged in for the purpose of secondary gains or extrinsic rewards.

The second tradition, represented in the work of White,[33] DeCharms,[9] and others, sees an alternative or additional motivational urge in humans. This tradition views motivation as intrinsically generated and as demonstrating tension-seeking properties. It is proposed that humans possess a drive for states of instability, challenge, and arousal that is located within the substratum of the nervous system. Thus, in contrast to the earlier tradition of viscerogenic drives, the effectance drive is neurogenic. In addition, the phenomenological aspect of human experience as a modifier of motivation is important in this view of behavior. The individual's experience regarding performance and its outcome influences future motivational urges. Humans are seen as conscious actors making choices to act based on their needs for exploration and engagement and their personal beliefs about their own abilities.

COMPATIBILITY WITH THE PREMISE OF OCCUPATION. In occupational therapy the concept of occupation is defined as goal-directed, active engagement. Such activity is observably conscious, planned, and pleasurable. Thus, the first tradition in psychology which stresses the motivational basis of activity grounded in unconscious, biologically-based tissue needs is largely inappropriate and incompatible with the accepted view of occupation. The second tradition, which proposes the intrinsic, neurologically based and conscious character of motivation is suited to and can be incorporated into the field's theory and principles of therapeutic intervention.

THE ORGANIZATION OF BEHAVIOR: ROLE THEORY

The second question respecting the application of social science knowledge concerns the integration or interface of occupational behavior with the social environment. The relationship between the individual's behavior and the social system is explained by the concept of role.[11] It is a broad concept included in the theories of several disciplines, and some of the premises that provided the foundations for its development are worth our attention.[27]

Symbolic interactionism, a tradition of thought represented in sociology explains the unique occurrences that result from two or more individuals interacting in a particular situation. This view can be contrasted with the perspective that defines situations as already existing in reality with specific properties or forces which will predictably affect the behavior of the individuals.[5] For the symbolic interactionist the determinants of behavior exist within and between individuals rather than outside of them. As two or more individuals become involved in a specific situation, they define it. Their definition is based on the past experiences and knowledge of each person as well as an interpretation of the present.[5] In this tradition roles are a source of defining the situation and can be located in the typical ways that individual actors construct behavior.

George Herbert Mead[22] is closely associated with the theory of symbolic interaction. In his view all behavior is shaped, motivated, and directed to social interaction and, in turn, such interaction is the basis for the development of the self.[25]

This dynamic process between the self and the environment can be illustrated through the developmental learning that occurs for the child involved in organized games. Games provide an opportunity for children to develop the capacity to assume attitudes and roles of others in order to evaluate their own behavior and that of other participants:

> The child must not only take the role of the other, as he does in the play, but he must assume the various roles of all the participants in the game, and govern his action accordingly. If he plays first base, it is as the one to whom the ball will be thrown from the field or from the catcher. Their organized reactions to him he has embedded in his own playing of the different positions, and this organized reaction becomes what I have called the 'generalized other' that accompanies and controls his conduct. And it is this generalized other in his experience which provides him with a self.[25]

These concepts are embedded in the symbolic interactionist view of role. Sarbin encompasses this dynamic interplay between intra-individual and extra-individual determinants in his concept of role:

> In role theory, the person as the broad sociological unit of interaction is retained, but a somewhat finer unit, the role is added. Thus role theory embraces reciprocal action between persons, but these actions are organized into roles . . . In broad perspective, contemporary role theory regards human conduct as the product of the interaction of self and role.[28]

Roles take on meaning as actions performed by persons in order to validate their positions within society.[28] The concept of role as informed by symbolic interactionism conceptualizes interaction as defined by the roles that actors are filling at the time of interaction. Role is a context of personal behavior which influences both self-perception and perception of the other. Stated another way, all interaction has a dynamic and emergent character born of the mutual interpretations and actions of actors, and the process of interaction is as much an interaction of roles as it is of persons.

Not all perspectives on role are supported by the premises of symbolic interactionism. Less dynamic views such as the Gestaltist perspective see roles as stable elements of an external order into which persons fit themselves. A similar perspective, informed by behaviorism, offers the view of a role as an inventory of specific behaviors or conditioned responses contrasted with an explanation of role as strategies for mixing habitual and improvised behaviors to meet the demands of a situation.[31]

CHOOSING CONCEPTS FOR OCCUPATIONAL THERAPY. The appropriateness of role theory for our definition of occupation can be decided by using the criteria employed to select motivation theory. The concept of role was examined in order to answer questions regarding the individual in interaction with society. More specifically, our concern was with how this interaction is determined and maintained. The concept of role as defined by symbolic interactionism gives us an understanding of this interaction.

THEORETICAL TRADITION. The concept of role grew out of a combination which sought to understand the interface between an individual and society. Gestaltist and Behaviorist perspectives viewed roles as behaviors influenced by forces outside of the individual and as conditioned responses. The symbolic interactionist viewpoint seeks to identify role behaviors as unique to each situation and each individual within the situation. Roles are thus broad definers of individual action based on normative guidelines that correspond to biologic, social and occupational criteria. However, the enactment of the role within a specific situation is defined by intra-and inter-individual determinants. In other words, all men do not interpret and enact their roles as fathers in the same way, all teachers do not conduct their classroom duties in the same manner, and all sisters and brothers do not interact in similar relationships.

COMPATIBILITY WITH THE PREMISE OF OCCUPATION. Occupation is concerned with productive participation of members of society within the social system. The symbolic interactionist concept of role offers a means of understanding how an individual's productive efforts are channeled and defined in social life; thus it is recognizable as an appropriate concept for delineating occupation. It is also compatible with our chosen theory of motivation which focuses on self-determined action. Gestaltist theories which stress predetermined patterns of behavior for the person in the social world and behaviorist theories which stress conditioned responses for interaction present a picture that does not fit because of the emphasis on mechanistic, unconscious origins of behavior. The symbolic interactionist view is consistent with the belief that an individual is consciously motivated to have an effect in the environment. This means that the individual seeks to occupy certain positions or roles in society, interprets desired roles within the parameters of normative behavior appropriate to those positions, and derives satisfaction and the desire to continue to interact from role performance.

CONTENT, VALUE AND SIGNIFICANCE OF OCCUPATION: CULTURE

The third question requires identification of the source of the content, value, and significance of occupational behaviors. It directs us to examine how an individual's repertoire of performance and his or her perception of those performances come into existence. A very useful concept in this regard is that of culture.[6]

Many views of culture exist. One early perspective saw culture as a stable external order determining the individual's life. More recent views acknowledge culture as a shaping influence of deep significance, while also recognizing the individual's contribution to elaborating and changing the culture.[19,29]

Hall[17] views culture as more than a catalogue of customs—as different ways of giving meaning to and organizing one's life that are communicated from generation to generation. In his view culture controls individuals' lives in subtle, unsuspected ways. The way a person arranges his or her personal environment, interacts with family, friends, and strangers, prepares meals, uses time and space and engages in special celebrations reflect a profound cultural influence.

Cohen[8] views culture as an instrument of adaptation, a tool that ensures the human fit to the environment. Culture, in his opinion, is made up of such distinct components as the organization of social relations, values and ideologies, and customary behaviors. Components of culture are transmitted to each individual in order to maintain life in a particular habitat and elaborate on the basic characteristics of the biological constitution.[8] Cohen views adaptation in humans as their fitness for reproduction and survival. This is not wholly a genetic explanation, rather, it implies an ability to utilize energy potentials that are present in the physical environment; for example, the importance to humans of recognizing the need for a shelter and utilizing their problem-solving abilities to harvest wood and other materials as building materials. This utilization includes the organization of individuals to form an ongoing culture. The resulting order of social relations dictates how messages will be communicated within the group, who will make important decisions, and how they will be carried out.

The view of culture as an adaptive mechanism is supported by the perspectives of evolution. Some writers point out that the evolution of human beings involved a process of growing plasticity in the human brain accompanied by more and more complex cultural traditions.[6,13,18] The role of culture in such a perspective is to preserve information for survival which had previously (i.e., earlier in the evolutionary timetable) been encoded in the brain. Simply put, culture replaces instinct as the source of information about survival.

Another view of culture stresses that much of its elements are superfluous to survival. In this perspective culture is viewed as an environmental element which elaborates and increases demands for performance beyond those required for survival.[7,19] Here culture is an end in itself, not simply a means to a biologic end. The implication of such a perspective is that as culture changes, demands for the individual change.

These views of culture are not incompatible, and many writers acknowledge the role of culture both as an adaptive mechanism and as an environmental order creating its own performance demands. From both perspectives it is possible to see how culture shapes the content and significance of occupational behaviors. Culture carries information necessary for performance; it supplies the technology for occupational behaviors. Secondly, culture is a carrier of value and meaning which gives each activity its particular significance. Culture is both shaper and definer of everyday life.

An example of this pervasive cultural influence on everyday occupational life is time. Culture provides a way of perceiving and valuing time; it creates the meaning of time. In Western cultures time is generally perceived to be a commodity which can be saved or wasted. It is perceived to be a progressive, absolute, and limited resource which can be allocated, demarcated, and anticipated.[17] In these and many other subtle ways culture provides its members with ways of experiencing and thinking about time.

Culture also provides the technology and order for using time. The cycles and rhythms which dictate the regulation of activities such as mealtime, playtime, and work time are connected with culture. The culture also instructs members how early or late they may be, and how to sequence behaviors. Within the culture are the artifacts for measuring, predicting, and scheduling time.

Time thus provides a useful example of how culture allows persons to adapt by providing them with tools for control of their environment. It also illustrates how culture creates its own requirements for performance. The content, value, and significance of time and those behaviors which fill it are deeply influenced by culture.

CHOOSING CONCEPTS FOR OCCUPATIONAL THERAPY. The concept of culture was examined in order to determine its utility for augmenting understanding of how the content, value, and significance of occupational behaviors evolved. The concept of cultural tradition offers a greater understanding of how people act within a given cultural group, how they define and value occupational activities, and how they organize their daily behavior.

THEORETICAL TRADITION. The study of culture appears to embody fewer varying premises than other concepts reviewed above. While there have been some structuralist views of culture, most writers see culture as a dynamic medium which informs and instructs members. The individual, in turn, uses the cultural heritage to order actions and to derive their meaning. As an accumulation of interrelated beliefs and know-how, the culture provides the information which the individual eventually acquires as his or her way of daily life. Culture also creates purposes beyond those required for survival. The combined perspectives view culture as a source of meaning and technical information for survival and as a source of further demands for performance.

COMPATIBILITY WITH THE PREMISE OF OCCUPATION. The purpose of focusing on occupation as an intervention strategy is to facilitate the person's successful interaction with and adaptation to the environment. The concept of culture provides an account of how the individual goes about that process and of how some further environmental demands are created. Thus, it is viewed as a useful formulation for the definition of occupation. Further, the concept of culture is compatible with the concepts of motivation and role. All recognize the conscious and interactive processes which support occupation.

ACQUIRING OCCUPATIONAL BEHAVIOR THROUGH SOCIALIZATION

The final area to be addressed in the interdisciplinary definition of occupation is how persons acquire occupational behavior. For this information we will turn to the concept of socialization.

Individual action is not idiosyncratic; rather, it is highly coordinated to the attitudes and actions of others. Individuals come to organize their behavior with reference to other social actors through a process called socialization.[20] Socialization begins in childhood as individuals learn basic attitudes and behaviors from adult role models and continues through adulthood as persons enter and must learn to fill new and changing roles. In socialization, expectations and knowledge of relevant reference groups (e.g., family, co-workers) influence and instruct the new member who learns to take on appropriate thoughts and behaviors. Thus, socialization is a process which results in individual acquisition of practical skills, information, and problem solving abilities.[20]

Socialization also plays an important role in the development of a sense of personal competence.[30] Through the processes of parental approval, support, and guidance children become confident of their own abilities. Styles of behaving are also a function of socialization; both children and adults are inducted into the ambience of social institutions through the process of socialization.[20] All socialization involves interactions with others. Role models are important for socialization since identification with the other or with the social group is a factor in socialization. Through socialization persons internalize an image of themselves as belonging to the group, and this serves as a guide to conscious decision-making. The socialized person conforms to the norms and values of the social group in order to belong. This view of socialization is influenced by the symbolic interactionist perspective.

In summary, socialization is a process of transmission of knowledge and personal identity to the new member of any institution. Socialization begins in childhood and continues throughout life as persons enter new social groups. Socialization results in a fit between the person and the new social environment he or she has entered. Since socialization is the process that transmits practical abilities, basic information, and problem solving skills it is well suited as a concept for therapy. These prerequisite behaviors are minimal requirements for adaptation to changing environments encountered during the occupational career.

CHOOSING CONCEPTS FOR OCCUPATIONAL THERAPY. The concept of socialization was reviewed to examine its utility for explaining how persons acquire occupational behavior. Socialization offers the useful perspective that persons acquire behavior in a process of being exposed to role models, expectations, demands for performance, and information about performance. Socialization aids development of new and appropriate thinking and behaving throughout the life span and thus serves the process of occupational ontogenesis.

THEORETICAL TRADITION. The process of socialization has close ties with the concept of role and is influenced strongly by the symbolic interactionist tradition. Socialization theory stresses how actors come to take on the behaviors and attitudes of their surroundings.

COMPATIBILITY WITH THE PREMISE OF OCCUPATION. In defining occupation attention must be given to the methods used to communicate external demands to the individual. As in the matching of other concepts, it is necessary to insure that the view of the individual is maintained as one of conscious, self-reinforcing and self-generating interaction with the environment. The concept of socialization does this by focusing on the general rules of social conduct transmitted to an individual which provide a framework for environmental interaction. The concept of socialization thus illuminates occupation as a behavior resulting from the expectations and informational input of others which is organized into a personal set of attitudes and abilities.

A DEFINITION OF OCCUPATION

The final criterion of interdisciplinary thinking illustrates the interrelationship of concepts by integrating them into a statement concerning the subject matter of the field. This review was oriented to deriving a statement concerning occupation. By starting with an appreciation for its complexity it was possible to begin to identify interdisciplinary knowledge to provide a more complete view of occupational behavior. This view included: (1) an individual's motive to be effective in the environment; (2) the concept of role which describes the interface between the individual and the environment; (3) the cultural traditions which influence each persons' life adaptation; and (4) the socialization processes that shape the individual as a social participant. Based on this interdisciplinary input we can acknowledge *occupation as a behavior which is motivated by an intrinsic, conscious urge to be effective in the environment in order to enact a variety of individually interpreted roles that are shaped by cultural tradition and learned through the process of socialization.* Thus, the importing of concepts from these fields provides occupational therapy with a definition of occupation that results in more precise and specific assessments of dysfunctional patterns of interaction. Appropriately logical, direct confrontation is possible regarding problems of disruption in motivation, feelings of effectance and internally originating behavior; difficulties in maintaining role performance; disorganization in culturally determined behaviors and habits that are part of each individuals daily routine; and inabilities to meet societal requirements that insure a useful and valued position in society.

The concepts suggest a profile of occupational therapy patient intervention programs designed to provide opportunities to practice competent and efficacious behaviors; develop skills that support desired role enactment; provide strategies that insure socialization to cultural group requirements and support satisfying daily life routines.

REFERENCES

1. ALLEN, VL: *Psychological factors in poverty.* Markham Publishing Company, Chicago, 1970.

2. BERLYNE, DE: *Conflict, arousal and curiosity.* McGraw-Hill Book Company, New York, 1960.

3. BOLLES, RC: *Theory of motivation.* Harper Row, New York, 1967.

4. BRUNER, J: *Play is serious business.* Psychology Today, 8:80, 1975.

5. CARDWELL, JD: *Social psychology: a symbolic interactionist perspective.* FA Davis, Philadelphia, 1971.

6. CHAPPLE, E: *Culture and biological man—explorations in behavioral anthropology.* Holt, Rinehart and Winston, New York, 1970.

7. CHERFAS, J and LEWIN, R: *Not work alone: A cross-cultural view of activities superfluous to survival.* Sage, Beverly Hills, 1980.

8. COHEN, Y: *Man in adaptation, the cultural present.* Aldine Atherton, New York, 1968.

9. DeCHARMS, R: *Personal causation.* Academic Press, New York, 1968.

10. ENGELHARDT, HT: *Defining occupational therapy: The meaning of therapy and the virtues of occupation.* American Journal of Occupational Therapy, 31: 666, 1977.

11. FARIS, R: (ED): *The discipline of sociology. Handbook of sociology.* Rand McNally, Chicago, 1964.

12. GAGNE, R and FLEISHMAN, E: *Psychology and human performance.* Henry Holt and Co, New York, 1959.

13. GEERTZ, C: *The interpretation of culture.* Hutchinson, London, 1975.

14. GILETTE, N: *Practice, education and research. In* Occupational Therapy: 2001 AD, 1979.

15. GREEN, M and LEPPER, S: *How to turn play into work.* Psychology Today, 49:54, 1974.

16. GURIN, G: *An expectancy approach to job training programs. In* V. Allen (ED), *Psychological Factors of Poverty.* Markham Publishing, Chicago, 1970.

17. HALL, E: *The silent language.* Fawcett Publications, Greenwich, Conn, 1959.

18. HALLOWEL, AI: *Culture and experience.* Schocken Books, New York, 1971.

19. HENRY, J: *Culture against man.* Random House, New York, 1963.

20. INKELES, A: *Social structure and the socialization of competence.* Harvard Educational Review, 36: 265, 1966.

21. McCLELLAND, DC: *The achieving society.* Van Nostrand, Princeton, NJ, 1961.

22. MEAD, GH: *Mind, self and society.* University of Chicago Press, Chicago, 1934.

23. MOGFORD, K: *The play of handicapped children. In* TIZARD, B AND HARVEY, D (EDS), *Biology of play.* JB Lippincott Company, Philadelphia, 1977.

24. PIAGET, J: *Play, dreams and imitation in childhood,* WW Norton, New York, 1963.

25. RECK, AJ: Selected writings of George Herbert Mead. Bobbs-Merrill, Indianapolis, 1964.

26. REILLY, M: *The modernization of occupational therapy.* American Journal of Occupational Therapy, 25:243, 1971.

27. REILLY, M: *Occupational therapy can be one of the great ideas of 20th century medicine.* American Journal of Occupational Therapy, 16:1, 1962.

28. SARBIN, TR: *Role theory.* In G. Lindzey (ED), *Handbook of social psychology.* Addison-Wesley, Menlo Park, Calif, 1968.

29. SCHUSKY, EL: *The study of cultural anthropology.* Holt, Rinehart & Winston, New York, 1975.

30. SMITH, MB: *Competence and socialization.* In Clausen, JA (ED), *Socialization and society.* Little, Brown and Company, Boston, 1968.

31. TURNER, RH: *Role: Sociological aspects.* A reprint from *The International Encyclopedia of the Social Sciences.* Crowell Collier—Macmillan, New York, 1968.

32. WHITE, RW: *Competence and the psychosexual stages of development. Nebraska Symposium on Motivation.* University of Nebraska Press, Lincoln, 1960.

33. WHITE, RW: *The urge towards competence.* American Journal of Occupational Therapy, 25:271, 1971.

CHAPTER 5

OCCUPATIONAL THERAPISTS AS TECHNOLOGISTS AND CUSTODIANS OF MEANING

H. Tristram Engelhardt, Jr.

EDITOR'S INTRODUCTION

The preceding chapters introduced a number of themes pertaining to knowledge in occupational therapy—all from the perspectives of occupational therapists. Those chapters have raised the issues of what knowledge is relevant, how knowledge is to be integrated, and the impact of knowledge for the practitioner's role. This chapter synthesizes these issues into a coherent and persuasive argument from the perspective of a physician-philosopher. It relates the issues of what the therapist must know and be able to apply in practice to the unique roles that occupational therapists play in the health care arena. Once again it is demonstrated that seemingly disparate roles are not only compatible but must coexist for effective actualization professional roles. This should not be construed to mean that professionals have absolute freedom to plot their own courses and define at will their own practices. Instead, it is noted that the mission of a professional group is defined at the level where society and the profession interact.

The chapter also places in clearer perspective the major issue that the field must return to its original principles and not be limited by the reductionist thinking which predominated theory and practice in the past. This proposition is often misconstrued to mean that therapists will have to leave behind their hard-earned technology in order to embrace the humanistic values and practices reflected in the field's early ideology. The chapter suggests the alternative that both may be embraced and that together they form the field's practice. The danger that one conceptual current may undermine another also is acknowledged. The idea that occupational therapists' special role in the health care system is dependent on their management of the meaning that patients experience through their activity is introduced. This theme, the importance of how patients experience and interpret their existence, is one that will resonate through the chapters that follow.

GK

It takes rare gifts and talents and rare personalities to be real pathfinders in this work. There are no royal roads; it is all a problem of being true to one's nature and opportunities and of teaching others to do the same with themselves. I went though the occupation departments of a large institution the other day and was profoundly impressed by the wide differences of the personnel and the manifold ways of approach leading to success with the work. It takes, above all, resourcefulness and an ability to respect at the same time the native capacities and interests of the patient. (Meyer, The Philosophy of Occupational Therapy)

THE AMBIGUITIES OF PROFESSIONS

Professions develop under the pressures of numerous and often contrary social forces. Professions are the ways in which complex sets of skills are taught to individuals so that they can support themselves, sustain those skills, and have status in their communities while serving an important social need. Professions therefore have both internally and externally directed goods and goals. To the extent that the skills of a profession are seen as elements of art and science, they give joy to the practitioner. A skill well mastered and well practiced is a good in itself, or it is at least an occasion for satisfaction for the one who possesses the skill. The development of such skills along with the financial and status rewards of the profession, and the profession's own views of altruistic acts, will inspire its members. Since professions also serve publicly defined goals, society will share a concern that they are not only well practiced according to the criteria of the profession, but also that they help to advance those goals. Since the goals of professionals and of societies are likely to be varied, a profession is unlikely to have a single raison d'etre. As noted in Chapter 8, occupational therapy may find its application within diverse sectors of health care. This is apparent if one considers the complex roles of physicians or lawyers. Physicians play a sacerdotal role in reassuring patients; they play the role of scientist-technologists in curing diseases; they give caring support to patients during illness; and they certify individuals as ineligible for the draft. So, too, lawyers serve as officers of the court, and as advocates for particular clients. They also play roles as counselors, judges, and arbitrators. Some of these roles have been fashioned primarily by the profession, others by society. Neither profession has a single conceptual or philosophical base, nor does either have a single cluster of goals that characterize all of its activities. This is as one would expect. Particular professions are the deliverances of social forces acting through history. As a result, individuals with titles such as "physician" or "lawyer", assume distinct social duties. What is true about physicians and lawyers is true about occupational therapists as well.

Occupational therapists shift within various roles, some similar to those of the technologist applying scientific theories, and others more like those of the healing priest. This heterogeneity of roles is often clouded by the need for a sense of professional identity. Consider, for example, the ways in which physicians harken back to an ethic that is articulated in the Oath of Hippocrates. The oath signals a professional unity, though it was written, not by Hippocrates, but rather by neo-Pythagoreans,[4] and though the Greek views of medicine have been displaced by modern understandings of the physician's charge.

This should give no one pause if it is recognized that professionals must inevitably assume various roles. It would not be at all incompatible for occupational therapists, on the one hand, to make use of a "reductionist" approach to many treatment problems, while on the other drawing upon conceptual and ideological roots found in the statements of Adolf Meyer and William Rush Dunton. Indeed, if the two modes of approach were mutually exclusive explanatory frameworks, there would be a question of a choice between them. However, as shown in Chapters 1 and 2, the issue is one of integrating conceptual modes. There is also the question of integrating roles. Professionals such as occupational therapists and physicians are engaged not only in explaining reality as scientists, but also in conveying complex services of care and guidance. They function as priests, or custodians of meaning, as well as technologists. Far from being competitive, the roles are complementary.

Actual circumstances usually invite both roles. The danger lies in onesidedness. On the one hand, occupational therapy requires a "reductionist" account in terms of a theoretical base grounded in the internal, organic, and psychic conditions of the organisms. That is, occupational therapists function as scientist-technologists, appealing to muscular skeletal status, sensory motor and nervous system function, and intrapsychic states to aid individuals to regain and maintain as much independent function as possible. On the other hand, this is not incompatible with the traditional understanding of occupational therapy as supporting pleasure in activity. Seeing these roles as exclusive and incompatible is an error, yet it is one to which health care in general is drawn. It is a particularly consequential error for occupational therapy since, as Chapter 1 illustrates, its history is one of abandoning a "holistic" tradition in order to acquire technical skills.

Many of the complaints lodged against contemporary medicine have focused on medicine's preoccupation with the merely technical and the short shrift it has given to those more holistic elements of medical practice that focus on the whole patient and his or her orientation in illness and therapy. Humans constantly seek meaning and significance. They hunger for more than technical or scientific accounts of why things happen and the significance of their condition in the world. They want *both* a scientific account *and* an account in terms of their functioning in their everyday life. Contemporary medicine has often failed to offer both, or has done so in a fragmented fashion because of the pressure to provide competent, specialized technical services.

It is not unexpected that occupational therapists are moved by the same forces that have encouraged physicians to cast themselves as scientist-technologists. Occupational therapists practice within a context dominated by high technology medicine. However, unlike medicine, occupational therapy as a recent profession can draw more unambiguously upon its original understandings of its diverse but complementary roles of service to patients. It has not fragmented into autonomous specialties, although the structure of health care, influenced by the structure of medicine, tends to invite such fragmentation. In fact, occupational therapy is subject to the same problems of defining its professional identity as is medicine. It is therefore useful to re-examine some of the original conceptions of occupational therapy in order to better chart its position in the last half of the 20th century.

THERAPY AS WOOING MEANING

The Greek $\theta\epsilon\rho\alpha\pi\epsilon\iota\alpha$, from which the English "therapy" is derived, ranges in meaning from a service paid to the gods, a medical or surgical treatment or cure, a courting or flattering, to that of wooing. In providing therapy one usually does more than engage in technical procedures. One attempts to aid patients in understanding their situation in illness or as subjects of treatment. One is not only doing something to patients, but aiding them to see the meaning of their situation, for it is only within a context of meaning that treatment can take place—that a patient can cooperate, that care givers or care receivers can understand the purpose of the activities taking place.

The classic account of occupational therapy's contribution to meaning in the life of patients was provided by one of the major figures in American psychiatry, Adolf Meyer (1866-1950). In an address, "The Philosophy of Occupational Therapy" to the fifth annual meeting of the National Society for the Promotion of Occupational Therapy (now the American Occupational Therapy Association) in Baltimore in October, 1921, he gave an account of occupational therapy in terms of its support of the appreciation of activities in time. He saw occupational therapy as affording a pleasureable engagement in activities. His account presumed a sense of the importance and significance of work: "A new step was to arise from a freer conception of work, from a concept of free and pleasant and profitable *occupation—including recreation in any form of helpful enjoyment as the leading principle.*"[6] Work was an engagement in reality, a mode of laying claim to meaning. To appreciate fully this focus on work, one has to see it in terms of the 19th century's understanding of work and activity as not only good, but health-giving and obligatory. Thus, Meyer quotes from an 1882 report by Dr. Henry M. Hurd concerning occupational therapy in European mental institutions: "Employment of some sort should be made obligatory for all able-bodied patients."[5] However, the point should be seen as signaling the ways in which humans, as organisms evolved to engage in activities, find pleasure and purpose in them. Even seemingly trivial activities can endow time with meaning. We might recall the etymology of occupation, from *occupatio*—a seizing, a taking possession of—to provide a gloss on Adolf Meyer's appreciation of occupational therapy as affording meaning by aiding patients to retake possession of their capacity for activity.

Adolf Meyer stressed the importance of an appreciation of time in the engagement of activities. Through activities individuals are able to structure time and to give meaning to their endeavors. Activity offers an opportunity for regaining a pre-reflective meaning in time which had been disrupted by sickness and disability. As Meyer argued, "The great feature of man is his new sense of time, with foresight built on a sound view of the past and present. Man learns to organize time and he does it in terms of *doing* things, and one of the many good things he does between eating, drinking and wholesome nutrition generally and the flights of fancy and aspiration, we call *work and occupation*."[5] Meyer was interested in aiding individuals to recapture "pleasureable ease" in the rhythms and performances of daily life. Directed activity, which helped to structure time, was seen to be therapeutic in supporting the well being and adaptation of patients.

Thus, Meyer outlined a set of presuppositions which clearly distinguish occupational therapy from physical therapy. The focus is not simply on maintaining certain physical capacities, but on aiding those capacities as human activities. Here a distinction is offered between physical behavior and the activities in which humans engage. The latter, no matter how routine, are embedded in an appreciation of time and of life. This difference draws the line between the maintenance of physical capacities and the support of the capacity to engage in activities. Meyer observes:

It had long been interesting to see how groups of a few excited patients can be seated in a corner in a small circle of two or three settees and kept wonderfully contented picking the hair of mattresses, or doing simple tasks not too readily arousing the desire for big movements and uncontrollable excitement, and yet not too taxing to their patience. Groups of patients with raffia and basket work, or with various kinds of handwork and weaving and bookbinding and metal and leather work, took the place of the bored wall flowers and of mischiefmakers. A pleasure in achievement, a real pleasure in the use and activity of one's hands and muscles, and a happy *appreciation of time* began to be used as incentives in the management of our patients, instead of abstract exhortations to cheer up and to behave according to abstract or repressive rules. The main advance of the new scheme was the blending of work and pleasure—all made possible by a wise supplementing of centralization by individualization, and a kind of re-decentralization.[5]

Individuals were learning that they could be active, could engage in life. They were not simply having physical capacities sustained.

On this point it is worth stressing the argument by J. Sanbourne Bockoven[1,2] that occupational therapy in America draws upon the traditions of the moral treatment movement in early 19th century mental hospitals. This movement developed in the McLean hospital in Massachusetts and the Frankfort asylum in Pennsylvania, among other hospitals. Modalities such as lectures in the arts and engagement in manual labor were used to adapt individuals to the mores and values of their culture. It was believed that through the development of regular habits, engagement in activities, and by learning about their culture, the mentally ill could regain normal function.[3] Bockoven[1,2] has asserted that the moral treatment movement's commitment to seeing patients as whole persons and to treating them through a range of human activities has continued in occupational therapy. This is a convincing argument in light of Adolf Meyer's elaboration of the wholesomeness of human activities.

In short, when we look to the early history of occupational therapy, we see it embedded in a matrix of views about the importance of patients as individuals and the significance of activity for health in a broad sense, including joy in performing physical tasks. The emphasis is not simply on restoring physical function, but on pleasure in activity. There is also a presupposition that activites endow time with meaning. Though adequate treatment will require a detailed appreciation of patients' psychologic and sensory motor capacity in order to enable them to live as normally as possible, the skills to achieve these ends must be placed within an occupational therapy commitment to human well being.

ACTIVITIES, RITUALS, PRACTICE

The attention of occupational therapists to overcoming the disorganization of habit structure and to reconditioning the body to normal living must thus be seen within the broad functions traditionally assigned to health care. As indicated above, health care professionals claim not only the roles of curers and carers, but sacerdotal roles in which they aid individuals in orienting themselves within the changing circumstances of aging, illness, and disability. Occupational therapy's interest in activities can be best appreciated in this light. Somewhat tendentiously, it involves a suggestion that weaving and lacing should be seen as rituals used not simply to recapture habit structures, but to recapture as well pleasure and significance in activity. Rituals are, after all, traditional activities through which one finds meaning and the health of salvation. Such disciplines are probably important in aiding many individuals in recapturing a sense of place, purpose, and function. The ritual and meaning-rich character of occupational therapy activities is emphasized throughout this book.

However, as with all professions in changing cultural circumstances, occupational therapy must maintain a commitment to the importance of its original concerns. It must resist the temptations within a highly technologic health care system to see itself as simply the bearer of technical skills. In particular, it must not see the choice as one between developing good skills or discharging more traditional commitments to broader senses of human health and well being. Instead, occupational therapy will need, like all health care professions, to see its charge to be skillful, as well as more attentive to the complex meanings that accompany the use of skills.

In order to flourish, a culture must offer the opportunity to learn about the importance and value of human enterprise. Occupational therapy thus has an opportunity to instruct beyond the confines of the clinic. It can offer models of therapy which take into account not only physical capacities, but the virtues of human adaptation in recreation and in physical and mental activities generally. If therapists remain not only technically skilled, but also able to support a view of the whole person in function and adaptation, they will make a significant intellectual as well as practical contribution to the goal of quality health care. They will have realized the promise of their profession seen by Adolf Meyer more than sixty years ago.

SUMMARY

To continue to develop as a profession encompassing both technical skills and attention to the meaning of activity will require avoiding two misconceptions. It must be recognized that there need be no competition between a technical or scientific account of therapy, human function, and habits, and accounts in the spirit of Adolf Meyer. These must instead be seen to be complementary, as integral to two distinct but inseparable elements of the profession of occupational therapy. The first is a part of developing skills and techniques, the second is part of a disciplined exploration of the importance of those techniques for patients. The last misconception is closely allied to the first. It would portray the role of the occupational therapist as a singular one, thus forcing an unnecessary choice between the roles of technologist and meaning-giver. However, these roles are intimately bound in health care. Attending with care to the conceptual relation between these roles will help to orient therapist and client, demonstrating that one is dealing with two different terrains that are part of the geography of one profession.

REFERENCES

1. BOCKOVEN, JS: *Legacy of moral treatment—1800's to 1910.* American Journal of Occupational Therapy, 25:223, 1971.

2. BOCKOVEN, JS: *Moral treatment in American psychiatry.* Springer Press, New York, 1963.

3. BRIGHAM, A: *Moral treatment of Insanity.* American Journal of Insanity, 4:1, 1847.

4. EDELSTEIN, L: *The hippocratic oath: Text, translation, and interpretation.* In Temkin, O and Temkin, CL (EDS): *Ancient Medicine: Selected papers of Ludwig Edelstein.* Johns Hopkins Press, Baltimore, 1967.

5. MEYER, A: *The philosophy of occupational therapy.* Archives of Occupational Therapy, 1:1, 1922.

PART 2

THE ENVIRONMENT OF OCCUPATIONAL THERAPY PRACTICE

CHAPTER 6

AUDACIOUS VALUES: THE ENERGY SOURCE FOR OCCUPATIONAL THERAPY PRACTICE *

Elizabeth J. Yerxa

EDITOR'S INTRODUCTION

The theme of Chapter 6 is more fully appreciated in the context of the chapters that preceded it and those that follow. It identifies perennial values of occupational therapy as expressed in the field's writing and practice, showing that these values were present from its beginnings and have persisted despite their inconsistency with the dominant values of medicine. Inasmuch as occupational therapy existed within a system controlled by medicine, its maintenance of these humanistic values is labeled by the author as audacious—a well-earned compliment.

Two important issues are raised by the author. The first pertains to occupational therapy's success in maintaining the ability to sustain these values in clinical practice. The history of occupational therapy suggests that it has encountered substantial difficulty in maintaining its commitment to these values as it has been subject to pressure from the values of mainstream medicine. Thus, one might conclude that while occupational therapy's heart has been in the right place, its actions have occasionally been diverted or thwarted by circumstances of a semi-political nature. It might be said that occupational therapists maintained their commitment to humanistic values while being obliged to accept reductionist, mechanistic theory borrowed from medicine that viewed humanistic values as secondary to

---

*A small amount of the content of this chapter originally appeared in the *American Journal of Occupational Therapy,* volume 34, 1980, in a paper titled "Occupational Therapy's Role in Creating a Future Climate of Caring." Some content was also presented at the First Annual Research Symposium in Occupational Therapy sponsored by the Occupational Therapy Department at Washington University at St. Louis in 1980, and has been submitted for publication in the Proceedings of the Symposium.

scientific-technical concerns. The argument of the first four chapters for a commitment to the field's traditional orientation to occupation and to day-to-day quality of life shows a potential for rejuvenation of the capacity to express these values in clinical practice. The authors call for the development of a theory base in occupational therapy that will give direct support to the values identified by this chapter as salient to health and indigenous to occupational therapy.

The second issue addressed by the author is the viability of humanistic values in future health care systems and social contexts. Drawing upon the work of futurist Alvin Toffler, the author foresees a climate in which such values will flourish, permitting occupational therapy to establish a broader and more definitive role in society.

Since this chapter speaks to values (the ruling domain of all human endeavor), it sets an orientation which is echoed in following discussions. While all of its themes are important, one is perhaps especially worthy of consideration. The author points to occupational therapy's appreciation for the patient's or client's subjective experience as a common thread reflected in all other values of the field. This existentialist or phenomenological orientation of occupational therapy, which gives weight to the subjective in an arena dominated by concern with objective science, is the most significant aspect of the field's audacious values.

The author offers thoughtful guidance to educators who must make value decisions about what to teach students, to clinicians who daily face questions of value in their patients' and clients' circumstances, and to students who are shaping their own professional values. Readers should carefully heed the chapter's message: It is worth the effort to be committed to unpopular ideals if they are in the best interest of clients and patients.

GK

Truth loves its limits, for there it meets the beautiful. Rabindranath Tagor, *Fireflies.*

The word "value" has eight senses according to a recent edition of *Webster's New Collegiate Dictionary* (1980). Small wonder that confusion exists about the meaning of this elusive term, couched as it is in an aura of mystery. Yet, values underlie all behaviors, philosophies, belief systems and professional practice, in short, all of life's most vital activities. Values may be hidden, even to those who possess them, while at the same time generating significant amounts of energy for behaving or thinking. In this covert sense values seem to fit into the viewpoint of de Saint-Exupéry who observed that "what is essential is invisible to the eye"[7].

Value is defined here as that which is perceived as intrinsically good or desirable. For example, a student might decide to enter the occupational therapy profession because he or she values helping other people and is consciously aware of that value and its role in the occupational choice process. On a less overt level, an individual might pursue a scientific career because of valuing certainty over uncertainty, yet be unaware of the real reason for such a choice.

Values, then, are strong motivators which exist at varying levels of consciousness for those who possess them. This chapter will identify those values which I believe underlie the current practice of occupational therapy and those supporting medical practice, compare the two sets of values, project the future direction of occupational therapy practice based on Toffler's prediction of changing social values, and finally highlight the challenges faced by occupational therapists as they attempt to implement their values in practice. My discussion of current values is based upon observations of occupational therapy practice as well as value statements appearing in our literature[29].

VALUES UNDERLYING OCCUPATIONAL THERAPY PRACTICE

Occupational therapy began in a climate of caring. Its roots grew out of reform in the treatment of "the insane" and the transformation of prisons and pest houses into hospitals. Otherwise devalued, mental patients were perceived humanistically by the pioneers in occupational therapy as people worthy of dignity who needed a balance of work, rest, and play in their lives for healthfulness, and who had the *right* to a pleasant, friendly and normal environment[22]. Thus the valuing of a person's essential humanity, in spite of severe and sometimes chronic disease, was central to the practice of the original occupational therapists. This value was somewhat unique in an industrial society which stigmatized, closeted, and otherwise deemed chronically disabled persons as useless and subhuman entities.

The historical values of the profession have been transmitted to modern occupational therapists, as may be seen in current patient advocacy efforts, as well as in occupational therapists' traditional provision of services to the most severely and chronically disabled patients. Such patients are often seen as "beyond help" by many other professionals because of extensive and irreversible pathologies. However, occupational therapists perceive and value the right to a satisfying life for each person regardless of the presence of quadriplegia, athetosis, developmental delay, chronic schizophrenia, or any other disability.

Rather than focusing exclusively upon pathology, occupational therapists have been concerned with health, facilitating and strengthening the healthy aspects of individuals, particularly in enabling such persons to engage in the activities they might wish to do. As presented in Chapter 1, pathology was always considered secondary to the patient's ability to function in daily life. Thus, occupational therapists are not limited to concern with the "body machine" but also with the effects of the environment and goals of the individual upon health[30].

Both the philosophic and pragmatic approaches of occupational therapists demonstrate a valuing of the individual's ability to do for himself and take responsibility for his own health. As Mary Reilly has stated it, a primary hypothesis of the profession is "that man, through the use of his hands as they are energized by mind and will can influence the state of his own health."[15]

The occupational therapy model of education, practice, and thought has been, for many years, that of a generalist. Thus, occupational therapists value perceiving the patient as a unified entity rather than fragmenting the person into body parts separated from a mind.[3] In their concern for the individual as a total being, occupational therapists are equally at home dealing with motion or emotion as long as it relates to the patient's ability to function with satisfaction as a whole person in the environment.

One of the unique contributions occupational therapists make to hospitalized patients is the recognition, regardless of the presenting medical problems, of their uniqueness, their potentials and their need to adapt to community environments. Such a focus is somewhat rare in the hospital milieu in which most attention is often given to a small part of the person and little to the individual's home situation or "natural" environment.

The mode of patient-therapist interaction employed in occupational therapy reflects the valuing of "mutual cooperation" with the patient, rather than patient passivity.[20] It appears that occupational therapists agree with the physician and physiologist, Hensel, that a therapeutic relationship has the primary goal of helping "the patient to regain autonomy."[9] Offering patients choices, or encouraging the child to "take over" his or her own treatment, are central to occupational therapy thought.[1,27]

Occupational therapists seem to reside in the philosophic camp of such nondeterministic, nonmaterialistic thinkers as Lauenstein,[14] a philosopher who views the individual primarily as one who acts on the environment. Thus patients are viewed, not as at the mercy of the environment, but as capable of responding to environmental stresses by developing adaptive skills.[12]

As observed elsewhere, occupational therapists value the potential existing in every person, disabled or not.[29] The occupational therapy process is concerned with teasing out, facilitating, and releasing that potential, whether for overall self-determination or for a task as seemingly simple as feeding oneself. Each patient is viewed as the person he or she might become, rather than as a damaged nervous system or a deranged psyche.

Occupational therapists value productivity and participation of the patient in the stream of life. Productivity is esteemed, not necessarily to benefit society economically, but rather as being intrinsically satisfying to the person. In this sense productivity is seen as engagement in that which has meaning to the patient. Thus, occupational therapists seek to avoid the "specialist effect" in which professionals tend to perceive patients' needs only according to the service which they can offer.[2]

Occupational therapists value play, rest, and leisure activity equally with work. Play is viewed as spontaneous, joyous, risk-taking in a safe place, and games as means of learning rules, values, and traditions.[17] Leisure activity is seen as a necessity for creating a balanced life. Leisure pursuits may even create a means of productive participation in society which work in the 20th century often fails to offer. By developing skills in the use of one's hands and raw materials, a person can revive a sense of competence and be connected once more with the natural environment, finding new purpose and meaning in self-initiated activity. Occupational therapists' concerns for a balanced life also lead to a valuing of temporal adaptation, demonstrated by helping patients learn how to use their time in satisfying ways.[11]

Finally, woven throughout all of the values identified thus far, is an appreciation of the subjective. Occupational therapists are often more concerned with patients' perceptions of their particular realities than with "objective" observations of behavior.[27] Since occupational therapy cannot take place without the patient's active participation, and since the focus is the *patient's* environment, not the medical milieu, understanding patients' views of themselves, their worlds and their sources of satisfaction is central to the therapeutic process. Moreover, patients are often seen as the most valid sources of information about themselves.[4]

In summary, occupational therapy intervention is founded upon a rather unique blend of values that exists at varying degrees of awareness for the individual occupational therapist. Values identified were those of belief in the essential humanity of patients and their right to life satisfaction; concern with health and enhancement of the healthy aspects of the person; fostering patients' self-directedness and ability to take responsibility for their lives; employing a generalist rather than specialist perspective; fostering a therapeutic relationship based on mutual cooperation; viewing the patient as one who acts on the environment rather than being determined by it; having optimistic faith in each patient's potential; encouraging patient productivity and participation; recognizing the healthfulness of play, leisure activities, and a balanced life; and seeking to understand the subjective perspectives as well as objective characteristics of patients and their worlds.

VALUES SUPPORTING MEDICAL PRACTICE

Since the majority of occupational therapists work with physicians in medically oriented environments,[10] it should be of some benefit to explore the current status of the medical profession with particular emphasis on the values underlying its science, practices, and role in society.

Siegler and Osmond refer to the physician-patient relationship as one based upon "Aesculapian authority."[21] (Aesculapius was the Greco-Roman god of medicine.) According to these authors, three types of power conveyed by this authority are significant in conferring certain rights upon the physician in clinical practice. "Sapiential" authority conveys the right to give advice and to be heard by reason of knowledge and expertise. The right to control and direct the patient is based upon "moral" authority, or the "rightness" and "goodness" of the medical ethic. Finally, "charismatic" authority means that the physician possesses a right to control and direct by virtue of God-given grace as a healer of disease or occupant of a "priestly role." The source of Aesculapian authority is the patient's fear of death.

A major function of the physician's power is to confer the "sick role" upon the patient. This role requires that the patient admit to being ill, submit to treatment, and curtail his or her usual activities while being exempted from normal responsibilities. It also relieves the patient of responsibility for the illness, since neither the patient nor anyone else is to be blamed for it.[21] The patient may leave the sick role through getting well, dying, or getting over the illness while remaining impaired (as in the case of a person with a permanent disability).

According to this view the "doctor's role ends when the illness ends, for Aesculapian authority does not cover the state of impairment."[21] Once further improvement is not to be expected, treatment of the person with an impairment is inappropriate. Since the well but impaired patient no longer fears death, a major foundation of Aesculapian authority is gone and the physician's role with the patient is therefore finished.[21] Thus, the physician values freedom from disease, conferring of the sick role, control and direction of the patient, and an expectation that the patient conform to a treatment regimen designed to reduce pathology. The physician's superior knowledge, ethical principles, and healing skills are the sources of power supporting these values which are in effect as long as the patient is sick.

If use of Aesculapian authority could be posited to correlate with social prestige, some empirical evidence exists to support Siegler and Osmond's views. Shortell, in a complex study,[20] correlated medical specialties' prestige ratings with the type of patient-physician interaction they employed. The three modes of interaction studied were "activity-passivity," in which the physician actively does something to the patient who is a passive recipient of treatment, "guidance-cooperation," in which the physician tells the patient what to do and the patient cooperates, and "mutual cooperation," in which the physician helps the patient to help himself and the patient is an active participant in the partnership. Only three out of twenty medical specialties were classified as employing the "mutual cooperation" model. These (physiatry, preventive medicine and psychiatry) tended to receive lower prestige scores than the specialties, such as neurosurgery, employing the "activity-passivity" model. Perhaps such prestige ratings were related to the medical specialty's use of Aesculapian authority, with its power to convey the sick role, while those medical specialties employing the mutual cooperation model tended to exercise such authority less, if at all, and to be associated more with prevention of illness and reduction of impairment than with curing acute disease. Thus, the use of Aesculapian authority does seem to be related to the degree of social prestige afforded various medical specialties.

Finally, in its desire to be more knowledgeable in the face of an information explosion in the physical and biological sciences, medicine has increasingly valued a specialist rather than a generalist approach to the patient[6]. As medical specialists have expanded their understanding of physics and chemistry they have focused increasingly on the ill person as a "body machine," often perceived as a reactive organism, whose status is determined by the combined effects of genes and the environment[8].

In summary, the traditional values underlying the practice and science of medicine include freeing the patient from the threat of death; eradicating disease and pathology while conferring the sick role; expecting patient compliance to orders due to moral authority; employing a specialist approach as a means toward possessing greater knowledge; engaging in an activity-passivity mode of interaction with the patient based upon Aesculapian authority; viewing the patient as more or less of a "body machine" determined by the environment; possessing faith in science and the competence of the healer; relieving the patient of everyday responsibilities; being concerned with recovery from illness rather than with patients' daily activities; and emphasizing the objective, observable, and palpable aspects of the patient.

COMPARISON OF OCCUPATIONAL THERAPY'S VALUES WITH THOSE OF MEDICINE

As displayed in Table 1, the values supporting the practice of occupational therapy are considerably different from the traditional values of medicine. The Aesculapian authority conferred on the physician seems to depend on society's need to ward off the fear of death, be relieved of responsibilities during illness, and be assured of competent curative medical technology. If Seigler and Osmond's[21] views are correct, medicine's responsibilities and authority end with the termination of the illness and do not extend to the state of "impairment" which may follow. By contrast, occupational therapy's values seem to focus more upon the individual who may have a chronic, severe, and lifelong disability and who will never be "cured." Thus, occupational therapy's values seem to be consistent with the therapeutic goal of "reduction of incapacity"[16] since they translate into concern for all aspects of the life of the person with a disability. They are thus focused

TABLE 1. Comparison of Traditional Values Supporting Practice of Occupational Therapy With Those of Medicine

Occupational Therapy	Medicine
Essential humanity of patient; obligation to provide life satisfaction for severely disabled	Freedom from threat of death; responsibility limited to illness
Maintain and enhance health; support healthy aspects of person	Eradicate disease, pathology; confer the sick role
Self-directedness and responsibility of patient	Of patient compliance to orders; moral authority
Generalist, integrated view of patient	Specialist, reductionistic emphasis on organ systems
Therapeutic relationship of mutual cooperation with patient; shared and sapiental authority of physician	Therapeutic relationship of activity of physician, passivity of patient: Aesculapian and sapiental authority of physician
Patient acts on environment rather than determined by it	Patient as determined by environment and "body machine"
Faith in patient's potential	Faith in science and healer's competence and charismatic authority
Patient productivity and participation	Patient relieved of all responsibilities except getting well
Play, leisure activities as essential components of balanced life	Recovery from illness, freedom from disease as major concern
Understand subjective perspectives of patient	Emphasis on objectivity, analysis, observation and diagnosis

upon developing patient autonomy as necessary for survival and adaptation, rather than patient compliance. From this perspective the values of medicine and those of occupational therapy may be seen as complementary, with medicine's appropriate to the period in which a person is ill, and occupational therapy's to that following illness when no "cure" has been accomplished, and disability persists in the form of incapacity which may be lifelong.

Some critics, many from within medicine itself, do not agree with perpetuation of the traditional medical values as outlined in Siegler and Osmond's analysis of Aesculapian authority. In 1977, *Toward a Man-Centered Medical Science*[18] appeared. It contained papers written by an internationally recognized group of scientists, physicians, and philosophers who criticized the traditional medical approach in attempting to create a new medical science and practice based on the uniqueness and wholeness of human beings.

Rene Dubos warned that medicine would become "irrelevant" unless it integrates its knowledge of the "body machine" with factors such as the physical environment, the history of the human species, and the goals of each individual. He cited these areas as essential to the quality of life of persons served by medicine.[8]

The medical profession was also criticized for adopting an exclusively "reductionistic" scientific approach. This approach was said to focus on pathology, teaching medical students to ignore the individual, while concentrating on the natural science analysis of the molecular structure of organs.[19] Reductionism is defined as "a theory that reduces complex data or phenomenon to simple terms," that is, oversimplification.[25] Attempting to explain how Beethoven composed his *Ninth Symphony* on the basis of synaptic patterns in the brain would be an example of reductionism.

Social demands were seen for a new partnership between the patient and the doctor. Dr. John Knowles, former president of the Rockefeller Foundation, believed that the next major advance in the health of the American people would result from what the individual was willing to do for himself. He felt that perpetuation of high cost, "after the fact" medicine would only result in higher costs and more frustration.[13] These authors seemed to be saying that unless the traditional medical value system shifted dramatically, the medical profession might turn out to be "irrelevant" to health.

An outgrowth of the emphasis upon the molecular level in medical science and practice was the increasing proliferation of specialties. Carlson[6] reported that at least 50 percent of physicians in the United States were specialists. The rationale for increasing the number of specialists was that by having the opportunity to study a part of the body in depth, they would gain greater knowledge and produce higher quality treatment. However, Weiss, a biologist, was skeptical about the possibility that true knowledge and understanding of the human person could ever be achieved through specialization. Instead, he believed that it would lead to "learning more and more about less and less."[26]

As has been seen, medical practitioners often view the patient as more or less the passive recipient of treatment provided by a physician, who if effective, "cures" the patient. Such passivity has been explained as required by the "sick role" position of the patient.[5] However, Lauenstein argued for a deeper explanation of the physician's expectation of patient passivity.[14] Because of adopting a Cartesian view of the world, in which the mind was split from the body, medicine saw human behavior as determined by the combined effects of genetic material and the environment. The result was that the human being was viewed as an "object" to be treated by the physician from a materialistic approach, using primarily drugs or surgery.

However, Lauenstein argued against this view by citing the significance of the person *acting on* the environment. He observed that no conscious thinking or even perception occurs without the will and intention of the individual. Interest is the basis for attending to a particular aspect of the sense perception out of the myriad of sensory information presented. The philosopher concluded, "If this self-fulfilling prophecy of materialism [in medicine] is to be avoided, men will have to become aware of themselves as intentional agents, as willing beings who actually insert themselves into their environments by intending it and self-conscious beings who, by self-intention, are self-creative as well."[14]

Looking now at the patient-physician relationship, Hensel believed that it should be characterized by ". . . the voluntary collaboration of autonomous individuals," making it a specifically human relation.[9] "No matter whether the patient is unconscious and unable to help himself, the idea of a free person remains always in the background of the relationship."[9] Hensel thus viewed the physician's primary activity as that of helping "the patient regain and realize his autonomy."[9]

The current status of medicine and its underlying value system have been viewed as being in rather "critical condition" by some observers both from within and outside the medical profession. In contrast to occupational therapy's value configuration, medicine has been described as failing to take into account the effects of the environment and the goals of the individual upon health, assuming a reductionistic philosophy of science which teaches medical students to focus on organs and pathology; which in its prolification of specialties has been unable to produce a unified knowledge of the human; which views the patient as the passive recipient of curative technology; and which may be in for trouble from an increasingly frustrated and disappointed society.

Many individual physicians practice contrary to the traditional values criticized. They are deeply concerned with the individual and understanding the person in a social context and as a whole. However, if the critics are correct, such physicians display these behaviors *in spite of* rather than *because of* their education and socialization into the medical profession and its values. In addition, authors such as Seigler and Osmond would counter that medicine's values are appropriately based on the Aesculapian authority that society needs to protect itself from the fear of death.

In spite of occupational therapy's proximity to the traditional medical model and its values, the profession has not adopted those values nor has it been incorporated into that model of practice. Occupational therapy remains ideologically separate from medicine in retaining a contrasting style that contributes unique values and practices to health care. Owing to these differences, occupational therapists have sometimes had difficulty implementing their values in the traditional medical setting. Their approaches, based on these values, have not been well understood by some physicians and other professionals steeped in the medical science view of health and illness. Yet, interestingly, many of occupational therapy's values are viewed, by some experts both within and outside of medicine, as those which *medicine* should adopt in order to regain relevance and survive in the world of the future.

The word "audacious" in the title of this chapter means "intrepidly daring." Occupational therapy has been sufficiently audacious to create and sustain its own unique model of practice while surviving within, and contributing to, health in the medical milieu. In many respects this persistence of professional values and a singular philosophy, in the midst of conflicting ideals and philosophies, has been intrepidly daring. One wonders what might have happened to all of those who had tuberculosis, poliomyelitis, schizophrenia, cerebral palsy, or spinal cord injuries had it not been for the occupational therapy value system and its translation into practice designed to help develop life satisfaction, meaning, and autonomy for disabled persons? Remarkably, occupational therapy has recognized and valued its role in reducing the incapacity of persons no longer ill, but disabled. That it has, for over sixty years, successfully resisted strong pressures to adopt the prestigious, ubiquitous, and widely accepted values of medicine is evidence of its belief in, and society's need for, such a perspective.

FUTURE OCCUPATIONAL THERAPY PRACTICE BASED ON TOFFLER'S VIEWS OF CHANGING SOCIAL VALUES

Alvin Toffler, futurologist, characterized the post-industrial, future era as the "third wave."[24] The first wave was that of the agricultural revolution and the second marked the rise of industrial civilization. The second wave, which Toffler believes is in its final crisis, is characterized by such values as centralization, specialization, synchronization, maximization, concentration, and standardization, all in "the service of the factory."

The third wave, already beginning, will signify the end of industrialism and the beginning of major changes in all social systems. Some of Toffler's predictions are of particular relevance to future occupational therapy practice.

Toffler called the third wave the "new age of synthesis."[24] He believes that the future will be characterized by large scale thinking, general theory, holism, and an attempt to put the pieces back together again after such a long period of emphasis on fragmentation. Occupational therapy's refusal to fragment or split the individual and its valuing of holism in practice seem congruent with Toffler's predictions of third wave thinking.

Toffler envisions people of the future enjoying a wide diversity of work opportunities. Since control and dissemination of information will be a primary vocation, he predicts that many persons will work in their own homes in control of computers. Occupational therapy's valuing of the person-environment fit will certainly lead to interventions designed to better prepare persons with disabilities to both live and work in their own homes. This change could remove many of the barriers currently preventing the employment of severely disabled persons.

The valuing of self-care in both medicine and health maintenance will increase dramatically in the future, as more and more persons "leap on the bandwagon" of taking care of themselves. Toffler believed that this movement reflects a substantial change in social values, definitions of health and illness, and perceptions of body and self. The desire to be more responsible for one's health seems to reflect occupational therapy's valuing of self-determination as reflected in Reilly's major tenet.[15]

Toffler foresees a major change in the role of the professional from that of "the objective, impersonal expert, who is assumed to know the answers, to that of a listener, teacher and guide" who works with the patient or client.[24] Occupational therapy's valuing of the "mutual cooperation" mode of interacting with the patient appears to have anticipated this change by relating patient participation in treatment to the desired outcome of patient autonomy.

Toffler also anticipates a rise in the "do it yourself" movement. Consumers will use their leisure time to become more involved in the production of goods for their own use. He foresees the development of a generation of persons "eager to use their own hands" and an ascendency of respect for good craftsmanship. If Toffler is correct, occupational therapy's traditional valuing of productivity, leisure activity, and craftsmanship will come into its own.

As the third wave engulfs society, Toffler anticipates an increasingly complex life style with a concomitant need for structure and meaning. He predicts the need to create a cadre of "life organizers" to help people "pull their daily lives together."[24] Such professionals could study "the structure of everyday life, the way time is allocated, the personal uses of money, and the places to go for help" in an extremely complicated society.[24] With occupational therapy's valuing of autonomy, self-direction, temporal adaptation, and a balanced activity pattern, occupational therapists would seem prime candidates to become "life organizers" for nondisabled persons as well as those with disabilities. These competencies have already been convincingly demonstrated in independent living skills programs conducted by occupational therapists for persons with a wide range of severe disabilities.

Currently, occupational therapists are educated to help patients seek and use community resources, solve physical and cognitive problems in the environment, plan their uses of time, conserve energy and increase their efficiency in carrying out the tasks of daily living, manage money, and otherwise develop competence in their ability to perform social roles. Occupational therapists, in other words, are experts in the knowledge and skills of human adaptation, especially as applied to the complex environmental challenges presented to disabled persons. Such background provides excellent preparation for assuming the role of a "life organizer" in Toffler's complex world of the third wave.

The values supporting the practice of occupational therapy seem to be congruent with Toffler's view of the future. In fact, occupational therapy practice appears to reflect more "third wave" than "second wave" values. In contrast to medicine, the values held by occupational therapy practitioners appear to reflect needed changes in how professionals relate to patients in order to preserve patients' essential humanity, dignity, uniqueness and autonomy. In many respects occupational therapy has been, audaciously, far ahead of its time.

CHALLENGES REMAINING

Occupational therapists must continue to be daring, strengthening their unique contributions to health care and society. What occupational therapy values is what society has been seeking increasingly: a grasp of the whole picture, person and environment; encouraging persons to take responsibility for their own bodies and destinies; and recognizing the potential, dignity, and autonomy of each individual. Occupational therapists need to recognize this contribution and their advanced thinking, resisting strong pressures to emulate medicine, while at the same time valuing their medical knowledge and cordial relationships with physicians.

Occupational therapy educators and practitioners need to strengthen and preserve the knowledge base that supports general rather than specialized practice. Even in such seemingly specialized occupational therapy practices as hand rehabilitation or sensory integration, the generalist understanding of the entire person is what enables occupational therapists to be so effective; not just knowledge of the hand or nervous system. The future will bring increasing numbers of persons with one or more chronic diseases, along with strong economic pressures to keep such persons out of institutions. Occupational therapists who are generalists concerned with environmental adaptation can be at the forefront of the movement to prevent the institutionalization of persons with chronic disabilities.

Occupational therapy has been characterized as a "feminine" profession.[28] In the past, femininity has been associated with compliance, lack of assertion, and "semiprofessionalism." As has been shown here, occupational therapy values translated into practice may be far ahead of their time. Occupational therapists need to speak out clearly and unmistakably about what they have to offer. We will be needed by society even more in the future due to the increasing complexity of life styles and the numbers of persons who will require help in developing adaptive skills.

Occupational therapy can have a powerful impact on creating a climate of caring not only for patients, but for nonpatients as well, in the complex world of tomorrow.

That climate will be characterized by a reaffirmation of the individual's right to dignity, a sense of mastery, and self-respect gained through engagement in leisure activities, play, self-maintenance, and work that restore meaning and structure to life. If Toffler's predictions of the future are valid, society will seek and nurture the values of occupational therapy as never before.

SUMMARY

A value is that which is perceived as intrinsically good or desirable. The unique blend of values supporting the practice of occupational therapy was seen to include belief in patients' humanity and rights to life satisfaction, enhancement of the healthy aspects of the patient, fostering patient autonomy, employing a generalized perspective, relating to patients in a "mutual cooperation" mode, viewing the patient as an actor rather than reactor, holding optimism about each patient's potential, recognizing the healthfulness of a balanced participation in activities, encouraging productivity, and seeking to know the subjective perspectives of the patient.

By contrast, the values supporting medical practice included freeing the patient from the fear of death, eradicating disease, conferring the sick role, expecting patient compliance with orders, employing a specialist approach to knowledge, relating to the patient in an "activity-passivity" mode, viewing the patient primarily as a "body machine," having faith in science and the healer's competence, relieving the patient of everyday responsibilities, being concerned with recovery from illness rather than resulting impairments, and emphasizing the observable, objective qualities of the patient.

The values of occupational therapy and medicine were found to be different and, in a sense, complementary to each other. Some physicians and philosophers have urged that in the future medicine adopt values that are similar to the traditional values of occupational therapy. Occupational therapy's values were seen as "audacious" since they have been created and sustained within the medical milieu, but have persisted in remaining ideologically separate from medicine's since their inception.

Occupational therapy's values demonstrated compatibility with Toffler's predictions of "third wave" social values. It was suggested that owing to their education and demonstrated skills, occupational therapists should be prime candidates to become "life organizers" for both disabled and nondisabled persons.

Finally, occupational therapists were presented with challenges for the future. These included recognizing the importance of maintaining their values, strengthening their generalist knowledge base, making their usefulness more widely known and helping to create a future climate of caring in a society which will increasingly nurture their values.

REFERENCES

1. AYRES, AJ: *Sensory integration and learning disorders*. Western Psychological Services, Los Angeles, 1972.

2. BELCHER, SA, CLOWERS, MR, AND CADARAYAN, AC: *Independent living rehabilitation needs of post-discharge stroke persons: A pilot study*. Archives of Physical Medicine and Rehabilitation, 59:404, 1978.

3. BING, R: *Occupational therapy revisited: A paraphrastic journey.* American Journal of Occupational Therapy, 35:499, 1981.

4. BURNETT, S AND YERXA, E: *Community-based and college-based needs assessment of physically disabled persons.* American Journal of Occupational Therapy, 34:201, 1980.

5. CALLAHAN, E, ET AL: *The "sick role" in chronic illness: Some reactions.* Journal of Chronic Disability, 19:883, 1966.

6. CARLSON, R: *The end of medicine.* John Wiley and Sons, New York, 1975.

7. DE SAINT-EXUPÉRY, A: *The little prince.* Harcourt Brace, New York, 1943.

8. DUBOS, R: *Foreword.* In SCHAEFER, K, HENSEL, H AND BRADY, R (EDS): *Toward a man-centered medical science.* Futura, Mount Kisco, 1977.

9. HENSEL, H: *The limits of scientific methods in medicine.* In SCHAEFER, K, HENSEL, H AND BRADY, R (EDS): *Toward a man-centered medical science.* Futura, Mount Kisco, 1977.

10. JANTZEN, A: *The current profile of occupational therapy and the future—professional or vocational?* Occupational Therapy: 2001 AD. American Occupational Therapy Association, Rockville, MD, 1978.

11. KIELHOFNER, G: *Temporal adaptation: A conceptual framework for occupational therapy.* American Journal of Occupational Therapy, 31:235, 1977.

12. KING, LJ: *Toward a science of adaptive responses.* American Journal of Occupational Therapy, 32:429, 1978.

13. KNOWLES, J: *Wallstreet Journal,* March 22, 1976.

14. LAUENSTEIN, D: *The idea of human individuality: A critical review.* In SCHAEFER, K, HENSEL, H AND BRADY, R (EDS): *Toward a man-centered medical science.* Futura, Mount Kisco, 1977.

15. REILLY, M: *Occupational therapy can be one of the great ideas of 20th century medicine.* American Journal of Occupational Therapy, 16:1, 1962.

16. REILLY, M: *The educational process.* American Journal of Occupational Therapy, 23:300, 1969.

17. REILLY, M: Play as exploratory learning. Sage, Beverly Hills, 1974.

18. SCHAEFER, K, HENSEL, H AND BRADY, R (EDS): *Toward a man-centered medical science.* Futura, Mount Kisco, 1977.

19. SCHAEFER, K: *Introduction.* In SCHAEFER, K, HENSEL, H AND BRADY, R (EDS): *Toward a man-centered medical science.* Futura, Mount Kisco, 1977.

20. SHORTELL, S: *Occupational prestige differences within the medical and allied health professions.* Social Science and Medicine, 8:1, 1974.

21. SIEGLER, M, AND OSMOND, H: *Models of madness, models of medicine.* Macmillan, New York, 1974.

22. SLAGLE, EC: *Training aids for mental patients.* Archives of Occupational Therapy, 1:11, 1922.

23. TAGORE, R: *Fireflies.* Collier, New York, 1975.

24. TOFFLER, A: *The third wave.* Bantam, New York, 1981.

25. *Webster's New Collegiate Dictionary.* Merriam, Springfield, 1980.

26. WEISS, P: *The system of nature and the nature of systems: Empirical holism and practical reductionism harmonized.* In SCHAEFER, K, HENSEL, H AND BRADY, R (EDS): *Toward a man-centered medical science.* Futura, Mount Kisco, 1977.

27. YERXA, E: *Authentic occupational therapy: 1966 Eleanor Clark Slagle lecture.* American Journal of Occupational Therapy, 21:1, 1967.

28. YERXA, E: *On being a member of a feminine profession.* American Journal of Occupational Therapy, 29:597, 1975.

29. YERXA, E: *The philosophical base of occupational therapy.* Occupational Therapy: 2001 AD. American Occupational Therapy Association, Rockville, MD, 1978.

30. YERXA, E: *The present and future audacity of occupational therapy.* Manuscript submitted for publication, 1980.

CHAPTER 7

THE CHANGING MEDICAL MARKETPLACE AS A CONTEXT FOR THE PRACTICE OF OCCUPATIONAL THERAPY

Jerry A. Johnson

EDITOR'S INTRODUCTION

Those who support theory and scholarship in a practice profession are not strangers to questions concerning the marketability of those ideas. "That's a nice idea, but how do I get paid for it" and "I do such and such because it is easily justified and no one questions billing for it," are the predictable responses of practicing therapists. Such perspectives are both sobering and challenging for those who perceive their major concern as the creation and elaboration of concepts.

Most chapters in this volume implicitly follow the theme that concerns of reimbursement must always be secondary to honest and informed appraisal of patient and client needs. Theory seeks to elucidate those needs and the best means to address them. This chapter takes a different tack which is sure to get the reader's attention. The author addresses the economic issue head-on with an appropriately calculating business sense. The reader will find an almost dizzying collection of facts concerning shifts in people and institutions and the billions of dollars involved in a rapidly changing health-care marketplace. A number of realities emerge with sobering impact. Such forces as deregulation, takeovers by the private profit-making sector, and increasing competition make health-care delivery systems look less and less like the benevolent institutions of the past and more and more like big business. As the reader absorbs these realities, the author explains their implications for occupational therapy.

It becomes clear that the field can no longer rely upon its traditional place in the medical retinue to ensure inclusion in health care delivery settings. Rather, it is incumbent on individual therapists and on the profession as a whole to think seriously about the *value* (in both humanistic and economic terms) of its service.

The author concludes that the most marketable kind of occupational therapy service in the future will be a theoretically grounded and empirically tested one which is neatly packaged for consumers and corporate decision-makers alike. By taking a very hard-nosed view of economic reality the author accomplishes what proponents of theory have for some time desired to articulate: A truly good idea or concept—well formulated and practical—is the easiest and best assurance of being reimbursed in the long run.

GK

Today's growth product is tomorrow's buggy whip—and often management does not seem to realize it. A company must learn to think of itself not as producing goods and services but as buying, creating, and satisfying customers. This approach should permeate every nook and cranny of the organization; if it doesn't, no amount of efficiency in operations can compensate for the lack. Marketing myopia is not easy to overcome, but unless it is, an organization cannot achieve greatness. . . . The railroads did not stop growing because the need for passenger and freight transportation declined. That grew. The railroads are in trouble today not because the need was filled by others (cars, trucks, airplanes, even telephones), but because it was not filled by the railroads themselves. Levitt, *Marketing Myopia*

The 1980s promise to be a period of upheaval produced by major changes occurring throughout all segments of society. Changes are evident in government legislative, funding, and regulatory decisions; in international competition for sources of energy and other resources; in economics, changing values, and in the necessity for higher productivity and more efficient operations in all businesses; in technological advancements and re-emergence of the private sector as a dominant force in society as government leadership declines. These changes are producing intense pressures for reorganization throughout our social structure, including the medical marketplace.

THE CHANGING HEALTH CARE INDUSTRY

Health care is now a 240 billion-dollar industry[8]. It is seen as big business, and there are numerous efforts to remove government regulation and introduce competitive forces similar to those in the private sector. In this changing environment, it is apparent that neither hospitals nor health professionals can continue to operate in traditional patterns. Drastic changes are occurring as hospitals search for methods to survive.

This chapter will identify major changes evident in the medical and health care marketplace and will examine their implications for the occupational therapy profession. Strategies for the design and implementation of occupational therapy services and proposals for marketing these services will also be outlined.

Emerging and proposed changes in medicine and in health care services affect almost every component of the health care industry. Elements responsible for change include better informed consumers; state and local governments in which health care legislation, funding, and regulations are being questioned and reordered; improved medical technology that affects hospitalization and direct patient services; and proposed legislation that would introduce competition and deregulation to the health care industry. Detailed articles about the medical and health care industry are increasingly found in publications such as *The Wall Street Journal* and *The Harvard Business Review* as various experts in fields outside of medicine seek to extend their services to the health care industry.

To appreciate the size and complexity of the health care industry, it is necessary to be aware of its major components and the extent of their financial investments. Six major groups are readily identifiable: government, hospitals and health care institutions, business and industry, insurance companies, medical and health professions, and consumers. A brief description of each force will provide an understanding of its investment in, and concern for, the health care industry.

GOVERNMENT

The first component is the government, whose agencies and departments spend 10 billion dollars annually to provide services to Eskimos, Aleuts, Indians, servicemen and their dependents, veterans, and merchant seamen. Government sources also provide 60 billion dollars annually to the private sector for Medicare and Medicaid services. Additionally, billions of dollars are allocated annually for biomedical and health services, and research and manpower development.[1] Government not only serves as a source of funds for services, but through legislation and regulatory activities its control and restraint mechanisms affect cost, supply and demand, manpower, and service delivery in the health care marketplace.

HOSPITALS AND HEALTH CARE INDUSTRIES

The second major component consists of hospitals and other health care institutions. This is the most rapidly growing force in the medical marketplace.[1] In 1978 the hospital industry employed 3.2 million workers and expended over 71 billion dollars. Problems confronting hospitals and their administrators have multiplied over the past fifteen years as the costs of care have escalated beyond the rate of inflation and as government efforts to regulate costs have increased competition among hospitals. In the same period significant external competition has arisen. As prime determinants of hospital utilization, physicians are competing with hospitals as they offer the same services in their private offices at lower cost (e.g., x-ray, laboratory analysis, physical therapy). Advances in medical technology also make it possible for many services, once available only in hospitals, to be offered on an outpatient basis (e.g., chemotherapy for psychiatric patients, kidney dialysis, outpatient surgery).[7] A recent Blue Cross study showed an 18.6 percent decline in inpatient days and a 137.6 percent increase in outpatient visits between 1968 and 1978.[7]

Hospitals are aggressively expanding their services to counter losses from these trends as well as changes brought about by reductions in government funding, opposition to costs by consumers, and declines in charitable contributions. Large for-profit corporations are purchasing and operating hospitals, nursing home management firms, clinical laboratories, and kidney dialysis centers. Services and financial structures are scrutinized to reduce costs, overlap and overstaffing, and financial and management controls are being adopted.[7]

In growing numbers hospitals, medical schools, and health care plans (such as Kaiser) are hiring physicians as staff employees. This action increases income, assures a steady flow of patients, and reduces competition by removing autonomous physicians—who might refer patients to any one of several facilities—from the open market. Physicians, especially young graduates who have incurred considerable debt to acquire their medical training, are willing to accept positions as "physician-workers."[19]

Other methods to reduce losses include mergers with other hospitals; organizing health prevention programs for sale to employers; providing services to manage weight loss, alcoholism, smoking, and stress; operating medical supply and laboratory services, subsidizing housing projects, operating health spas; and owning rental property. Profits of these various businesses are returned to the parent hospital as contributions. One executive of a holding company formed by a hospital board of trustees is quoted as saying, "The hospital of the future must be a full-service health corporation, not just a hospital."[20] If the concept of competition and free enterprise gains acceptance in the medical marketplace, it may replace government as the primary force in the health care industry.

BUSINESS AND INDUSTRY

The third major component is represented by business and industry, which annually purchases about 50 billion dollars of health insurance premiums and spends another 45 billion dollars for workmen's compensation, pensions, and health benefits for retired workers and their families.[1]

HEALTH INSURANCE INDUSTRY

The insurance industry, advocates of self-insurance, and administrative services organizations comprise the fourth component. These groups compete among themselves as potential insurors, as contract administrators for Medicare and Medicaid, and even as direct service providers.[1]

MEDICAL AND HEALTH PROFESSIONS

The medical professions and health-related professions compose the fifth major component. Services provided by these groups now have price tags, and there is growing concern that members of these disciplines are being co-opted by other components of the health care industry.[1] The number of physicians practicing independently is declining, and the American Medical Association reports that the number of physicians in group practice more than doubled between 1969 and 1980, increasing from 40,093 to 88,290. Others are being employed by hospitals. Reasons cited for the decline in private practice and the accompanying increase in group or hospital-based practices are costs of establishing an office and practice, the high costs of malpractice insurance, and the attraction of regular hours and guaranteed free time.

Many physicians see the federal government as the enemy of traditional fee-for-service patterns, and they are under pressure from third party payers to cut costs, sometimes at the expense of quality health care. The American Medical Association now declares that its primary task is the "representation of physicians," a step many see as a move toward unionization of physicians.[19] This force is not yet well organized or cohesive, although physicians exert powerful influence through their control of hospital utilization, drug prescriptions, and referral for most services for which reimbursement is available from Medicare, Medicaid, and other health insurance plans.

There is growing support for the health professions to regroup as a force for competition and for assuming responsibility for their missions and for issues requiring their consideration. However, there is conflict within the professions over their appropriate functions and responsibilities, and even over the meaning of medical care and health care. Kass[10] argues that health is the end goal of medicine, making a strong case for medicine to attend to health promotion and maintenance, just as it does to diagnosis, treatment, and curing disease. He states that medicine should redefine its boundaries and recommit itself to a broader perspective of health as proposed by Socrates and other great philosophers. Kass suggests that Western medicine's reductionist approach has created confusion about medicine's proper ends and purposes. Adding to this confusion are societal demands for medical help to provide happiness and gratification, to address social or judicial problems through biologic manipulation, and to alter human nature. For example, Kass suggests that physicians attend to happiness and gratification when surgery is performed to remove a normal breast because it interferes with one's golf swing or when, following amniocentesis, an abortion is requested because the fetus is of the wrong gender. Problems of social adjustment or civic virtue reflected in juvenile delinquency, crime, and indolence may be "treated" by physicians using biologic manipulations such as psychosurgery, behavior-modifying drugs, or genetic screening to detect genotypes that may predict violent behavior. Advances in technology make possible pharmacologic reduction of aggressiveness in political leaders, drug induced peace of mind, and laboratory grown babies. Consumers generate demand for these services. However, Kass sees these services as aimed at personal gratification or indulgence, *not* at health. Thus, they represent false goals that are perpetuated by delegation of responsibility to physicians to biologically manipulate the body.[10] While Kass presents compelling arguments that medicine should renounce its false goals and concern itself with health and illness, his presentation suggests that medicine cannot easily retrace its steps because society expects and demands access to such services.

Cassell agrees that current medical care is concerned with sickness, not with health:

> American medicine has done a first class job of taking care of diseases. We do more—cure more, repair more, return more people to function from more conditions than ever before in the world's history. . . . American medicine is not a health care system. It is expensive, it is overly devoted to its technology, it cares more about diseases than sick persons . . . but it is effective.[3]

Cassell states that we do not know what health is, how it can be achieved, or how to define it. Furthermore, he feels that health education has failed to bring about changes in life-style. Finally, he acknowledges that the research methodologies that are so effective in medicine and care for the sick are not applicable to a study of health.

Obviously, physicians are subject to strong pressures, but they nevertheless exert a powerful influence over the health care industry. Even though other health professionals are eroding some of this power as they acquire new authority and increasing responsibility to diagnose and treat certain problems, their ability to influence the health care system is limited.

THE CONSUMER

The sixth component to be considered is the consumer. Noting this force in *The Aquarian Conspiracy*,[6] Ferguson argues that consumers wish for "holistic health" while a new collection of entrepreneurs seeks to deliver it:

> The autonomy so evident in social movements is hitting the old assumptions of medicine hard. The search for self becomes a search for health, for wholeness—the cache of sanity and wisdom that once seemed beyond our conscious reach. If we respond to the message of pain or disease, the demand for adaptation, we can break through to a new level of wellness.
>
> For all its reputed conservatism, Western medicine is undergoing an amazing revitalization. Patients and professionals alike are beginning to see beyond symptoms to the context of illness: stress, society, family, diet, season, emotions. Just as the readiness of a new constituency makes a new politics, the needs of patients can change the practice of medicine. Hospitals, long the bastions of barren efficiency, are scurrying to provide more humane environments for birth and death, more flexible policies. Medical schools, long geared to skim the cool academic cream, are trying to attract more creative, people-oriented students. Bolstered by a blizzard of research on the psychology of illness, practitioners who once split mind and body are trying to put them back together.
>
> No one had realized how vulnerable the old medical model was. Within a few short years, without a shot being fired, the concept of holistic health has been legitimized by federal and state programs, endorsed by politicians, urged and underwritten by insurance companies, co-opted in terminology (if not always in practice) by many physicians, and adopted by medical students.[6]

While Ferguson cites many examples of changes occurring within medicine, her referent seems to be health. Many of the changes she describes emphasize personal responsibility and the recognition that one may indeed influence one's state of health. As part of this assumption, individuals seek to become more aware of their bodies, the status of their health, their treatment by physicians, and the relationship that exists between the individual and the environment. Health thus becomes a goal people seek to attain. Being healthy is defined as the freedom to live a satisfying life without constraints or awareness of the body and the limitations it can impose through fatigue, disability, and discomfort.

A society whose members are healthy has the potential for growth, creativity, productivity, and self-determination. Contrast this state with conditions in countries wracked by war and displacement, poverty, and malnutrition. In the first instance, people are able to care for themselves, to engage in work and play, to care for their families and to contribute to the society in which they live. In the latter instance, people must devote their full energy and attention to survival with little energy left for other purposes. Between these extremes are varying states of health common to cultures and to individuals. Health may thus characterize a whole society, and it also has a separate meaning for each individual.

The medical marketplace is being redefined by a changing perspective in which people no longer attend to their bodies only when they are sick and need medical care. Health is defined as quite apart from sickness and does not necessarily infer absence of all known disease. Consumers look to physicians for health as well as medical care. In striking contrast, many basic medical texts discuss regimes and treatments for known diseases while omitting any reference to regimes for becoming healthy or for maintaining health.

SUMMARY

Six major forces seek to influence the delivery of health care services: government, hospital associations, business and industry, insurance companies, the medical and health professions and consumers. As yet there is no broad consensus or dominant force that exerts primary leadership, although physicians currently control entry into the medical system. Consequently, those who work within health care must seek to understand the complexities, conflicts, and ambiguities that exist in order to plan for the future. Perhaps the only certainty is that the future will be marked by continuing change.

RESPONSE OF THE MEDICAL MARKETPLACE

Responses to these changes vary, although the most likely strategies can be predicted from those historically used by private corporations and business as markets mature:

(1) Aggressive competition (especially for physicians who control utilization of hospital and other services).

(2) Diversification of services (expanding from acute inpatient care to a broader mix of services).

(3) Developing captive distribution systems to control patient flow into hospitals.

(4) Promoting the institution's services (especially through the use of marketing techniques).[7]

In short, the medical marketplace may become a full-service health complex. Scientific medicine will probably continue its present course, focusing on sickness as the health care system expands. These changes will produce corresponding changes in occupational therapy and in the environments in which it is practiced.

It is difficult to predict with certainty how future delivery of health care services will differ, but a study of the evolution of professions and occupations indicates that those which significantly contribute to science, technology, or general welfare appear to be survivors. It can be foreseen that there will be increasing competition among health disciplines. Consequently, those which contribute to scientific knowledge and improvement of the human condition and which adapt to the changing marketplace will continue to exist and expand their influence. Others may remain viable under certain conditions, be absorbed into broader contexts, or disappear.

The impact of these changes may present extensive problems or new opportunities and challenges for occupational therapists, depending upon the leadership of the profession and the way in which puzzles and challenges presented by the changes are perceived and addressed. It is a perilous time for a discipline whose members only recently (in the 1970s) have made serious attempts to influence the political system by seeking state licensure; acquiring recognition for services through legislation and regulations at the federal level; and working with private insurance companies to promote coverage for patients and clients needing occupational therapy services. These efforts sought recognition of the profession's services in order to establish eligibility for reimbursement from third party payers. Eligibility for such reimbursement is a prerequisite for independent or private practice, and it is also essential to the ability of professionals to adapt their practice to the demands of a changing marketplace.

THE NEED FOR PRACTICE MODELS

New practice models, based on theory, must continue to evolve to promote survival in the rapidly changing health care marketplace. This section will focus on one theoretical approach underlying occupational therapy practice that offers promise for success within a changing context.

The early paradigm of occupational therapy had three underlying tenets about humans that seem to be universal and applicable throughout the life span. The first is that each individual has an occupational nature that is reflected in work, play, and self-care. Occupation is thus a fundamental need and serves as an organizing principle for an integrated life. The second is that disability, illness, or stress produced by environmental conditions, especially if severe or prolonged, disrupts occupation, thereby fostering dependency and some degree of social and personal disorientation. The third tenet is that occupation can be used to organize behavior, thereby enabling persons to become productive members of society. Occupation may be applied to a variety of problems, including lack of coordination, muscle strength, or range of motion, response to illness or disability, and reorganizing one's life to prevent stress-induced dysfunction.[9,11,16] The model of human occupation[12,13,14,15] is the first practice model explicitly based on these principles, and it represents both the potential for the principles to be applied in practice and for future models to incorporate the same principles. Within this perspective the occupational therapist seeks to diagnose the problems of occupational dysfunction and to establish regimes to restore functions, thereby contributing to the individual's social and behavioral organization and integration.

Bockoven identifies society's need for services which focus on the occupational nature of humans, asserting that occupational therapy is the discipline best suited to deliver those services:

> Thousands upon thousands of Americans are drifting about in a state of social disorientation, suffering the lot of displaced persons in their own country. They need concrete, tangible, highly visible activity programs to attract their interest, to help them discover their own selves, and to find their way out of demoralization. . . . It is my contention that moral treatment will never again be developed by medical men to meet the needs of the times. All of them, including psychiatrists, are too thoroughly possessed by the need to keep up with the latest technical knowledge in their specialized areas of endeavor.[2]

Dubos[5] supports Bockoven's thesis concerning the need of an occupationally-focused service in his argument that one of the great challenges confronting humankind today is the lack of meaning many experience in their everyday lives.

A theory focusing on occupation is consistent with the basic tenets of occupational therapy and aligns with the mood of the times. It is responsive to changes in the health care marketplace, offers a rationale for an efficient, clearly delineated practice model whose hypotheses can be subjected to research, and it should be attractive to consumers.

THE PRACTICE MODEL IN THE MEDICAL MARKETPLACE

Two themes that emerged from our examination of changes in the health care marketplace are consistent with the utilization of a paradigm of occupation. The first is that there is a more demanding and informed consumer. This person may be one who defines his or her own health needs and wants more personal control over these needs. The consumer may also be a third party payer, an employer who contracts for certain health care benefits, or a health care institution that employs professionals to provide specific services. Each of these consumers is concerned with costs, expectations, and results. The second theme is that a corporate or businesslike marketplace for the delivery of health care services is emerging and is often associated with national organizations or chains.

Within the context of these themes, therapists may use a theory of occupation to develop conceptual statements that provide an integrated framework and a rationale for models of practice that appeal to consumers, administrators, and third party payers. These should include the following concepts, each of which will be discussed in greater detail below:

(1) Clear statements of the service or product that respond rationally and logically to the needs of the consumer, corporate decision-maker, or third party payer.

(2) Descriptions of a packaged or standardized approach for delivery of occupational therapy services for specified clients or patients.

(3) Descriptions of the program's efficacy and its underlying rationale.

(4) Models of service delivery that can be developed in a variety of locations and environments, independently by occupational therapists or in conjunction with other health care providers.

The discussion that follows details the significance of each of these concepts, analyzing them in the context of relevant principles of marketing services or products. Marketing is a complex activity that is basic to the success of any product in a competitive environment. It may include such activities as public relations or advertising, but it is far more extensive in scope, as it is concerned with product or service management, consumer expectations and needs, pricing, availability, communications, and packaging of the product or service to make it appealing to prospective buyers. Marketing is basic to the concern of occupational therapists in a changing marketplace: how to make available services that will improve the lives of persons with disabilities.

(1) *Crisp, clear statements of the service or product that appeals to, and meets the needs of, the consumer, the corporate decision-maker, or the third party payer.*

Statements should describe the goal of the service or product and its anticipated results so that the prospective user may determine whether it is consistent with the institution or corporation's goals and mission.

It has not been common practice for occupational therapists to conduct feasibility studies of populations served or services provided or planned by a health care facility in which they may be applying for a position. It also is relatively uncommon for therapists applying for positions to prepare proposals detailing recommendations for occupational therapy programs to be offered in a particular institution or group of institutions. However, as the job market shrinks, and as hospitals and health care facilities shift their focus, it may become necessary for the therapist as job applicant to submit a proposal along with an application and resumé. The ability to design a program for an institution or corporation will be as important as selling oneself to a prospective employer. Need, cost, anticipated results, and expected return on investment will be covered in the prospectus.

(2) *Description of a packaged or standardized approach for delivery of the service or product.*

This approach may be difficult for many health care providers, including occupational therapists, who stress the exclusiveness of services based on evaluation and diagnosis of individual problems. By contrast, this may be of critical importance to purchasers of services who are less concerned with individual needs, but who are in need of services for homogeneous groups (e.g., learning disabled children, alcoholics, stroke patients, or clients with hand injuries).

A standardized plan of occupational therapy must be consistent with the needs of the populations served by the institution in which the therapist seeks employment. It will be prudent to consider how the facility is coping with, and adapting to, the changing medical and health care marketplace so that the programs proposed are suited to those changes. For example, a facility might have a large inpatient population or a large number of beds, but be located in an area that has an excess of hospital beds and considerable competition for patients. The therapist must be aware of these possibly conflicting elements and anticipate what kind of program might best fit the facility's prospects.

Within the context of humans' occupational nature and the need for a balance of work, play, and self-care, programs can be designed for "workaholics," children who cannot play and who are thus deprived of sensory and cultural input, those whose daily lives are disrupted by disease and disability, and those who are unable to occupy themselves to their own satisfaction. Such programs should identify the unique and useful ways therapists conceptualize human problems and the ways they can be effectively remediated through occupation.

(3) *Statements describing the efficacy of the program and the rationale underlying the program.*

Ideally, research data, financial implications, and documented results of treatment all provide backup information that support the effectiveness of treatment. These data must, of course, be developed through the efforts of occupational therapists, with the object of making statements more persuasive. In developing evaluation and treatment programs consistent with the missions of health care facilities the relevance of theory, or scientific knowledge, becomes apparent. Scientific knowledge basically aims at description and explanation. Frequently it provides a typology or method of classification, predicting what can be expected under certain conditions, explaining past events, and providing for control of events.[18] A highly developed body of scientific knowledge concerning occupational therapy will enable therapists to better explain their practice. It will facilitate prediction of outcomes under certain conditions; it will provide better explanations of how and under what conditions therapeutic approaches have been effective; and it will give therapists, clients, administrators, and third party payers a better understanding of results and the conditions that bring them about.

A theory-before-research approach, a research-after-theory approach, or a composite of both approaches may be used to further the development of a body of scientific knowledge and its application to problems. Reynolds[18] suggests that there are three stages of scientific activity and describes them as follows:

(1) Exploratory research to examine the parameters and composition of a phenomenon. In occupational therapy such research into the occupational nature of humans was begun early in this century. It has not progressed significantly since then. However, the rationale and basis for a science of occupation are presented in this volume.

(2) Description of patterns found in or hypotheses emerging from exploratory studies can be developed to create generalizations about the phenomenon explored or observed. This process is in its infancy in occupational therapy. The principles identified in this chapter and the postulates articulated in the following chapter are steps in this direction.

(3) Activities that may provide explanations are conducted. The results of these activities (or research) often facilitate the development of generalizations found in stage two. There should then be a continuous cycle of theory construction, testing, and reformulation.

This process will ultimately promote stronger theoretical formulations about the contributions of occupational therapy to the processes of prevention, health promotion, restoration, and curing. Therapists can then more readily develop proposals detailing the efficacy and rationale of occupational therapy.

While it may not be feasible for every therapist to be involved in research, all can support such activity by encouraging the major professional organizations to support research and development, and by making financial contributions to further research. Linkages with universities will also promote research and make available some of the resources and qualified personnel to undertake needed study. Research endeavors should be oriented toward understanding, explaining, and predicting the results of occupational therapy treatment methodologies, and moving the profession in new directions by being in the forefront of knowledge development.

Successful industries consider their investment in research and development to be critical support for survival and future growth. An overall marketing plan aims toward distributing and selling current products or services and continually scans the horizon for new products and services in order to remain in the strongest competitive position. By being aware of new occupational dysfunctions and by exploring new applications of occupation to health problems, occupational therapists can pursue such a strategy.

(4) *Establish models of service delivery that can be developed by therapists in a variety of locations and environments, independently or in conjunction with other health care providers, or in health care facilities.*

Occupational therapy services can be organized within the context of three basic principles: (1) the human need for occupation that calls for a balance of play, work, and self-care; (2) the implications of occupational dysfunction to humans and to society; and (3) the employment of occupational methodologies to restore or develop a balanced life style and foster one's contributions to others.

Services may differ depending upon the framework within which they are offered and the population for which they are designed. Thus, the availability of services in an acute care hospital, in specialized outpatient programs attached to hospitals, in a private practice setting, in an occupational workshop designed and staffed by occupational therapists, in a school system or industrial setting, or in some of the more traditional long-term rehabilitation or residential facilities may require differing therapeutic modalities. Within these differences, however, the goal is to enable participating clients or patients to assume social and occupational roles and functions appropriate to their capacities.

Basic to such services are efficient occupational evaluative and diagnostic procedures to provide information for treatment planning and implementation. As noted earlier, the focal point for occupational therapy should be occupational dysfunction.

To "diagnose" the meaning of occupational dysfunction to a given individual, the therapist must analyze the sensorimotor, cognitive, social, and emotional skills of the individual in combination with the emotional and motivational values the occupation has in that community. This is done through histories obtained by interviews, by standardized testing and observation, and by collaborative efforts of client, therapist, and family. The client must become an active participant and partner in this stage of occupational diagnosis.

Bockoven[2] sees occupation as central to our social institutions and to individual existence. In terms of the person, occupation is a component of individuality. It is of central importance not only for individual human behavior but also for community development.

OPERATIONALIZING A MODEL IN THE MEDICAL MARKETPLACE.

Achieving a level of independence to market services in a corporate framework will impose requirements on the profession: a stronger sense of professionalism and professional identity; extended periods of higher education to achieve competence in diagnosis, testing, program development and implementation, evaluation of results, and handling interdisciplinary collaboration and referral mechanisms; acquisition of the knowledge and skills to manage a business operation; and development of a strong ethical code of behavior.

For many disciplines professional associations provide resources and guidelines for developing specific models of practice (e.g., private practice, group practice, or institution-based practice). These guidelines are inclusive, covering such topics as conducting feasibility studies to determine the type of service most needed in a particular area; financial, legal, and organizational advice; marketing and public relations; and ongoing evaluation of the services being provided.

This chapter has emphasized that health care professionals must acquire new perspectives regarding their services and the delivery of those services in a marketplace that is undergoing rapid changes. This may create conflict for those who have a highly personalized approach to the delivery of health care and who resist what they perceive as regimentation or Madison Avenue approaches to salesmanship. However, in an era of economic crisis and hardship, professionals who fail to consider some of these methods may not survive.

A theme that has resounded in the health care field in recent years and one to which occupational therapists have responded has been the attempt to reduce overlap among the various health care disciplines, primarily in an effort to reduce costs. Various disciplines have sought to find the unique quality or aspect of service that differentiates them from other disciplines, while also, at the level of practice, individuals have often adopted modalities or techniques of other disciplines to obtain reimbursement or to round out their services. Licensing laws have sought to define the areas for which each of the disciplines has competence and authority.

With concepts such as supply and demand and competition becoming more acceptable within the health care field, and with reduction in federal regulation and control, it is conceivable that more overlap may occur. Marketing experts in the private sector acknowledge that the consumer is always in the position of choosing one product over another. Competition, combined with supply and demand, causes producers of similar products or services to consider them as a package: "The 'product' . . . is the total package of benefits the customer receives when he buys."[4]

Marketing experts consider several elements when marketing a service or product: the generic product, the expected product, the augmented product, and the potential product. The generic product is the fundamental, substantive product or service that makes it possible for a business to participate in marketing. For the auto industry, this item may be steel; for banks, loanable funds; for a realtor, property. The generic product in occupational therapy is the health-giving potential of occupation.

The expected product includes the generic product and also terms and conditions that are of critical import to the purchaser: delivery of the product or service, including the possibility of preferential treatment; the terms for purchasing the product and service, including pricing and time specifications; supporting efforts such as advice, consultation, and backup support when needed; and finally, new ideas, such as more efficient ways of using the generic product, new types of fabrication (as in the case of splinting), and new applications. It is well known that the consumer purchases a generic product only when it also fulfills his or her criteria for the expected product.[17] At this point models of practice in occupational therapy that articulate the generic product and its relevance to a set of needs or problems is critical.

The augmented product is best described as a product or service which exceeds the requirements *and* expectations of the consumer. For example, the company that not only sells its product, but helps consumers to explore new uses for it, or trains personnel in its use or to expand its use, is providing an augmented product. Augmentation may even include cost and price reduction in a mature market.[17] As indicated in Chapter 1, the idea that patients may not only have dysfunction remediated, but develop new interests and aptitudes, fits into this category of augmented product.

Finally, the potential product includes all that can be done to attract and hold consumers, purchasers, or customers. In marketing products, activities associated with the potential product may involve redesign of the product to reduce weight, increase strength, add flexibility, or enhance safety; market research to learn more about the customers' preferences and attitudes toward the product or service under consideration; introduction of new methods or technologies that in some way enhance the product or service; and new applications or uses of the product or service.

In general, a product is defined by economic conditions, business strategies, customers, competition, and by managing marketing so that the purchaser readily sees a distinct advantage to purchasing one product or service rather than another. For many well known companies, such as IBM or Xerox, it is not the product, but the process of marketing the product that is differentiated and that makes the product competitive.[17] Such a process in occupational therapy involves identifying why occupational therapists are best suited to deliver certain types of services.

It may be most profitable for occupational therapists to give more serious consideration to those activities in which therapists excel. By adopting an assertive approach, it will be possible to focus the profession's efforts toward developing guidelines for effective models of practice supported by theoretical frameworks and substantive documentation. Historically, occupational therapists have done one thing very well: they have used occupations to enable persons to regain health, to find meaning in their lives, and to minimize the effects of permanent disability. They thus offer a viable product that is needed and can be supported by a theoretical rationale.

Models of practice based on concepts of occupation have particular relevance during this time of change. By using an organized and integrated service delivery approach, combined with the use of sound marketing principles, occupational therapists can provide a service uniquely adapted to society's needs at a time of great change.

REFERENCES

1. Alumni Council/Harvard University Program for Health Systems Management. *Competitive Strategies in the Health and Medical Market of the 1980's*. Updated, unpublished program, 1981.

2. BOCKOVEN, JS: *Moral treatment in community health*. Springer Publishing, New York, 1972.

3. CASSELL, EJ: *Our sickness care system*. The Wall Street Journal, March 3, 1980.

4. COREY, E: Key options in market selection and product planning. *Harvard Business Review*, September-October 119, 1975.

5. DUBOS, R AND ESCANDE, J: *Quest: Reflections on medicine, science, and humanity*. Harcourt Brace Jovanovich, New York, 1979.

6. FERGUSON, M: *The aquarian conspiracy*. J.P. Tarcher, Los Angeles, 1980.

7. GOLDSMITH, JC: *Corporate health care: Threat or challenge?* The Wall Street Journal, June 15, 1981, 40.

8. IGLEHART, JK: *Drawing the line for the debate on competition*. New England Journal of Medicine, 305:291, 1981.

9. JOHNSON, JA: *Old values—new directions: Competence, adaptation, integration*. American Journal of Occupational Therapy, 35:589, 1981.

10. KASS, L: *Regarding the end of medicine and the pursuit of health*. ADLER, M. (ED): *The great ideas of today*. Encyclopedia Brittanica, Chicago, 1978.

11. KIELHOFNER, G: Occupation. In HOPKINS, H. AND SMITH, H., (EDS): *Williard & Spackman's Occupational Therapy*, Ed 6, JB Lippincott, Philadelphia, In Press.

12. KIELHOFNER, G. AND BURKE, J: *A model of human occupation, Part one. Conceptual framework and content*. American Journal of Occupational Therapy, 34:572, 1980.

13. KIELHOFNER, G: *A model of human occupation, Part two. Ontogenesis from the perspective of temporal adaptation*. American Journal of Occupational Therapy, 34:657, 1980.

14. KIELHOFNER, G: *A model of human occupation, Part three. Benign and vicious cycles*. American Journal of Occupational Therapy, 34:731, 1980.

15. KIELHOFNER, G, BURKE, J AND IGI, C: *A model of human occupation, Part four. Assessment and intervention*. American Journal of Occupational Therapy, 34:777, 1980.

16. KING, LJ: *Toward a science of adaptive responses*. American Journal of Occupational Therapy, 32:429, 1978.

17. LEVITT, T: *Marketing success through differentiation of anything*. Harvard Business Review, January-February: 84, 1980.

18. REYNOLDS, PD: *A Primer in theory construction*. Bobbs-Merrill, Indianapolis, 1971.

19. SCHWARTZ, H: *The decline of the independent physician continues*. The Wall Street Journal, August 11, 1981.

20. WALDHOLZ, M: *Some hospitals are entering diverse businesses, often unrelated to medicine, to offset losses*. The Wall Street Journal, August 12, 1981.

CHAPTER 8

OCCUPATIONAL THERAPY IN THE HEALTH CARE SYSTEM OF THE FUTURE

**Jerry Johnson
Gary Kielhofner**

EDITOR'S INTRODUCTION

Preceding chapters have offered a range of themes that are bound to raise questions for some readers concerning their relevance to the circumstances of health care. This chapter takes several themes from Part One and relates them to the changing realities of the health care delivery system and cultural forces which impact the system and the need for occupational therapy services. The authors acknowledge traditional services and propose new directions for occupational therapy. Because it portrays the health care system in a state of flux paralleled by extraordinary changes on the world scene, the chapter is a crystal ball in which the reader may glimpse a different set of circumstances that will both constrain and offer future opportunities for clinical practice. Educators who must prepare students for practice in coming decades, students who must be secure in their identity yet flexible enough to survive in a turbulent system, and clinicians who must keep abreast of changing times will find in the formulations of this chapter some food for thought. Even those who do not agree with the authors' predictions should find it a stimulus to their own visions of the future.

In presenting an argument for the place of occupational therapy in health care, the authors consider the respective roles of physicians and occupational therapists, predicting a more democratic and mutually respectful relationship between the two. This may provide some insight to the perennial problems of working with, rather than under, physicians. The authors also address the question of whether occupational therapy is a medical service and what its relationship is to health care outside the domain of traditional medicine. The authors suggest ways of approaching these questions, proposing where occupational therapy fits into traditional and emerging health care arenas.

The themes and issues of earlier chapters are formulated into a set of postulates concerning the health needs occupational therapy is suited to address, forming a rationale for proposed efficacy. The themes identify occupation as a remedial, restorative, preventive and health promoting factor. Thus they reflect the argument for a practice that addresses a broader range of health needs and problems than in the past. The authors point to the need for diversification in occupational therapy practice and suggest the manner in which this may be accomplished without fragmenting the field. Thus themes of earlier chapters which stressed the unity and cohesiveness of theory and practice are allied with the need for diversity. The authors follow the dictum that differentiation of practice is possible only when diverse parts are integrated into a coherent whole.

Finally, a number of strategies are proposed that are deemed necessary for the field to actualize its postulates in theory, research, and practice. While not everyone will agree with the proposed changes, the chapter should help to stimulate dialogue concerning how the field can best prepare for the future.

GK

The medicine of the future won't necessarily invent a mechanical substitute to replace a lost organ, but will teach the individual to function without that organ. Rene Dubos, *The Mirage of Health: Utopias, Progress and Biological Change*

This chapter addresses occupational therapy as it may be practiced in the health care system of the future. A brief introduction to the historical roots of modern medicine and occupational therapy's relation to it will lead to our proposals for the current and future practice of occupational therapy.

Most organized bodies of knowledge in the Western World have their roots in Greek philosophy. Early philosophers observed and contemplated the natural world, human nature and its relationship to the physical environment, and the meaning of their interpretations of the objects and events of that world. The philosophers sought to penetrate both internal and external reality. They attempted to accomplish this through the use of logic and reason and the careful formulation of important questions for empirical observation.

Physical science and its method evolved from early philosophical thought as individuals sought to discover and explain the natural laws of observed events and objects of the inanimate world. The issues with which the earliest scientists were concerned were primarily those of the physical world since it was more readily observed and comprehended than the inner mechanisms of the human body and mind. Thus physics, astronomy, and geometry were some of the earliest investigatory traditions to emerge from philosophy as independent sciences.

Western philosophers were, however, concerned with the human body and mind. They shared with Eastern philosophers a belief in the unity of mind, spirit, and body, and the unity of the human being with the environment. Thus, they viewed health and illness in the same way. Socrates argued, "As you ought not to attempt to cure the eyes without the head or the head without the body, so neither the body without the soul, and this is the reason why the cure of many diseases is unknown to the physicians of Hellas, because they are ignorant of the whole . . . for the part can never be well unless the whole is well"[13] He associated health with moderation, recognizing that individuals were responsible for maintaining their own good health. While illness and its cure was often believed by early philosophers to be connected with physical phenomena, it was also understood to be influenced by the degree of harmony between the individual and the environment.

The influence of these reflections on medicine is seen in scientific-religious traditions. For instance, the ancient Greek ideal of medicine was embodied in two mythological gods. One was Hygeia (from whom we derive the modern term, 'hygiene') and the other was Aesculapius, who, according to legend, became the first physician in the 12th century B.C. and later was raised to the status of a god.[5] Hygeia represented the laws of natural living that prevented disease and assured the well being of the individual and the populace. In the Hygeian tradition health was primarily a feature of humans' adaptive struggle to live in harmony with their nature and their environment. Disease was believed to emanate from failure to abide by laws of nature or from problems in the adaptive struggle to achieve harmony with one's environment. It was believed that persons could find relief from misery and pain of disease by accepting the wisdom of healthful living and by striving to adapt to the environment. Aesculapius represented the idea of a healer who mastered the use of the knife and employed the curative powers of plants. This ancient practitioner presaged the healing powers of the modern physician.

Hippocrates, the Greek physician from whom the modern physician takes pride and identity, believed that both Hygeian concepts of adaptation and Aesculapian curing comprised medicine. According to Dubos:

> Hippocrates regarded disease as the result of infringement upon the natural laws . . . his writings are pervaded with the concept that the life of the patient as a whole is implicated in the disease process and that the cause is to be found in a concatenation of circumstances rather than in the simple direct effect of some external agency.[5]

Among those features of life and environmental circumstances Hippocrates included occupation and its effect on the total health of the person.

Because the physical sciences had an earlier start in the evolution of Western knowledge, they became the sciences par excellence and their methods came to be regarded as *the* scientific method. As other disciplines emerged they sought to emulate the methodology of the physical sciences. This was no less true in the emergence of medicine. Though medicine originally grew out of philosophic thought that included concepts of mind-body and person-environment unities, in the course of its development it adopted a scientific attitude that imitated the methods of the physical sciences which stressed simple cause and effect agency.[1,24] It consequently ignored the early Western and Eastern philosophies that stressed wholeness and connectivity.

Through careful study of the cause and effect relationships between biophysical phenomena, medicine built a powerful diagnostic and healing technology. Knowledge of the causative agents of disease, their impact on the human body, and possible courses of introducing other agents and events into the disturbed order has made possible a vast and complex technology for curing a plethora of disorders. However, as Riley notes:

> The development of Western medicine must be understood not only in terms of the knowledge and technology inputs from science itself, but also in terms of the ideology of scientism—the belief that science is a pre-eminent way of dealing with reality. Scientism has been a rather consistent ideology, even though the meaning of science itself has not been consistently agreed upon.[24]

The disagreement about science to which Riley refers is the growing awareness that the methodology of the physical sciences is only one way of being scientific. The term 'reductionism' has been used to describe the vast scientific technology that grew out of the physical sciences and that sought to reduce phenomena to their constituent elements in order to discover their cause and effect relationships.[1,19] While recognizing the efficacy of this approach to science many modern writers have been pointing to the importance of more holistic approaches to the study of empirical events.[1,2,19] In short, they call for a return to early Western philosophy and a recognition of Eastern ideas which acknowledge the connectivity of mind and body and the interrelationship of the person and the environment. This emerging trend in science is influencing all modern inquiry and, most certainly, the area of health and health care.

Kass writes that "the fruitful marriage between the ancient art of healing and the new, vigorous sciences of physiology, microbiology, biochemistry, pharmacology, genetics, and molecular biology"[16] required a shift from inquiry of appearances, from perceiving the world as it appears to our senses, to a search beneath the surface in order to understand the laws of matter and motion and acquire mastery over this aspect of nature. In so doing, medical science ceased to be concerned with broader questions of health. Increasingly, it became less possible for medicine to retrace earlier steps and to adopt a different paradigm.[16] The irreversibility of medicine's deep plunge into the internal workings of the human organism via physical science methodologies means that expanding contemporary perspectives of health will require the contributions and leadership of other sectors of the health care system.

Medical philosophies and practices that embrace reductionist science and the Aesculapian curative tradition in our estimation form an incomplete or partial approach to health care that represents only one of many possible approaches to health and illness. Modern medicine best serves acute, remedial or manageable pathologic problems that may threaten the integrity of functioning parts of the person or life itself. However, in such instances medicine frequently offers the patient a tradeoff of life for loss of some part or function, resulting in a permanent condition which threatens health in a larger sense. Medicine thus saves lives, but in so doing frequently neglects a broader concept of health which demands that one address quality of life as well as longevity.

Unfortunately, in many societies and particularly in the 20th century, medicine has been viewed as an end in itself and as the major, if not sole means, to health[5,24] rather than as part of a larger context of health. However, medicine's status and authority in health care are giving way and must continue to give way to a pluralistic health care system in which a variety of professionals address rapidly changing health needs and problems. These changes in views of health and illness make it appropriate to ask what might be the role of other professionals in the health care system of the future, and what kind of leadership must be exerted in a more pluralistic health care delivery system. In considering the role and possible leadership capacity of occupational therapists, the following questions are posed and will structure our remaining discussion:

(1) To what extent is occupational therapy a medically related discipline and to what extent are its services oriented to a broader concept of health?

(2) What anticipated changes in the social environment, in the demographics of our society, and in the health care system will place demands on occupational therapy in the future?

(3) What strategies of change should we as occupational therapists pursue in order to prepare for our functions in the health care delivery systems of the future?

HEALTH, MEDICINE AND OCCUPATIONAL THERAPY

When viewed in terms of its philosophic origins, health implies a proper balance of mind, body, and environment. Increasingly, there is recognition both by the public and by scholars that health is more than the sum of disease-free parts. Health is a dynamic, complex condition in which the parts contribute to an organized whole and in which the whole functions to preserve the integrity of the parts. Moreover, the condition of health involves an interaction between individuals and their environments which affects the dynamic processes within each person. According to Dubos[5] health is always a struggle, a dynamic process in which human beings seek to actualize their own values. Newly emerging definitions of health suggest that it is not only a state of being but also an observable feature of one's activity and which, importantly, requires and involves activity.

Kass defines health as a "state of being that reveals itself in activity as a standard of bodily excellence or fitness, relative to each species and to some extent individuals, recognizable if not definable, and to some extent attainable".[16] More simply, he says, "health is the well-working of the organism as a whole," or again, "an activity of the living body in accordince with its specific excellences."[16] Montagu and Matson define health as "the ability to live, to work, to play, and to use one's mind critically."[22] Rene Dubos defines health as "primarily a measure of each person's ability to do what he wants to do and become what he wants to become. Good health implies an individual's success in functioning within his particular set of values, and as such it is extremely relative."[6] Dubos adds that one's state of health reflects the degree of success in adapting to environmental challenges and involves an interplay between that human being and his or her environment.[6]

A myriad of factors may interrupt the process of health at any point along the continuum from conception to death. Internal and external circumstances can lead to illness or create dysfunction, thereby disrupting internal order and the relationship of the person to the environment. If one addresses such health problems with medicine's technology alone, the options, though often successful, are limited. If medicine cannot effect a cure, arrest disease, or provide temporary respite from its ravages, the person is left short of a healthy condition. Further, if the procedures of medicine leave the individual with residual disability as a result of either the pathologic problem or the treatment itself, a gap remains between the person's status and health. Hence, restoration of health must go beyond the process of disease eradication and control to include reconstruction of lifestyles within the constraints of residual disability. This restorative process lies outside the domain of medicine. Finally, medicine, though often successful in the cure of existing disease with its methods of diagnosis and treatment, offers less significant contributions to disease prevention and promotion and maintenance of health.

SECTORS OF HEALTH CARE

Within the context of health there is an identifiable need for four service sectors: the curative or medical sector, the restorative sector, the preventive or health maintenance sector, and the health promotion sector. The curative sector concerns itself primarily with disease that can be controlled or eradicated. The restorative sector of health involves a process of enabling individuals who are left with residual physical, mental, or social problems to succeed in the struggle to adapt and change themselves or their environments or both. Prevention of disease (also referred to as health maintenance) is a classic theme in Western concepts of health. Prevention focuses on potential dangers to health that are inherent in a variety of situations. Finally, health promotion recognizes that health is more than the absence of disease. Ideas such as high level wellness and self-actualization characterize the concerns and efforts of a health promotion sector.

THE CURATIVE SECTOR

The processes of curing involve primarily those techniques developed by and for physicians through application of knowledge and methods acquired from the biological and physical sciences. Chemotherapy and surgery are the primary approaches to management of disease processes. Ancillary to the curative process physicians require the assistance of many disciplines whose members apply specific measures for the diagnosis and management of the course of disease and recovery. Within the curative sector occupational therapists contribute occupations to positively influence the course of recovery from disease. As such, occupational therapy is, in part, a medically related discipline.

THE RESTORATIVE SECTOR

Since restoration follows intractable internal problems, it focuses largely on the relationship between chronically disabled persons and their environment. It involves the facilitation, enhancement, and modification of function. In the restorative sector medicine makes more limited contributions. Restoration—or rehabilitation—implicitly acknowledges that the absence or eradication of disease is *not* a prerequisite to health. Medicine can deal with the problems of managing a chronic condition (e.g., decubiti or kidney infections in spinal cord injury). However, beyond these interventions are often chronic residual mental, emotional, or physical limitations.

In the restorative area the major problems center not on the affected parts of the system, but on the overall balance of body, mind, and spirit, and on the harmony of the person with the environment. It is within this restorative area that occupational therapy most fully functions, in contrast to medicine's more limited contribution. Physicians, supported by others who shared their perspectives, first recognized the value of occupation and supported the development of occupational therapy. These persons also recognized the limited contributions of medicine to the restorative process and the importance of the organizing processes that occurred through engagement in occupation. Thus, while occupational therapy's roots are in medicine, it is an outgrowth of the recognition of the need for another discipline in the context of restoration. The reasons why medicine is central to the curative area do not apply in the restorative context. Occupational therapy is not properly a discipline ancillary to medicine in the process of restoration. There are good reasons, as we will note below, why occupational therapy may be best suited to be the leading discipline in the field of restoration.

THE PREVENTIVE SECTOR

Current approaches to prevention emphasize such processes as health education, regarding the dangers of illness-producing agents as behaviors, the regulation of harmful chemicals and organic substances, and the control of disease through immunization.[11,12,20] There is also a growing recognition of the importance of stress and related factors in the etiology of illness.[21,27] In the area of health maintenance there has been renewed awareness that lifestyle, including the individual's balance of work and play, are important factors in health.[7] Further, boredom and lack of meaningful activity are recognized as major sources of stress-producing threats to health.[5,7]

Occupational therapy makes two major contributions to the preventive, or health maintenance sector in enabling individuals to modify health-threatening lifestyles and in restoring or constructing healthy patterns of work and play to replace unsatisfactory patterns, disrupted function, disorganization, or unnecessary dependency.

THE HEALTH PROMOTION SECTOR

The World Health Organization has emphasized that health is more than the absence of illness.[21] Healthy living is often considered only a means of avoiding the ravages of disease, rather than an end in itself, and indeed, as Cousins[3] points out, even longevity may be an offshoot of a self-actualizing lifestyle. However, there is growing recognition that health and its satisfactions are worth pursuing and promoting.

Because occupational therapy has always devoted its practice to improved quality of life, it is uniquely suited as profession to contribute to the promotion of health. The field's understanding of work and play satisfaction, the creative and self-expressive processes, and the importance of a balanced life for happiness, is a major asset in its long-standing support of health promotion. There may be a substantial role for occupational therapy as occupational life style consultants or life planning experts who assist individuals to seek greater satisfaction in their everyday lifes. Therapists may also contribute to urban and industrial planning by designing environments to optimize work and play experiences.

CONTRIBUTIONS TO THE HEALTH CARE SECTORS

Occupational therapy also has the potential for significant contributions in the preventive, restorative, and promotion sectors of health care. The relevance of occupational therapy to medicine in the curative sector is limited and in the future less important than in sectors concerned with restoration, prevention, and promotion. The extent of its contribution to medicine must, in our opinion, be primarily oriented to the use of occupation as the treatment of choice. Efforts of some therapists to extend their roles in the curative and restorative sectors by employing methods which are not occupational in nature, appear shortsighted when measured against occupational therapy's potential to exert leadership in the larger health arena.

While occupational therapy and medicine share areas of mutual concern, there are areas in which their objectives, methodologies, and approaches to health differ, and therapists and physicians should recognize and appreciate their common ground and their differences. Whereas the physician is a specialist in diagnosing and treating pathologic conditions, the occupational therapist is concerned with the ability of individuals to competently interact with the environment. The therapist who understands the effect of pathologic conditions on function and what it means to be deprived of occupation is able to provide an environment in which occupation enables patients and clients to bridge the gap between dependency and health to reassert control of their lives. In essence, the occupational therapist establishes a laboratory for transition from the sick role to re-engagement in life and its tasks, responsibilities, and activities. The importance of this contribution in future health care depends, in part, on a number of changes now emerging.

CHANGES IN THE SOCIAL ENVIRONMENT, HEALTH DEMOGRAPHICS, AND THE HEALTH CARE SYSTEM

Human life and the culture systems which sustain it are currently involved in a pace of change hitherto unknown. In their respective works, Toffler[30] and Salk[26] suggest that civilization is entering a new epoch of major ideological, economic, and political change. They see reorganization of the concept of health and illness and of health care accompanying these changes. We believe this change should be viewed with caution and optimism: caution, because of the realization that failure to move forward in concert with change may mean the demise of occupational therapy as a health service; and optimism, because coming changes promise a climate which supports and demands the type of service that is the essence of occupational therapy.

THE PRO-HEALTH FUTURE

In *The Third Wave,* Toffler sees civilization on the brink of replacing the industrial society which had earlier replaced an agricultural way of life. He predicts movement beyond the way of life brought about by the industrial revolution. The focus of the 19th and 20th centuries on technological solutions and large scale consumption of goods conveyed the message that people would need to rely less on their own efforts than on technology for problem-solving and adjustments to change. Moreover, individuals were to be relieved of the burden of assuring their own well being and survival because the products which assured these states could be purchased. This ideology also dominated the health care industry. Medicine and the drug industry promised to cure headaches, acid indigestion, and all pain and anxieties stemming from self-indulgent living or misfortune.

In addition, the industrial revolution resulted in a fragmentation of thought and action. Much of the success underlying technical progress was based on the reductionist strategy of searching for the elementary building blocks of nature and their causal relationships. Elementary causation dominated thinking of the past three centuries, and while it greatly advanced human knowledge and technical control over the environment, it also fragmented the former, making it more difficult to deal with global problems.[30] As noted above, medicine achieved its success as a scientific and technical discipline by following this pathway.

Toffler identifies elements of today's emerging change as global recognition of the essential unity of mind and body, person and environment, and reduction of passive consumerism, with increased individual participation in the production of one's own goods, including those necessary for health.

Salk predicts a transformation from Epoch A to Epoch B (phenomena present in all living ecological systems) which he believes will have the following impact:

> Epoch B seems to be what might be called pro-life and pro-health-oriented while in Epoch A the orientation seems to have been more anti-death and anti-disease. Obviously attention must be given to both, from the viewpoint of survival and evolution. There is a considerable difference in a balanced view, compared to one in which there is a preponderant preoccupation with death and disease. . . . Less preoccupied by the possibility of his own early demise, it is understandable that a preoccupation with health for each individual will develop that he may be able to live a full and contributing life and not become a burden, to his own BEING and to others.[26]

According to the views of these two authors, the social climate in which occupational therapists are likely to be working in in the not-so-distant future will be one in which people will seek to regain control over their own affairs and the satisfaction of their own needs. It will also be one in which individuals will live in harmony with the environment, rather than in antagonistic exploitation of it. Ferguson[9] sees such a transformation occurring quietly but powerfully among individuals, and beginning dramatically to alter our way of life.

Along with these trends there is growing recognition of the limited contribution of medicine to health. The reliance of the populace on what Dubos[5] termed the "magic bullet of medicine" to cure all disease will be transformed into an awareness of the importance of individual control in maintaining one's health. Because of its atomistic focus on parts and their disruption and repair, medicine offers a service almost exclusively oriented to curing sickness[5] and only secondarily to happiness and personal gratification.[16] Medicine will likely need to adhere to its primary commitment to atomistic concerns to continue offering a highly technical service for curing disease. A more pluralistic health care system seems both unavoidable and desirable in the future. Fox[10] proposes a reorganization of the structure of health services with reduction of physician autonomy and controlled growth of alternative modes of health delivery. In such a system professionals other than physicians will assume an expanding role in offering services necessary for health.

FUTURE HEALTH PROBLEMS

In coming decades many of the demands of health care will result from casualties of the industrial revolution and the separation of production from consumption and the worker from control over the conditions of work.[7] Alienation of the worker from work and inability to achieve satisfaction in the marketplace are major sources of ill health, according to these writers. Dubos more recently proposed that one of the conditions most threatening to the survival of the human species is the growing inability of persons to achieve satisfaction in their play and work, accompanied by resulting biologic and moral deterioration.[7] As they enter the struggle for a more autonomous lifestyle many persons will be found unfit for such a task by virtue of having been programmed to consume, having lost basic skills of production and self care, and the ability to cope and adapt in a rapidly changing world. One of the greatest problems facing American society in the near future will be increasing numbers of persons who cannot find meaning and purpose in their lives—the sick, the aged, the alienated, the disabled, the incompetent. Drucker[8] sees this problem in terms of changing technology and the job market, with increasing numbers of routine and repetitive tasks requiring attention, but little thought and no creative ability. There is no sense of completion and no sense of craftmanship in such work. The assembly line worker and middle management become extensions of the machine. Products used in our daily lives are constructed to be serviced only by trained technicians and mechanics, with parts replaced rather than repaired.[8] Persons experience less control and competence in their own households, where many tasks once useful for self-maintenance of the living-space are now outmoded. Individuals whose educational experiences have not equipped them with basic academic skills have increasing difficulty finding employment that provides a sense of dignity or the opportunity to be upwardly mobile.

In addition, the notion of the importance of struggle in life has eroded in American culture. The emergence of a drug culture that emphasizes chemical control of feelings and sensations and withdrawal from complex problems signals the coming of generations whose mode of coping is to avoid struggle, commitment, and attempts to solve problems. These conditions create a tremendous need for services to restore health to individuals and to entire groups; but the service is not one of curing, not one currently offered by medicine. In attempting to enter this arena of problems, medicine has added to the passivity, the helplessness in the face of suffering, the escapism of drug users.[14] The rising services will be those which enable persons to regain competence in their daily lives and to struggle with complex problems and find satisfaction in the struggle. Another major requirement will be the involvement of professionals in the systematic alteration of social, work, and play environments so that they provide the necessary conditions and resources to enhance individual development. The restoration of playfulness, craftsmanship, and sportsmanship to life tasks, the marketplace, and social systems will be a major task for health restoration and health promotion and maintenance in the future.

THE FIELD'S HERITAGE: HYPOTHESES ABOUT THE HEALTH-GIVING POTENTIAL OF OCCUPATION

Much of the original enthusiasm for occupational therapy grew out of observations of its effectiveness for enhancing patients' recovery. As noted in Chapter 1, the balance of work, play, and leisure, the harmony of a normal schedule, and the organizing influence of purposeful and culturally-meaningful pursuits were all part of the health-giving properties of occupation.

However, before it was possible to fully explore the power of occupation to alter disease and restore or maintain health, the Depression and a series of wars taxed the resources of the fledgling profession. Its efforts then focused on job security and service provision.

As rehabilitation became a viable force in American society, success in reconstructing injured servicemen encouraged renewed efforts to rehabilitate disabled civilians and to put greater emphasis on children. The economic value of preventing disabled children from becoming handicapped adults dependent upon society and government for their care and upkeep was stressed. Throughout this period, occupational therapy was closely allied with medicine. Most occupational therapy services were provided in hospitals, and very few therapists boasted more than a bachelor's degree or certificate (a credentialing mechanism originally designed to permit certification in occupational therapy).

In the 1960s and 1970s, major shifts occurred throughout the country. Medical services were expanded by legislation to provide for the disabled. Training of professionals was upgraded and funds for graduate education became more readily available.

At the same time there was increasing demand for more accessible health care services, especially for the poor and for minorities who lacked ready access to hospitals. Consumers asserted their rights to have some part in the decisions affecting their medical care. Giant hospital complexes that for years had housed the chronically ill were ordered to disperse their patients to community settings, and a variety of small, localized health centers were developed to provide preventive services and outpatient care. Within a short span, numerous problems apart from physical or emotional sickness were relegated to the medical community for care and treatment.

These factors led to the creation of jobs outside the traditional hospital, and occupational therapists found that they had contributions to make to the promotion of health, often in environments that had little connection with medicine or the curative arena.

Events moved so swiftly that members of the profession had little time to assess the relevance of occupational therapy services in these new environments, to systematically test assumptions regarding diagnosis and treatment, or to evaluate the effectiveness of methodologies. Indeed, there were few occupational therapists qualified to do so. Perhaps too frequently, therapists moved out of hospitals into community positions to obtain better salaries or to escape the physician-dominated hospital environments in which occupational therapy, nursing, and physical therapy were held in low esteem. The activities of occupational therapists and the results of their efforts during this period are only now being described and fully analyzed. We would like to propose that from these experiences, four important themes, or postulates, are emerging.

OCCUPATION AS A REMEDIAL MEASURE

The first theme concerns the nature of disease processes and their remediation. There has always been and is now growing recognition among occupational therapists that the course of disease, and especially its arrest or cure, involves many elements. In short, a unified mind-body, person-environment, view of the curing enterprise has been accumulating. Recognition of this feature of the healing process is growing in many disciplines, but it has been essential to occupational therapy's perspectives since the early 1900s. As noted in Chapter 1, the principle that engagement in occupation maintained the morale needed for recovery from both physical and mental disease was important in the field's early practice. As Chapter 2 pointed out, the incorporation of systems theory into occupational therapy by the occupational behavior school has greatly enhanced the field's ability to understand how the disease process and recovery is part of the dynamic problem of a much larger system. Systems theory recognizes the existence of a relationship between all parts of any entity and acknowledges that the system is maintained through interaction with the environment. The myriad of forces interacting with an individual must consequently be considered in the understanding of disease and recovery. In other words, it cannot be expected that a drug, surgery, diet, or other form of treatment acts upon an isolated condition in an isolated manner. Rather, systems within the individual, and the person as a whole, are subject to a variety of influences, which, if appropriately harnessed to work with and for the client, can act to provide additional support. If not, they may counteract, disrupt, or impede the process or goal that one is trying to achieve through the treatment of choice. This theme yields the first postulate concerning occupational therapy practice. It asserts that *used as a remediative measure, properly guided occupation can produce reorganization of pathologic bodily and mental states. This reorganization includes changes to bring about reality-based thinking, stress reduction, increased motor coordination and other functions which involve mind-body, person-environment unity.*

OCCUPATIONAL DYSFUNCTION IN CHRONIC DISABILITY

The second theme concerns the role of occupational therapy in the health care of the chronically disabled. Occupational therapists have always recognized that chronic illness requires a holistic approach which acknowledges the complex relationships between mind and body and between the person and environment. It has been increasingly acknowledged that many chronic problems must be viewed not only from the perspective of pathologic processes, but in terms of social, economic, and family consequences.[15,17,23,31] The major problem of chronic illness centers on the way in which a person can continue to live and function as a member of a family unit or community.[29] This requires long-range planning and long-term health maintenance efforts. We believe occupational therapy is naturally suited to provide a holistic service based on principles of mind-body unity and person-environment interaction. The historical basis of the field supports such a perspective. The traditional uniqueness of occupational therapy is that in occupations, the patient or client engages in a process requiring active participation of the body, mind, and spirit, as well as interaction between the person and environment. The early philosophical principles of the Western world concerning human nature and health are embodied in the occupational therapy process, making the field uniquely suited to offering care to the chronically disabled.

In the restorative phase, occupational therapy focuses on restoring inner balance to harmonize with the environment. The prescription and training with adaptive equipment, activities of daily living, styles of coping, and skills of managing an altered body or social role comprise an important part of this phase. Occupational therapists can be active in helping the client or patient and their families maintain a balanced level of activity, including work, play, rest, and leisure. Therapists assist persons to organize their daily activities, schedules, and routines to maintain physical and emotional endurance and strength while providing meaning and satisfaction and a continuing sense of competence and contribution to family, neighborhood, and other relevant social systems. The therapist also supports maintenance of the client's health by assuring his or her continued investment in daily living and the continued availability of resources necessary to maintain harmony with the environment. This may include assisting with the reorganization of the living space to permit maximum function and mobility of the client; adapting the work environment to permit continued employment, if possible; and assisting the client and family with social and recreational activities which still permit the client to be an active participant. Changes in roles, long-term life-style planning and related forms of activities that assist the family and the client with managing their daily living are also addressed. Finally, it is necessary to assist the family and friends with planning activities in which the client or patient is a participant, and to identify options whereby the family has some relief from the stress and burdens of caring for a member who is increasingly dependent. The theme of restoration in chronic disabilities thus yields the second postulate: *Chronic disease and residual dysfunction disrupt occupational patterns. When this occurs, an occupational dysfunction is recognized. Occupational therapists can intervene in such cases, enabling persons to regain confidence, to seek new alternatives, and to establish new patterns of everyday living to replace old ones.*

HEALTHY OCCUPATION AS A PREVENTIVE MEASURE

The third theme concerns the role of occupational therapy in preventing disease and dysfunctional processes. There is a growing recognition that lifestyle, especially patterns of work and play, may be a major factor in the etiology of disease and disability. Ennui, a loss of engagement and meaning in life, creates a whole new arena for the genesis of medical disease.[5,26] The viruses, trauma, and carcinogens of the twentieth century may be less significant than boredom, incompetence, indolence, and disengagement from daily life as major health problems in the future.

Occupational therapists have long recognized their unique contributions to reducing such problems. As noted in Chapter 1, the early literature of the field foresaw the impact of the industrial age on the workaday world as occupational therapy leaders lamented the progressive dehumanization of work and its implications for threatening individual health. They argued for a balanced lifestyle in maintaining health, asserting that loss of a balanced use of time, including leisure and recreation, was a major etiological factor in disease. Therapists in practice within the curative and restorative sectors, through their observations of circumstances that lead to injury, dysfunction, and failure continue to generate important hypotheses concerning the prevention of such problems.

There is a growing awareness among therapists that many of those in need of preventive occupational therapy services will not be referred through medical channels, since they are not diseased but are disengaged from daily life.[25,31] The failing student, the unemployed worker, the elderly person in retirement, and the widowed are examples of persons who may have occupational dysfunctions. The challenge of meeting the problems of these persons will require movement beyond traditional settings to the community, neighborhood, and family. In prevention, the new occupational therapy clinic will be the community.[4] The therapist will assume the role of managing resources, supports, and systems of productive exchanges in communities as part of the process of maintaining the dynamic balance between persons and their environments. Therapists engaged in preventive pursuits will assess jobs, roles, physical and social resources for activities, and other elements which could limit or enhance the occupations of persons. This will require therapists to develop more fully the profession's knowledge base concerning social systems and their impact on individuals. From this theme we derive the third postulate: *Occupation is a necessary prerequisite to health. When social systems or other conditions deprive the individual of satisfying engagement in occupation, there is a clear threat to the mental and physical integrity of the person. Occupational therapists can intervene in such situations to remediate the conditions of work and play, and the social, economic, and other factors that disrupt normal patterns of occupation.*

HUMANS AS OCCUPATIONAL CREATURES

The fourth theme in occupational therapy is one of its oldest. It concerns the very nature of human life and the most fundamental of human needs. As noted in Chapter 1, early occupational therapists saw humans as occupational creatures who derived satisfaction and pleasure from the exercise of their capacity to work and play. Human life is permeated with the results of generations of productive and ludic pursuits. The greatest of human achievements in art, architecture, religion, government, and science are manifestations of the occupational nature of humans and their drive to explore and master the world.[18]

Reilly[23] has pointed out that the fullest expression of life may be found in the work of human hands. She proposes that therapists have inherited the ability and right to serve this trait of occupation. Recognition of the importance of occupation for life constitutes the core of occupational therapy's ability to contribute to the health promotion efforts of the future. No other field is so uniquely suited to bring an appreciation of the need to nurture and support this human ability and need to the public. Over the years as some therapists observed the struggles of patients to reaffirm their existence by involving themselves in creative and productive processes, a deeper appreciation of the occupational nature of *all* persons grew. Furthermore, many therapists themselves found pleasure and self-actualization in the occupations used as therapy for their patients. The occupational therapist is a natural promoter, both personally and professionally, of the value of occupation for a good life. This theme is reflected in the fourth postulate emerging in occupational therapy: *Humans are occupational creatures who can find great satisfaction through their creative, productive and playful efforts and who flourish by engaging in them.*

SUMMARY

The postulates we see in occupational therapy reveal emerging roles for the field in health care. Changes in modern civilization and the health care system, combined with these postulates, point toward a vibrant and important role for occupational therapy. The field may well emerge with important solutions and perspectives for major health problems of future decades. Actualization of this role will require that the field carefully assess its assets, its pattern of change and growth, and its overall position in health care. Occupational therapists must rally their intellectual and clinical talents around their traditional concern for human occupation and its special relationship to health. The role of occupational therapy can be an exciting and vital one, but its future depends on the soundness of its strategies.

STRATEGIES OF INTERNAL CHANGE TO SUPPORT OCCUPATIONAL THERAPY'S FUTURE ROLE

Reilly[23] once proposed that occupational therapy's greatest enigma was the wide discrepancy between the complexity of patient problems confronted and the commonplace nature of the methods used to alleviate those problems. In addition, the field has chronically been haunted by the extreme distance between the complexity of the postulates underlying its practice and the scholarly tools available to therapists. It is not pretentious to assert that occupational therapy was an idea ahead of its time; it is a simple historical fact. When used to promote health, occupation is a complex agent whose breadth and depth requires sophisticated tools for research and theorizing. Occupational therapy has always existed in a climate where a more narrow and mechanistic science reigned supreme, and in this context, its postulates appeared unscientific. The narrow language of reductionist science was inadequate to the task of conceptualizing how occupation can affect health. Rather than approaching the topic in a holistic manner, occupational therapy narrowed the study of occupation to the effects of activity on discrete motor and mental functions. The most serious task facing the field today is the need to understand the difference between the postulates that assert occupation's impact on health, and the more narrowly conceived postulates which propose that activity can affect discrete variables. Both must be part of the science of occupational therapy, but the field cannot afford to continue its nearly exclusive focus on the latter.

Future intellectual and health care climates will be more disposed to support such holistic postulates. The public and the health care system will be searching for groups who can conduct research and develop services based on holistic concepts of mind-body unity and person-environment harmony. The future will both challenge and support occupational therapy's development of its original scientific postulate, "That man through the use of his hands as they are energized by mind and will can influence the state of his own health."[23]

The task of achieving an integrated theory which explains the organizing agency of occupation and which recognizes mind-body and person-environment unity will require that occupational therapy attend to and use scientific concepts which acknowledge and explain wholeness. This will require a major reorganization of knowledge and an integration of currently disparate bodies of knowledge, the kind of task begun in Chapter 2. Furthermore, occupational therapy must seriously begin the work of testing the postulates identified above.

Several approaches are necessary to test these postulates, to incorporate the findings into a theoretical formulation, and to implement services on the basis of research and theory. The first is that an attitude of critical thinking, holistic analysis and synthesis must be built into the fabric of our service programs, just as the preparation to engage in this conceptual activity must be part of the preparation for entry into the profession of occupational therapy. Future therapists must learn to give equal weight and importance to treatment and to scientific examination of that treatment. A second approach will be to employ experienced and knowledgeable investigators to provide guidance in creating appropriate research designs, and methodologies to implement them. Such programs could be established in university and clinical settings, utilizing occupational therapy faculty and clinicians, and involving collaborative investigation between institutions. Students could be involved in local research, thereby introducing them to this activity at an early stage in development of their careers.

Another approach may be to recruit professionals who hold doctoral degrees (psychologists, sociologists, anthropologists, and others with appropriate expertise and interest), provide special training and certification for them, and prepare them to help with the conduct of treatment programs and research. It will be necessary to recognize and accept the fact that the field requires and must acquire the surge of intellectual power necessary to confront the complexity of its postulates. Indeed, as the theoretical base expands, the field might seek to join forces and consolidate with other disciplines who share its professional perspectives and concern for activity as a means of promoting and maintaining health.

Immediate, thorough reorganization of the field's orientation toward theory and research is essential. There must be recognition of the need to organize the field's knowledge around concepts of occupation and to integrate and synthesize its diverse knowledge in terms of these central concepts. The educational requirements for entry into the field must be upgraded to permit sufficient grounding in theoretical principles and research methodology as well as the complex clinical technology of the field. Finally, there must be a commitment to theory and research as an integral part of good clinical practice and as a component of professional responsibility.

There are hazards inherent in each of these proposals. There will certainly be timidity and resistance from those who believe such change may impair personal status or function, or that change may jeopardize jobs or the field's relations with medicine. There will be embarrassment over a public commitment to the everyday tasks of life and over therapeutic occupations (arts, crafts, music, dance, sports, and the like) that appear on the surface to be of less value than the technology of medicine. There will be insecurity in facing the need, not merely to defend, but to assert the benefits to be derived from occupational therapy programs and methodologies, especially as such claims must be made to powerful, male-dominated professions of medicine and hospital administration.

There are risks in any course of change, risks that seem greater than the risk of maintaining the status quo. However, to do justice to occupational therapy, to the significant contributions that the field can make to health, and to the dreams and legacy of its founders, therapists must take those risks, make needed changes and claim, with justification, a rightful place with other disciplines that are committed to improving health for all.

REFERENCES

1. VON BERTALANFFY, L: *General system theory and psychiatry*. In Arieti S (ED): *American handbook of psychiatry*. Basic Books, New York, 1966.

2. BOULDING, K: *Ecodynamics: A new theory of societal evolution*. Beverly Hills, Sage, 1978.

3. COUSINS, N: *Anatomy of an illness as perceived by the patient*. Bantam Books, New York, 1981.

4. CROMWELL, F. AND KIELHOFNER, G: *An educational strategy for occupational therapy community service*. American Journal of Occupational Therapy, 30:629, 1976.

5. DUBOS, R: *The mirage of health: Utopias, progress and biological change*. Harper and Row, New York, 1959.

6. DUBOS, R: *Health and creative adaptation*. Human Nature, 1:74, 1978.

7. DUBOS, R AND ESCANDE, J: *Quest: Reflections on medicine, science, and humanity*. Harcourt, Brace & Jovanovich, New York, 1980.

8. DRUCKER, P: *Management: Tasks, responsibilities, practices.* Harper and Row, New York, 1973.

9. FERGUSON, M: *The acquarian conspiracy.* J.P. Gardner, Los Angeles, 1980.

10. FOX, R: *The medicalization and demedicalization of American society.* In Knowles, J (ED): *Doing better and feeling worse: Health in the United States.* W.W. Norton, New York, 1977.

11. FREEMAN, H, LEVINE, S, AND REEDER, L (EDS): *Handbook of medical sociology.* Prentice-Hall, Englewood Cliffs, NJ, 1979.

12. GOLDSTON, S: *Primary prevention and health promotion.* In Lieberman, EJ (ED): *Mental health: The public health challenge.* American Public Health Association, Washington, DC, 1975.

13. HUTCHINS, RM: (ED): *Great books of the western world (Vol 7).* Encyclopaedia Britannica, Chicago, 1952.

14. ILLICH, I: *Medical nemesis.* Pantheon Books, New York, 1976.

15. JOHNSON, J: *Occupational therapy: A model for the future.* American Journal of Occupational Therapy, 27:1, 1973.

16. KASS, LR: *Regarding the end of mecicine and the pursuit of health.* In Adler, M (ED): *The great ideas today, 1978.* Encyclopaedia Britannica, Chicago, 1978.

17. KIELHOFNER, G: *Temporal adaptation: A conceptual framework for occupational therapy.* American Journal of Occupational Therapy, 31:235, 1977.

18. KIELHOFNER, G AND BURKE, J: *A model of human occupation, part 1: Conceptual framework and content.* American Journal of Occupational Therapy, 34:572, 1980.

19. KOESTLER, A AND SMITHIES, J: *Beyond reductionism: New perspectives in the life sciences.* Beacon Press, Boston, 1969.

20. KNOWLES, J: *The responsibility of the individual.* In Knowles, J (ED): *Doing better and feeling worse: Health in the United States.* W.W. Norton, New York, 1977.

21. LIEBERMAN, E (ED): *Mental health: The public health challenge.* American Public Health Association, Washington DC, 1975.

22. MONTAGU, A AND MATSON, F: *The human connection.* McGraw-Hill, St. Louis, 1979.

23. REILLY, M: *Occupational therapy can be one of the great ideas of 20th century medicine.* American Journal of Occupational Therapy, 16:1, 1962.

24. RILEY, J: *The western medicine's attempt to become more scientific: Examples from the United States and Thailand.* Social Science and Medicine, 11:549, 1977.

25. ROGERS, J: *Order and disorder in medicine and occupational therapy.* In press, American Journal of Occupational Therapy, 36:29, 1982.

26. SALK, J: *The survival of the wisest.* Harper and Row, New York, 1973.

27. SELYE, H: *The stress of life.* McGraw-Hill, New York, 1956.

28. SLAGLE, E: *Training aides for mental patients.* Archives of Occupational Therapy, 1:11, 1922.

29. SUSSMAN, M: *A policy perspective on the United States rehabilitation system.* Journal of Health and Social Behavior, 13:152, 1972.

30. TOFFLER, A: *The third wave.* William Morrow, New York, 1980.

31. WEST, W: *The growing importance of prevention.* American Journal of Occupational Therapy, 23:226, 1969.

CHAPTER 9

THE DEMYSTIFICATION OF HEALTH CARE AND DEMISE OF THE SICK ROLE: IMPLICATIONS FOR OCCUPATIONAL THERAPY

Janice Posatery Burke
Shawn Miyake
Gary Kielhofner
Roann Barris

EDITOR'S INTRODUCTION

It is almost banal to state that modern health care exists in order to serve higher values that human beings cherish. Yet, it is the theme of this chapter that medicine has not always done so unequivocally. The institutionalization of healing and related processes appears to be a feature of every culture. It may be embodied in the person of the witchdoctor, shaman, midwife, or in any of a variety of medical professionals who function in modern cultures.

This chapter builds upon the argument of many modern writers that medicine is not as effective as it might be and that it unintentionally harms where it should be helping. These accusations are generally directed at the most obvious target in institutionalized medicine, the physician. However, on the assumption that they apply equally—if not intentionally—to all medicine professionals (including occupational therapists), the generic term 'medicine' is retained in this chapter as a reference for all health practitioners, including occupational therapists. The reader should be aware of this usage, since it differs from other chapters, in which 'medicine' refers exclusively to the domain of physicians. It should also be assumed that the term itatrogenesis, which means physician-induced illness or disability, may equally apply to patients' inability or helplessness resulting from occupational therapy procedures.

This chapter relates the overarching arguments of the critics of modern medicine to everyday realities. The critics whose viewpoints are examined assert that modern medicine creates helplessness in individuals and that, in so doing, it paradoxically takes away health. The authors identify the situational variables of this helplessness at the level of patient. By focusing on how patients experience the ministrations of health providers and how they are expected to behave, the authors reveal some tangible and thus manageable elements. The authors then propose solutions to the problem of unwanted side effects from medicine's efforts to cure.

The authors maintain that the creation of helplessness is most consequential in the area of chronic disability and that occupational therapy is suited to offer leadership in remediating the situation in care of the chronically disabled. Underlying their discussion is the thesis that modern medicine causes problems because it focuses on biomedical phenomena to the exclusion of the social domain (which includes the process of delivering the service). Occupational therapy, it is argued, has always sought a synthesis of the biologic and social domains and has traditionally organized its practice with attention to the social features of service delivery—the latter an essential part of the therapeutic process. The authors conclude by proposing a structure for occupational therapy's contribution to a changing model of medical service delivery. This is accomplished by suggesting a conceptualization of the client's role and a set of principles for the operationalization of that role.

GK

Later he would have to assume responsibility. He would have to take his body, in which he himself happened to be housed and which he had abused most dreadfully, treating it with a negligence he would not have shown to any other body in the world, and restore it as best he could. That would take rethinking and retooling, big changes in his life. But he didn't want to think about it yet. There was no need to do anything—anything at all; simply to float here cocooned in this soft postcardiac calm, observing how curious this familiar world looked from his new vantage point. (Lear, Heart Sounds.)

Modern medical practitioners operate with a deep and refined knowledge that allows them unprecedented prediction and control over events that affect illness. Bolstered by the methods of scientific inquiry, physicians and other health professionals employ exact knowledge of the causal and correlative nature of biologic phenomena to limit and arrest disease. It appears that medicine has approximated the ideal of assuring the total health of society's members.

Ironically, more than ever before, medicine finds itself beset with criticisms.[10,24] People are increasingly dissatisfied with the medical care they receive and increasingly taking things into their own hands.[2,29] In the face of its massive technical accomplishments, it seems paradoxical that medicine should be losing the trust of the public.

A careful examination of modern medicine reveals that more is at stake in health and illness than the scientific-technical competence of medical practitioners. Scientific-technical advances have greatly enhanced the ability of highly trained practitioners to control the *biochemical* elements of health and disease. However, they have neither kept pace with environmental concomitants of health, nor realized the extent to which they have unwittingly undermined social and cultural criteria of wellness and illness.[3,10,24] The major impact of this trend has been iatrogenesis in the health care system resulting from expanded boundaries of health and medicine, growing bureaucratic, consumerist structures, and creation of passive and helpless patients. Thus, modern medicine is accused of failing, not in the scientific-technical dimension, but in the domain of human relations and in its preventive impact on the health and illness of persons.

This chapter develops the argument that the critical problem generated by over-technicalization and bureaucratization of medicine is the pairing of the omnipotent medical professional with the yielding consumer in a relationship that is no longer adequate for health care delivery. It proposes an alternative sociological reality, predicated on a base of knowledge and motivation for health shared by both clients and professionals.

IATROGENIC HEALTH CARE

Two major themes appear in discussions of social iatrogenesis. In the first, the focus is on the structure of society and medicine with its promotion of passive consumerism; in the second, the overemphasis of the technical aspects of medicine at the cost of concern with the social domain is stressed.

SOCIOSTRUCTURAL ARGUMENTS

Illich and Navarro are the major proponents of the sociostructural arguments. Although they differ in locating the origins of the problems and in their proposed solutions, they agree on the problems' manifestations.

Illich, the best known critic of modern medicine, sees the negative effects of modern medicine as part of a larger tendency of industrialization to depersonalize and disenfranchise social members. He argues that social iatrogenesis occurs when

> . . . medically sponsored behavior and delusions restrict the vital autonomy of people by undermining their competence in growing up, caring for each other and aging or when medical intervention disables personal responses to pain, disability, impairment, anguish and death.[10]

Social iatrogenesis is abetted by increased industrialization since it trains the person as consumer to seek professional help for nearly every discomfort, illness, or stress.[21] As a result, the current generation has become powerless and does not accept responsibility for its own health. Illich[10] concludes that society's faith in its own ability to maintain well being is undermined by health care when it becomes a commodity. According to this argument, preindustrial societies view health as a state of living to be attained or practiced while modern generations view it as something to be purchased. The shift is from an active participant in health to a passive consumer of health care.

Illich uses the term cultural iatrogenesis to refer to the undermining of cultural definitions of health, illness, pain, and healing practices by the medical establishment. Throughout history, different cultures have evolved meaningful rationales and methods for their sick members to cope with illness:

> Suffering can be explained, for instance, as Karma accumulated through a past incarnation, or can be made valuable by interpreting it as a close association with the Savior of the Cross.[10]

Illich argues that responsibility for the care of sick members and acceptance of the chronically ill and disabled into the cultural group erodes as the ill are removed from the home and placed in the hospital for treatment. The process of transferring care of the ill to the medical center accompanies a transfer of people's beliefs in the efficacy of their own cultural traditions to the (often mistaken) belief that medicine can cure their ills—no matter what they might be.[3,10] This has the effect of reducing the natural coping abilities of cultures and their members.

Cultural erosion is further abetted by the expansion of medicine into nearly all facets of existence. Thus, as individuals begin to equate health with general well being, they attempt to purchase the services of medical practitioners to remove all sources of discomfort in their lives.[5,13,32]

While Illich accuses bureaucracy and industrialization of creating the need for consumption, Navarro argues that the drive for consumption has been created and is maintained by a capitalistic society based on class and sex distinctions. He states that

> . . . addiction and dependency on consumption . . . is the result of the basic needs of an economic system that requires for its survival . . . the creation of wants, however artificial or absurd they may be . . . and . . . replication of consumer ideology whereby the citizen is judged not by what he *does* (his work) but by what he *has* (his consumption).[22]

Navarro does not deny the effect of bureaucracy on consumption, but he attributes the problem to a different source. "Thus, to understand the *sphere of consumption* we have to understand the *world of production* . . . ."[22] His argument is critically relevant to occupational therapists. He argues that when most workers do not have control over their work, and when creativity and self-expression are not realized on the job, the worker becomes alienated and dissatisfied. This alienation then ". . . leads to the fetishism of consumption."[22]

Although Navarro's and Illich's ultimate implications for change are not the same, we find in both arguments condemnation of the marketing of health care, of the lack of opportunity to derive a sense of worthiness from daily life, and of a consumer orientation that seeks to replace this by shopping for health. Inherent to the consumer orientation is the existence of incompetence and helplessness in individuals' responses to illness. As consumers of health, people become externally directed in the health care system, yielding the management of their health to medical professionals.

THE OVER-TECHNICALIZATION OF MEDICINE

Other writers associate the loss of individual responsibility for health with medicine's increased technicalization. The crux of this argument is the underlying contradiction created when technological advances are used to measure progress in a field whose caring aspect is its least scientific and least technical, yet symbolically, most important part.[24] Riley suggests that medicine could be more successful in alleviating suffering by being more concerned with the sick person and less concerned with the disease process.

This concern was anticipated by Dubos, who argues that by focusing on its technological accomplishments, medicine has lost its perspective on the relationships between people and their surroundings. Instead of striving for harmony between persons and the environment, medical professionals have sought to reduce mortality. In this they have been successful. However:

> If one were to use as criteria the amount of life spoiled by disease, instead of measuring only that destroyed by death; or the number of days lost from pleasure and work because of so-called minor ailments; or merely the sums paid for drugs, hospitals, and doctors' bills, the toll exacted by microbial pathogens would seem very large indeed.[3]

The price for the public has been high—less concern for the individual's post-illness lifestyle, and with it, depersonalization of the relationship between professional and client.

Depersonalization has been facilitated by the ". . . 'age of the computer,' for what might be too embarrassing . . . in a face-to-face encounter can now be asked and analyzed impersonally by the machine . . ."[32] In addition, the increase in medical technology has led to a need for specialization and subsequent fragmentation in the delivery of services.[20] Goffman[8] elaborates on this theme in his characterization of the medical enterprise. He suggests that modern physicians, like industrial workers, have organized their work in a manner he refers to as the shop industry. In this context of service delivery, the physician (and by implication, the therapist), engages in tinkering—a term referring to the process of repairing and replacing parts, adjusting function and making use of tools which are foreign to the everyday commerce of the persons they service.

The shop model is greatly reinforced as practitioners select more and more specialized problems—or parts—to repair. Treatment that is repeatedly received in an environment that emphasizes technical and chemical intervention unwittingly denies the importance of the personal effort.

Whether one approaches the problem as large-scale phenomena related to industrialization and social structure, or chooses instead to focus within this structure on the growth of technology in medicine, the end result is the helpless patient, divested of responsibility for health care. Regardless of its source, iatrogenesis is experienced at the micro level, where individuals interface institutions. Specifically, iatrogenesis (i.e., creation of helplessness and its health-robbing effects) occurs through two processes: (1) the *mystification* of the patient when he or she experiences health care, and (2) the *expectations* for behavior which he or she encounters when entering the sick role.

MYSTIFICATION AND THE SICK ROLE

Modern medicine mystifies the patient who finds himself not only at the mercy of outside forces, but seemingly under the control of mysterious processes which require blind faith. Dubos adds in this vein:

> The common use of the word "miracle" in referring to the effect of a new drug reveals that men still find it easier to believe in mysterious forces than to trust in rational process.[3]

The symbolic value of the garb and technical apparatus of health care personnel and other unfamiliar objects and processes also convey the message that the health care system is mystically powerful. The impact of such an atmosphere on the person contributes to the belief that treatment is, as Dubos labels it, the "magic bullet" which will provide health. The combined belief in the miracles of medicine as well as the powerlessness of patients before the physician and other health care workers results in lay persons who return incessantly to the medical world for treatment, because they eventually "find it easier to depend on healers than to attempt the more difficult task of living wisely."[3]

The process of mystification has been greatly enhanced by the development of highly technical and esoteric knowledge, to which the professional alone is privy, and by the ever-widening scope of health.[5,13,18,32] Extending the domain of medicine by expanding the boundaries of health gives medical personnel powers over more and more aspects of life. When social adjustment or obedience falls into the purview of medicine, its practitioners can begin to intervene in legislative, moral, and ethical issues:[18]

Although sin, crime, and sickness are not related in a simple, invariant way, there has been a general tendency in the society to move from sin to crime to sickness. . . . [This] evolution has been most apparent with respect to the conditions that are now considered to be mental illnesses, or associated with serious psychological and/or social disturbances. These include . . . states of hallucination . . . that once would have been interpreted as signs of possession by the Devil . . . alcoholism, drug addiction, compulsive overeating, and compulsive gambling.[5]

The medical industry not only gains access to hitherto private parts of individuals' lives, but does so under the shroud of omnipotence. This is not necessarily a completely negative process. Much of medicine's success—historically and cross-culturally—can be attributed to its placebo effect, or the patient's belief that recovery is possible.[2,3,10,24] Believing that the healer has mystical powers strengthens the placebo. But when these magical powers no longer support the patient's own healing tendencies, the placebo has become a "nocebo":

To a large extent, social iatrogenesis can be explained as a negative placebo, as a *nocebo* effect. Overwhelmingly the nontechnical side-effects of biomedical interventions do powerful damage to health . . . Medical procedures turn into *black magic* when, instead of mobilizing his self-healing powers, they transform the sick man into a limp and mystified voyeur of his own treatment.[10]

Thus, the counterpart of the omnipotent, mystical healer becomes the impotent, ignorant client, unable ". . . to understand his case and too upset to use whatever information the professional might give him wisely."[16]

From this first encounter with the power and expertise of the medical profession, it is just a small step into the role of sick, helpless patient. Individuals entering the modern medical care system find themselves in a transformed world where they have literally lost control over their personal care:

Patients saw themselves as sojourners in a strange institution dominated by physicians, nurses, aides, orderlies, technicians, and administrators. Their illness forced them to submit to the orders and manipulations of the functionaries who ran the hospital. The patients realized they were reduced to dependency in this situation and had to adapt to the demands of those who controlled it. They often objected to hospital routine, complaining for example that, 'the nurse wakes me up at night to give me a sleeping pill.' Such behavior disturbed the patients, but they knew they could do nothing about it . . . the despair of the patient was revealed by their frequent references to the hospital as a jail and to themselves as its prisoners. For the panic stricken patient there was no way out of the dilemma that enmeshed him—he was a prisoner of his illness under the complete control of others.[4]

The concept of the sick role was developed by Parsons[23] as an explanation of the significant social changes a person experiences in the presence of illness and its care. Persons who enter the sick role are governed by four interrelated dimensions that alter the expectations and demands placed on them. Societal norms dictate that a healthy adult should be employed in productive pursuits to earn the necessities of life and contribute to the group's welfare. When an individual becomes sick, a new set of definitions and expectations are present.[23] First, persons in the sick role are exempt from responsibility for the illness or incapacity they are experiencing. This is based on the principle that no one wants to be sick; those who are, are seen as suffering something beyond personal control.[25] Second, the sick role excuses the person from normal role obligations. The sick person receives a temporary respite from roles of a worker, parent, spouse, and so forth. Third, the sick person is responsible for seeking technical, competent help. In other words, the individual who is ill is expected to seek a physician for appropriate and necessary medical care. Fourth, the sick person is expected to cooperate in the process of getting well by compliance to the physician's prescriptions and prohibitions.

These sick role expectations result in a person becoming temporarily helpless, passive and submissive in order to insure cooperation and compliance from the medical and psychosocial professions who provide health care. Individuals are supposed to obtain a form of repair service from health professionals so that they may once more be productive members of society. For this repair the physician requires control of the person's body and mind. By relinquishing physiologic and conscious processes to the ministrations of the physician, the patient assumes a helpless position. This condition is a necessary one for certain medical procedures. For instance, a physician cannot perform surgery without having complete control over the patient's body.

However, the process of relinquishing control over self for care can have the paradoxical effect of destroying the individual's autonomy and ultimately his productivity.

THE FAILURE OF MYSTIFICATION AND THE SICK ROLE

People will continue to enter the medical system with a variety of illnesses for which they seek remediation. However, the traditional sick role which stressed compliance with the medical regimen and with its counterpart in the all-knowing professional, is slowly being replaced with another role in which persons assume mutual responsibility with medical personnel for their care and recovery. This shift in social relations is coming about largely because the sick role has proven to be inadequate, and even harmful, in the pursuit of health. Awareness of its inadequacy has grown for several reasons. First, the criticisms described above, levied by writers such as Illich, have contributed to a negative social perspective on the process of labeling people as ill:

> Casting persons in the sick role is regarded as a powerful, latent way for the society to exact conformity and maintain the status quo. For it allows a semi-approved form of deviance to occur which siphons off potential for insurgent protest and which can be controlled through the supervision or, in some cases, the "enforced therapy" of the medical profession.[5]

Even when "social control" is not the result, labeling is still acknowledged to lead to isolation of the individual and the sanctioning of a deviant lifestyle.[6]

Another reason for disavowal of the sick role comes from empirical evidence linking helplessness with higher death rates,[15,19] and recovery with positive attitudes and knowledgeable patients.[1,2,27,28] When patients begin to generalize the feeling of helplessness acquired during the course of treatment and institutionalization, they tend to give up on life. One example is the higher rate of mortality cited for older people who are shuttled to different nursing homes against their will, compared with individuals who participated in the decision-making.[15] Similarly, the Simontons suggest that while several studies document the relationship between the loss of a loved one and a predisposition to cancer, it is the individual's response to the loss—" . . . such that it engenders the feeling of helplessness and hopelessness"[27]—that is an even more critical determinant of whether the individual will eventually develop a malignancy. This premise led the Simontons to initiate a cancer therapy program of relaxation and mental imagery in which the patient visualizes the malignant cells being conquered and destroyed by healthier cells.[28] The body-mind connection has been noted by others, with Norman Cousins perhaps its most renowned spokesman. Cousins recovered from a disease diagnosed as progressive and incurable by laughing to combat pain, taking large supplements of vitamin C, and most importantly, not acquiescing to the dismal picture given him:

> . . . the will to live is not a theoretical abstraction, but a physiologic reality with therapeutic characteristics. . . . Since I didn't accept the verdict, I wasn't trapped in the cycle of fear, depression, and panic. . . .[2]

Further evidence for the insufficiency of the sick role concept is found in the case of chronic disability. The sick role appears to be particularly ill-suited for chronic disability because it is predicated on the assumption that sick persons will return to the roles that characterized their pre-morbid lifestyles. But ". . . the impossibility of resuming full role-participation at pre-illness capacity, the necessity of adjusting to a permanent condition rather than overcoming a temporary one, and the emphasis on retaining, rather than regaining an optimal level of role performance and autonomy . . ."[14] is incompatible with this assumption. The problem of making a transition into a new set of roles is ignored by the social process within the current medical-technical system. The medical community, with its focus on technical-scientific care, provides only limited and acute episode-oriented services:

> General hospitals treat chronically ill patients only for acute episodes and for important complications. After the emergency is over, general hospitals accept little or no responsibility for those needing continued out-patient care.[9]

The chronically ill are thus locked into a system that treats them as "normal" only when they have exacerbations. Even rehabilitation, with its avowed purpose of enabling persons to adjust to permanent disability, appears to be drawn into this mode. Shorter hospital and care periods and increasing emphasis on pathology-reduction (especially within occupational therapy) as the most efficient means of addressing long-term problems in a short-term framework, are indications that rehabilitation has not moved beyond the sick-role model of service delivery. And within this model, rehabilitation personnel are often as guilty as other medical staff in perpetuating the dependency of the chronically ill.[31]

Thus, in cases of chronic illness or disablement the current focus on technical-scientific medicine and relative neglect of social processes are major blocks to effective services; and in illness generally, the iatrogenic effect of helplessness has proven itself to be costly, both in terms of later social disability and in its impact on the recovery process itself.

BEYOND THE SICK ROLE: TOWARD A RESOLUTION OF IATROGENIC MEDICINE

A major problem which medical professionals must address is finding the balance that will allow them to administer processes that may reduce pathology without eliciting the unwanted side effect of helplessness. The health care system is changing; it is beginning to respond to the message that "people who . . . recover or . . . stabilize their conditions appear to do so by being sufficiently motivated to seek out answers."[1] Mystification implied keeping the patient largely uninformed about the disease, its course and treatment; demystification means educating patients. Although the success of placebos has often been linked to the patient's "blind faith," individuals who have overcome devastating diagnoses have done so because they made extraordinary efforts to learn about their illnesses and to understand various therapeutic options.[1,2] One change in this direction is the increasing information patients are being given concerning their condition, prognosis, treatment choices, and risks. This information enables persons to assume more responsibility for their own illness management and to make informed decisions about their care.[11,17] White[30] points out that good medical care is possible only if patients are able to articulate their circumstances and symptoms and collaborate with medical practitioners to define their problems. Furthermore, the best solutions are as likely to involve action by the patient as to require medical intervention. White thus describes the ideal nature of the health-seeking and health-giving process as ". . . essentially problem-solving encounters that take place in an open system."[30]

The changing attitudes of the public and the medical profession indicate the emergence of two health-related roles to replace the sick role. In acute phases of illness those persons undergoing the scientific-technical ministrations of health professionals will assume a personal *health manager* role. Rather than relinquishing control over themselves to the healer, they will retain—where appropriate—control over their bodies and the decisions affecting health and recovery from sickness, and will do so based on adequate information about their health and sickness conditions. Such persons will draw upon the cultural and social resources of their families and other institutions. They will use increased knowledge of their conditions, and the implications of the conditions, to assume a collaborative responsibility with health care providers for managing their illness and their response to it to enhance recovery.

In the case of chronic disability the health care system will need to provide a role that allows the patient to make a transition from the initial phase of onset or trauma to altered roles in the home and community. The psychological and social impacts of chronic illness require a broadened perspective for care that is not limited to medical and physical deficit states, but also includes consideration of patients' experiences and the role prescriptions they encounter.[9] To meet this perspective through a long-term, transitional role, we propose a new role, *the health apprentice*. The role of health apprentice would stress patients learning new skills and reorganizing life tasks around exploration of alternatives, decision-making, and problem-solving. The health apprentice role would also stress control so that patients could begin to manage their own difficulties, and set priorities for the constitution of their new lifestyles.

The condition of chronic illness is clearly a time for true rehabilitative treatment. Individuals require training for a host of new skills to support desired roles. Reorganization of the patient role requires reciprocal reorganization of the health professional role.

Instead of the traditional role of healer with the "laying on of hands" mystique, the health professional would assume roles of teachers, consultants, co-planners and resource managers. Furthermore, persons in this altered health provider role would convey a new set of social expectations. In the sick role patients are not expected to be productive or take control; their passivity, dependence, and nonproductivity is legitimized by the health professional who sanctions their entry into the sick role and symbolically absolves them of obligations for normal productivity. The health professional, seeking to assist patients to function within a health apprentice role, would convey active social expectations for these individuals, possibly including re-evaluation of life goals, finding alternative pathways of gaining control and participating in activities considered to be important.

Although occupational therapists will continue to be involved with acute-care medical problems, we believe that occupational therapy has much to offer in the realm of chronic care. The health apprentice role will find its major complement in the health care delivery system in the personage of the occupational therapist. In short, it will be the task of occupational therapy, in collaboration with other relevant disciplines, to begin the work of advancing the health apprentice role.

OPERATIONALIZING THE HEALTH APPRENTICE ROLE

Occupational therapy is particularly suited to guide the process of generating a health apprentice role because of its historical mandate and concerns. Occupational therapy has traditionally attempted to achieve a balanced view of the human as both a biologic and social being. This perspective was first articulated by Meyer[21] and echoed throughout the field's literature. As Shannon notes, occupational therapy has grown from the belief that "requisite skills for wholesome living are those competency behaviors demanded by the social environment and acquired in the reality and actuality of doing and practice."[26] Finally, as noted in Chapter 1, the field has consistently focused its efforts on chronic disability. Thus, as a field which has sought an integrated biosocial perspective on chronicity, and which conceptualized its treatment as a process of socialization, occupational therapy appears well equipped to begin the fabrication of a health apprentice role.

Implicit in this argument is the assumption that the directions for practice and theory in occupational therapy, proposed in Chapters 1 through 4, are necessary for the field to operationalize its historical mandate and to promote the health apprentice role. Thus, occupational therapy may continue to direct its practice in an increasingly sick-role mode, as outlined in Chapter 1, or recommit itself to its fundamental tenets and search for a new model of service delivery which we have termed the health apprentice role. Our preference and expectation is, of course, for the latter pathway.

The work of developing a health apprentice role is a substantial challenge for occupational therapy, and will require a long period of development. The remainder of this chapter outlines the sociological conditions which must support such a role in the occupational therapy clinic. They are stated as a series of principles designed to respond to issues raised in earlier discussions of iatrogenesis and the sick role.

The first principle is that the *occupational therapy clinic must embody the symbolic message that health cannot be purchased, but must be earned.* The clinic must not encourage false and demoralizing hope in the ministrations of the therapist. Rather, therapy and the physical and social setting must be organized to give the sometimes painful and unwanted message that patients must struggle, face pain and possible failure, and commit themselves to the process of attaining health through personal effort. To this end the occupational therapist must be a bearer of bad tidings (implicitly if not explicitly) that residual problems are likely to be permanent, along with the hopeful message that they can be accommodated and overcome.

The second principle complements the first. *The occupational therapist must acknowledge that patients are responsible for the outcomes of their illness.* While patients may not be culpable for their disease or trauma, their adaptation to it is their personal responsibility. Decline and degeneration may not be caused by the disease, but by failure to face the challenge that the disease posed. Along with this message, the therapist is obligated to provide the support patients need to overcome the problems posed by illness.

The third principle is that *therapists must believe in the intrinsic value of individuals as sources of their own health restoration and maintenance.* When applying this principle to individuals with chronic conditions, the person must be regarded first as worthy and valuable, and only secondarily as one needing help. This means that patients may share their goals and concerns with the therapist who in turn responds tangibly to their messages. The principle recognizes the person's ability to make decisions and sanctions dignified involvement in self-determined activity.

The fourth principle proposes that *a new collaborative relationship for the patient and therapist must exist, based on the value of individuals as equal participants in the health care process.* Unlike the traditional vertical relationship that places the therapist in a dominant role with the patient a passive recipient of care, a horizontal relationship stresses active involvement of patients in all aspects of their therapy. Therapist and patient take complementary roles with both participating actively in the healing process based on their abilities. In this situation therapists contribute their expertise regarding adaptation to chronic dysfunction, with the individual, as health apprentice, learning and practicing skills for decision-making and setting priorities that will affect his or her daily life and ultimate goals. Inherent in this principle is a commitment to preserve the autonomy of those receiving treatment. By recognizing the importance of the sick persons's opinion about his or her body and own set of values, the therapist opens the doors to a cooperative relationship as patient and therapist become allies in the recovery and rehabilitative effort.

The fifth principle is that *the occupational therapist must assume an advocate role in preventing processes that rob patients and clients of respect, control, and responsibility.* This will necessitate eliminating situations that contribute to the depersonalization of the patient. Individuals are depersonalized when they are referred to as diagnoses or treatments in order to discuss the course of their treatment, quality of their progress, and prognosis for therapy. Depersonalization diminishes when therapists interact with patients in a direct, sincere manner. This includes practices as basic as directing inquiries to the individual, rather than to other professionals or family members who may be present. More elaborate practices require including the patient in the decision-making process in the therapeutic program. This may mean allowing persons to choose an activity based on their interests and values, rather than giving a false sense of choice by allowing selection from a predetermined set of therapeutic activities, or rationalizing an activity as having some biologic efficacy.

Application of the first five principles requires a sixth: *The occupational therapist must be willing to allow the individual to have sufficient power in the form of knowledge* to truly participate as a partner in the health process. Informed and responsible choices regarding such things as planning objectives require information from the therapist. While the patient intuitively understands what is happening to his or her body, he or she may lack the objective knowledge of the disease process and the repercussions of treatment needed to make informed decisions. By educating the patient, the therapist demystifies the illness and helps the patient to avoid falling into the trap of uninformed compliance.

The seventh principle is that *the therapist's efforts to increase the patient's control must extend to the environment of therapy.* Demystifying the occupational therapy clinic will necessitate a decrease in such things as the amount of medical jargon used by therapists in explaining the goals and objectives of therapy, removal of high technology apparatus that tends to inspire awe and helplessness, and an increase in the availability of patient-controlled materials. With an increase in patient-controlled activities, opportunities for exploration and feelings of efficacy and competence are encouraged and rewarded.

CONCLUSION

It is no longer sufficient in occupational therapy to assume immunity from the process of rendering patients helpless merely because the field espouses patients' independence and self-control. Whether aware of it or not, health professionals are emissaries of society's expectations for the person who is sick or disabled. The social messages given by the current sick role and shop industry model of medicine have had, as we have seen, the effect of creating helplessness. The alternative of creating independence and control requires that attention be given to the construction of social parameters of health care.

The health care system of the future will probably have two health-related roles to replace the sick role: the health manager and the health apprentice. People with acute illnesses will become their own personal health managers, seeking an understanding of the disease and their bodies' responses that will allow them to collaborate in the recovery process. The health apprentice role will provide a means for individuals with chronic illness and disability to move toward organization or reorganization of their lifestyles. To achieve these changes in patient roles, occupational therapy must carefully examine its own practice for elements which may render patients helpless, while actively participating in building alternatives to old sociological models of delivery.

As the field becomes concerned with the technical competence of its practitioners, it cannot afford to make the mistake of eschewing its sociological role. If increasing competence of therapists is gained at the expense of patients' control over decisions about their own lives, opportunities to set priorities for their recovery or adjustment, and choices for their futures, such technical competence will undermine its own ends. As therapists become more sophisticated in techniques of practice based on neurologic, kinesiologic and psychologic principles, they must not lose sight of the much larger process to which the patient's independence will ultimately be owing. The physical, cognitive, and emotional skills for performance are important, but the belief that ultimate control is with the self is *all important.* And the latter is not achievable through the mysterious ministrations of the therapist. Patients must have something other than faith in the competence of the therapist; they must believe in their own competence.

REFERENCES

1. ACHTERBERG, J AND LAWLIS, GF: *Bridges of the bodymind.* Institute for Personality and Ability Testing, Champaign, Ill, 1980.

2. COUSINS, N: *Anatomy of an illness as perceived by the patient.* WW Norton, New York, 1979.

3. DUBOS, R: *Mirage of health.* Harper & Row, New York, 1959.

4. DUFF, RS AND HOLLINGSHEAD, AB: *Sickness and society.* Harper and Row, New York, 1968.

5. FOX, R: *The medicalization and demedicalization of American society.* In KNOWLES, JH (ED): *Doing better and feeling worse: Health in the United States.* WW Norton, New York, 1977.

6. FRIEDSON, F: *Professional Dominance: The Social Structure of Medical Care.* Atherton Press, New York, 1970.

7. FRIEDSON, E: *Disability as social deviance.* In FREIDSON E AND LORBER J: (EDS): *Medical men and their work: A sociological reader.* Aldine-Atherton, Chicago, 1972.

8. GOFFMAN, E: *Asylums.* Doubleday, New York, 1962.

9. HAMMERMAN, J: *Toward a social-health policy for the chronicaly ill and the disabled. Care of chronically ill adults.* American Hospital Association, Chicago, Ill, 1971.

10. ILLICH, I: *Medical Nemesis.* Calder & Boyars, London, 1975.

11. KASL, SV AND COBB, S: *Health behavior, illness behavior and sick role behavior.* Archives of Environmental Health, 12:246, 1966.

12. KASL, SV AND COBB, S: *Health behavior, illness behavior and sick role behavior. II, sick role behavior.* Archives of Environmental Health 12:531, 1966.

13. KAAS, LR: *Regarding the end of medicine and the pursuit of health.* In *The great ideas today, 1978.* Encyclopedia Brittanica, Chicago, 1978.

14. KASSEBAUM, GG AND BAUMANN, BO: *Dimensions of the sick role in chronic illness.* Journal of Health and Human Behavior, 6:16, 1965.

15. LAWTON, MP: *Environment and aging.* Brooks-Cole, Monterey, Calif., 1980.

16. LIGHT, D: *Becoming psychiatrists.* WW Norton, New York, 1980.

17. MACCOBY, N, et al: *Reducing the risk of cardiovascular disease: Effects of a community-based campaign on knowledge and behavior.* Journal of Community Health, 3:100, 1977.

18. MAGARRO, P, et al: *The mental health industry: A cultural phenomenon.* John Wiley & Sons, New York, 1978.

19. MAGILL, J AND VARGO, JW: *Helplessness, hope, and the occupational therapist.* Canadian Journal of Occupational Therapy, 44:65, 1977.

20. MECHANIC, D: *Ideology, medical technology, and health care organization in modern nations.* American Journal of Public Health, 65:241, 1975.

21. MEYER, A: *The philosophy of occupational therapy.* Archives of Occupational Therapy, 1:1, 1922.

22. NAVARRO, V: *The industrialization of fetishism or the fetishism of industrialization: A critique of Ivan Illich.* Social Science and Medicine, 9:351, 1975.

23. PARSONS, T: *Definitions of health and illness in the light of american values and social structure. Patients, physicians, and illness.* Jaco, EG (ED): The Free Press, Glencoe, Ill, 1958.

24. RILEY, JN: *Western medicine's attempt to become more scientific: examples from the United States and Thailand.* Social Science and Medicine, 11:549, 1977.

25. SEGALL, A: *The sick role concept: Understanding illness behavior.* Journal of Health and Social Behavior, 17:162, 1976.

26. SHANNON, PD: *The derailment of occupational therapy.* American Journal of Occupational Therapy, 31:229, 1977.

27. SIMONTON, OC AND SIMPSON, SS: *Belief systems and management of the emotional aspects of malignancy.* Journal of Transpersonal Psychology, 7:29, 1975.

28. SPRINGARN, ND: *My mind vs. my cancer.* The Washington Post, Sept. 13, 1981.

29. TOFFLER, A: *Future shock.* Bantam Books, Toronto, 1970.

30. WHITE, KL: *Health and health care: Personal and public issues. The 1974 Michael M. Davis Lecture.* Center for Health Administration Studies, Graduate School of Business, University of Chicago, 1974.

31. WILLEMS, EP: *The interface of the hospital environment and patient behavior.* Archives of Physical Medicine and Rehabilitation, 53:115, 1972.

32. ZOLA, IK: *Medicine as an institution of social control.* In Conrad P and Kern, R (EDS): *The sociology of health and illness.* St. Martin's Press, New York, 1981.

PART 3

FEATURES OF OCCUPATIONAL THERAPY PRACTICE AND THEIR IMPLICATIONS FOR CLINICS AND INTERVENTIONS

CHAPTER 10

OCCUPATIONAL THERAPY'S ROLE IN THE CLIENT'S CREATION AND AFFIRMATION OF MEANING

Gerald W. Sharrott

EDITOR'S INTRODUCTION

Occupational therapists are not strangers to the notion of *meaningful* activity. Despite universal recognition of meaning as an element of occupational therapy, it remains an elusive concept. In the years since the founders of occupational therapy postulated the health giving effects of meaningful participation in occupations, little has been done to extend the field's appreciation of meaning as a feature of human experience or to augment understanding of how meaning is created and trasmitted in human action and interaction.

There has been substantial interest in this problem in the field of philosophy and, more recently, sociology. This chapter brings the rich literature of those traditions to bear on the central problem of meaning in occupational therapy. The reader will encounter an exposition of important ideas and concepts that seek to explain meaning in human life, its creation in human action, and its transmission in the commerce of social interaction. These foci are then related to the specific case of occupational therapy, culminating in the author's identification of their implications for clinical practice. Because the author remains faithful to the terminology of the disciplines from which knowledge is borrowed, the reader will encounter a number of new and unusual terms and concepts. Rather than being perceived as onerous, these should be added to the therapist's repertoire of knowledge for clinical practice. They are clearly defined and clarified by examples to facilitate comprehension.

If occupational therapists are to fulfill their special role as custodians of meaning as articulated in Chapter 5, this chapter points the way to an important tradition of theory and application. By introducing the problem of meaning into occupational therapy as a perceivable and understandable phenomenon, the chapter serves the important function of stirring thought and dialogue about a critical concept. As noted in Chapter 2, meaning lies at the core of human experience and resonates from the social realm to the physiologic domain as part of a complex hierarchy of phenomena. When an array of knowledge in occupational therapy (from neurophysiology to adaptive equipment) is understood in terms of its relationship to human meaning, the field's effectiveness will be vastly increased.

Those who are particularly attracted to the therapeutic relationship (i.e., therapeutic use of self) as a major aspect of occupational therapy, found in earlier chapters a call to move beyond this psychodynamically based therapeutic role toward one which is more task oriented. If these readers found those proposals wanting in detailed outlines for a new kind of therapeutic relationship, this chapter will be perceived as a welcome addition to the volume, since it offers just that. Beginning with a general discussion of the role of occupational therapy in the reconstruction of patients' and clients' realities, the author goes on to propose a set of therapeutic guidelines. These provide instructive and provocative information which offers a new vision of the therapeutic enterprise and illuminates some time-worn clinical principles. While these principles will, of course, need empirical verification and elaboration, they form an important collection of instructions for how occupational therapy may offer meaningful (or more properly, meaning-giving) activities to patients and clients. Long overdue, this serious discussion of meaning and reality in occupational therapy should revive an important tradition of theory and practice from the early years of the field that has been dormant for several decades.

GK

I stand between two worlds.
I am at home in neither, and
*I suffer in consequence. (*Thomas Mann, *Tonio Kroger)*

The existence of emotionally and physically disabled persons can be described as bifurcated: one existence as disabled in an able-bodied world, and one existence as disabled in a world for the disabled; both are untenable. The philosophy of occupational therapy contends that every person, regardless of physical and emotional status, has the right to full and participatory membership in society. The thrust of rehabilitation is an attempt to reduce this bifurcation to a reintegration of the disabled into society at large. Rehabilitation, however, is often unsuccessful in this task.

Take, for example, two clients with whom I have been associated. One was a middle-aged woman hospitalized for acute depression with suicidal ideation. Though she had achieved maximal benefits by the hospital's criteria, she still expressed marked dissatisfaction with her life. With her husband deceased and her children grown and living out of state, her adult roles of wife, homemaker, and mother were no longer valid. Having no recourse, but still perplexed by her situation, the client was discharged by the staff. We received word one week later that she had committed suicide.

The other was a previously robust, outgoing, physically active adolescent male who sustained a C_5 cord lesion resulting in quadriplegia. Following onset of disability, his marriage engagement was broken, his friends began to abandon him, and he recognized his leisure interests and career objectives as physically impossible. Though his physical rehabilitation was proceeding successfully, his psychological status declined. Drug abuse as a coping mechanism continued upon discharge. His independence in functional activities and the integrity of his remaining physical capacity diminished markedly.

These cases represent the failure of rehabilitation—inadequate reintegration of the disabled into the prevailing social structure. The clients mentioned experienced a loss of meaning; significant occurrences in their lives had drastically altered their previous life styles which had validated for them their worth and value. No longer able to follow those lifestyles, and being unable to reorganize their lives for satisfactory and validating experiences, they engaged in maladaptation. Had there been some re-creation of meaning for these people, I do not believe they would have taken the paths they chose.

This chapter generates out of these clinical experiences, and is offered as an exploration of the phenomenon of meaning reconstruction in occupational therapy. Furthermore, principles for practice are provided by which clinicians may facilitate the reconstruction of meaning in clients as part of therapy, thereby achieving a better reintegration of the disabled into society.

A NEW PERSPECTIVE FOR OCCUPATIONAL THERAPY

Occupational therapists play a profound role in the creation, affirmation, and experience of meaning by the chronically disabled. From the early days of Slagle's habit training, in which occupational therapists imposed on clients rigid activity schedules reflecting the community at large, to these contemporary times when occupational therapists provide reality-testing experiences for clients to confirm or disconfirm their freely chosen therapeutic goals, occupational therapy has been influencing clients' acquisition of a socially confirmed constellation of meanings for their actions, or, in other words, the acquisition of socially constructed reality.

Theoretical and philosophical developments in occupational therapy have paralleled paradigmatic changes in sociological thought to the degree that the composite perspective of these two schools of thought provides the foundation for a new and insightful understanding of the impact of occupational therapy on the lives of our clients. The increasing embrace of existential thought in occupational therapy[26] first expressed in 1967 by Yerxa, the inclusion of a systems view of the human as a bio-psycho-social being inclusive of the transcendental level,[17] and the relatively new embrace of an ethnomethodological perspective[16,18] in occupational therapy, are providing a context for our discipline alternative to the essentialistic and reductionistic view of humans that characterizes our history and much of contemporary practice.[17] This burgeoning perspective in occupational therapy also represents a kindredness with significant changes in the field of sociology, thereby providing a greater store of knowledge from which to draw in an effort to enhance our understanding of the role occupational therapy plays in a client's existence.

Existential sociology, a relatively new sociological investigation of human existence from an existential stance, represents the most sophisticated component of sociology's knowledge base. The existential stance some sociologists and occupational therapists are endorsing rejects the belief that a person's subjective experiences have no impact on the self and everyday life. Only by acknowledging and addressing direct personal experience as a significant variable in the human being's existence can we begin to more fully understand the human experience,[10] including the experience of the chronically disabled person.

This chapter attempts to explicate the contribution of occupational therapy to the client's creation and affirmation of meaning by incorporating the phenomenological and ethnomethodological perspectives of existential sociology. The first step will be to explain what is meant by the existential sociological concept of "meaning." This section explores the relationship of meaning to reality as groundwork for the explanation of the sociological perspectives being utilized. Finally, the composite perspective developed will be utilized to analyze occupational therapy's role in the re-creation of clients' meaning. The thrust, however, will be a presentation of prescriptive principles by which occupational therapists may consciously foster the creation, experience, and affirmation of meaning by our clients as part of rehabilitation.

MEANING

What is meant by the concept "meaning"? As I began initial thoughts and research regarding this chapter's thesis, I encountered the problem of defining that concept. My first orientation to meaning derived from previous research in the manifestations of existentialism in occupational therapy.[26] A quest for meaning was associated with a quest for answering a fundamental question regarding human existence: "Why do I exist; what is the meaning of my life?" Existentialism does not provide an answer to that question; rather, it endorses the belief that one cannot know the answer as a solution or meaning derived from some absolute or objective source outside individual subjective experience. Some existentialists[2,27,28] go so far as to say that the meaning of one's life is created by the individual as his or her subjective experiences are shared with and validated by the community; in other words, one's life's meaning is created intersubjectively.

The existential sociological conceptualization of meaning is divorced from the almost metaphysical aura surrounding the existentialistic (philosophic) investigation of meaning; however, similarities between the two orientations abound. According to Cicourel, "the problem of meaning for the anthropologist-sociologist can be stated as that of how members of a society or culture acquire a sense of social structure that enables them to negotiate everyday activities."[7] In this quote, Cicourel identifies two major characteristics of the existential sociological perspective: meaning as pragmatic methods to accomplish goals, that is, everyday activities; and meaning as socially confirmed and shared knowledge of these methods.

MEANING AS PRAGMATIC METHODS FOR GOAL ACHIEVEMENT

It was Wittgenstein who told us that we can know the meaning of a word by looking at its use. The same dictum can be applied to physical actions as well. However, this does not mean that a word or an action will always carry the meaning associated with it in a particular situation. Meaning is contextually determined, that is, ". . . the context within which a given statement or action occurs is of fundamental importance in determining the meanings imputed to it by the members of society."[10]

An action is meaningful if it serves a practical purpose, and a person's competence is, in part, assessed by how well he chooses among various courses of action. The act or goal a person attempts to achieve provides the context within which each action or specific step to attain the goal is viewed as sensible. Therefore, for an individual action to be understood or regarded as sensible, that action must be viewed with an understanding of the intended act. The act or goal gives meaning to the actions or steps taken to achieve the goal.[1] In short, purpose becomes the context for meaning; the purpose of an action gives that action its meaning.

For example, Johnny is an autistic nine-year-old who is observed by two therapists as he repeatedly allows a ball to roll off a table. The first therapist, endorsing a behavioral theoretical perspective, views Johnny's behavior as yet another pathologic characteristic of autism, and would attempt to extinguish the behavior through extinction or reciprocal inhibition. The second therapist, endorsing an occupational behavior perspective, views Johnny's behavior as curious exploration of his environment to acquire rules of motion and rules of objects and attempts to foster even more exploratory behavior for rule acquisition. The second therapist recognizes the purpose of his behavior—to learn about the properties of a ball—and sees the behavior as meaningful. The first therapist, not recognizing the purpose, sees the behavior as meaningless. An understanding of the purpose of Johnny's behavior makes the specific behavior sensible, or meaningful.

MEANING AS SOCIALLY CONFIRMED AND SHARED KNOWLEDGE

According to Barrett,

> meaning is not, first and foremost, a mental phenomenon but an aspect of things within our daily world. Things have such-and-such a meaning as they point or refer to other things or to behavior that they elicit from us . . . . Signs, symbols, meanings—these do not enter as phenomena from a distinct realm of the mental but as aspects of the various things we encounter and have to deal with in our environment.[2]

The human environment is not composed of *objects* that possess intrinsic meaning. An object is defined as any thing toward which action can be organized or directed, and any unitary constellation of behaviors that can be designated as an event. As such, objects can be mental or physical structures or processes, things or events, such as a ghost, obtaining a college degree, and putting on one's clothes. The meanings given to objects arise from an organized interactional, or group perspective,[8] not from the ontological structure of the object.

The meanings we give to objects or actions and experiences in our lives constitute what Schutz refers to as the natural attitude, or a shared stock of knowledge essential for competent performance of day-to-day routines. It is this store of contextually determined, pragmatic, and socially shared meanings for our actions and experiences which constitutes reality.[3,5] For example, the occupational therapy patch does not inherently represent our profession, our sense of ethics, and our perspectives of mankind; the patch means all these things only because a group of people, primarily occupational therapists, have attributed these meanings to the patch and have created an interactional process, specifically education and intraprofessional functions, whereby new members learn and sustain those meanings.

What people know as reality is this common-sense stock of knowledge that enables them to function competently in their everyday lives. And, according to Berger and Luckman, ". . . It is precisely this 'knowledge' that constitutes the fabric of meanings without which no society could exist."[5] Consequently, to recognize how occupational therapists can foster the creation and affirmation of meaning in the chronically disabled, we must investigate the processes provided in the everyday world of occupational therapy for our clients that allow for the emergence of meaning.

THE WORLD OF EVERYDAY LIFE

Schutz's work is primarily responsible for the initial development of the existential, phenomenological, and ethnomethodological perspectives in contemporary sociology. He relied heavily upon the philosophical investigations of Husserl and agreed with the latter that consciousness is the generator of reality. Schutz believed that the nature of the social world and the source of shared meanings essential for communication in social life can only be understood as data of the life-world, or the everyday world. The problem of the origin of social life and shared meanings

> . . . is rather a datum of the life-world. It [the everyday world] is the fundamental ontological category of human existence in the world and therefore of all philosophical anthropology. As long as man is born of woman, . . . [the world of everyday life] . . . will be the foundation for all other categories of human existence.[25]

Consequently, Schutz established the world of everyday life as the primary source of sociological data. In response to this direction, Schutz attempted to develop a general theory of meaning grounded in everyday life to explain the relationship between an act, an actor, and a situation, or individuals and their behavior in a given situation.

Schutz's conceptualization of the world of everyday life is that of an *intersubjective* world, an organized world experienced as real or valid by most people. This world is interpreted or understood by a stock of common knowledge passed on to us by our predecessors and *modified* by our interactions with objects (human and nonhuman) in our environment. The most astonishing feature of this world is that it is taken for granted by people:

> As common-sense men living in the mundane world, we tacitly assume that, of course, there *is* this world all of us share as the public domain within which we communicate, work, and live our lives. . . . We naively assume . . . that the rough present in which we find ourselves is epistemically given to all normal men in much the same way. . . . We simply assume, presuppose, take it for granted that the daily world in which all of these activities [play, love, creation, suffering, death] go on is *there;* it is only on special occasions, if at all, that a serious doubt arises as to the veridical character of the philosophical signification of our everyday world.[20]

The world of everyday life is the paramount reality. Even though alternative realities exist—the child's playworld, insanity, art, dreams, intellectual pursuit—our point of reference is always the world of everyday life; it is the world in which we physically, and most often mentally, locate our bodies and minds. It is also the realm of existence that we can manipulate and change through bodily activities.[20,23]

The everyday world is a social world; the knowledge taken for granted regarding this world is assumed to be taken for granted by all participants in this everyday world. "The power of socially approved knowledge is so extended that what the whole in-group approves—ways of thinking and acting, such as mores, folkways, habits—is simply taken for granted; it becomes an element of the relatively natural concept of the world. . . ."[24] The taken-for-granted aspect of this world allows social interaction and physical activity to be executed without placing impossible demands on the cognitive capacities of individuals.[21] Day-to-day activities are addressed and executed via socially given and enculturated methods; the person does not have to attend consciously to these activities and to create new ways of accomplishing them each time the necessity of a given activity arises.

The stock of knowledge by which we know the everyday world is acquired through social learning and is necessary for competent performance of day-to-day activities. The shared operational procedures which we utilize to execute these routines, such as putting on our clothes, answering the phone, and knowing when to come in out of the rain, are known as *typifications*. Our knowledge of the social world is, for the most part, in the form of typifications. Typifications are extractions of the standardized, recurrent, and objective characteristics of any phenomena, such as life styles, dressing, crossing a street, and the establishment of types based on those extractions. Typifications are formed in relation to some purpose at hand.[24] An example of a typification would be how to make a ham sandwich, or how to get dressed. Although each particular instance of such acts will have its own unique features and a one-time-only unfolding nature, these are ignored and it is relegated to a class of typified sandwich makings or dressings. People designated as incompetent or insane act as though these routines or typifications are arbitrary or illegitimate.[1] People who incur physical disability find that their typifications no longer are legitimate.[21]

The exception to knowing the social world through typifications is knowing the world, or a person in it, through the *we-relation*. As a person interacts with another person, that person can experience the other in his or her uniqueness, not as a type. However, when one begins to reflect upon, or attend to, the we-relationship as it occurs, typifications emerge; one begins to interact with the other on the basis of types.[15,23] For example, most people as students establish one or more relationships with their teachers that are more personal than the typical student-teacher relationship. While interacting with that teacher on a personal basis, that is, within the context of a we-relation, the student acquires information and feelings about the teacher that are idiosyncratic to that person which would not ordinarily be obtained in the more formal relationship. However, when student and teacher are in a classroom situation, or when the student during the we-relationship attends to the person as a teacher, the student responds to, thinks about the teacher as a type, as a teacher and all that is entailed in that label.

Typifications or types of human behaviors important to this chapter's thesis are the personal ideal type and the course-of-action type:

> The course-of-action type serves as the objective meaning of an action, that is, the type is "what is being done" or "what has been done." The personal ideal type, on the other hand, tells us the subjective meaning in the mind of the person who executes a certain action.[15]

In other words, the personal ideal type is a typification or a model of a person performing a given task, for example, therapist, teacher, spouse. The course-of-action type is a typification of the expressive or behavioral process of that performance, the typical outward results of a process; for example, the typical behaviors enacted by a teacher or a spouse. The course-of-action and the personal ideal types are intimately related. An understanding of any personal ideal type is based on knowledge of the course-of-action type. In other words, you cannot define the ideal type of teacher without first having an understanding of what a teacher typically does.

The appropriate typifications are recognized by an actor and observer by imputing motives to behaviors, by understanding acts as means to specific ends. By employing motives to typify a person's behavior as a course-of-action type appropriate for a personal ideal type, we begin to understand why a person is emitting a given behavior or action:

> In the process of understanding a given performance via an ideal type, the interpreter must start with his own perceptions of someone else's manifest act. His goal is to discover the . . . motive . . . behind the act. He does this by interpreting the act within an objective context of meaning in the sense that the same motive is postulated as constant for the act regardless of who performs the act or what his subjective experiences are at the time. For a personal ideal type, therefore, there is one and only one typical motive for a typical act.[23]

Schutz also believes that what a person views as meaningful depends upon what is reflected upon in that person's stream of consciousness or experience. Schutz further states that "Our practical interest alone, as it arises in a certain situation of our life . . . is the only relevant principle in the building up of the perspective structure in which our social world appears to us in daily life."[24] Schutz is acknowledging that what becomes meaningful to a person is a function of what he or she attends to as pragmatic necessities within life situations of relevance to that person.

Finally, Schutz recognizes that the reality of the everyday world can become problematic, that the taken-for-granted aspect of existence can become suspect or questioned. "This will be the case, for example, if there occurs in the individual or social life an event or situation which cannot be met by applying the traditional and habitual pattern of behavior or interpretation. We call such a situation a crisis."[24] Schutz refers to these crises as imposed relevances, situations or events that become relevant to us not of our choosing. A primary source of imposed relevance is disease or disability which renders typifications illegitimate.

THE SOCIAL CONSTRUCTION OF MEANING

Berger relies heavily on Schutz's phenomenological perspective in his efforts to explain how reality is socially constructed. He views the construction of a social or objective reality as the process of the creation and reappropriation of typifications and language by the individual. This process is referred to as the *dialectic*.

> The fundamental dialectic process of society consists of three moments, or steps. These are externalization, objectivation, and internalization. Only if these three moments are understood together can an empirically adequate view of society be maintained. Externalization is the ongoing outpouring of human being into the world, both in the physical and mental activity of men. Objectivation is the attainment by the products of this activity (again both physical and mental) of a reality that confronts its original producers as a facticity external to and other than themselves. Internalization is the reappropriation by men of this same reality, transforming it once again from structures of the objective world into structures of the subjective consciousness. It is through externalization that society is a human product. It is through objectivation that society becomes a reality *sui generis*. It is through internalization that man is a product of society.[3]

Externalization represents the individual's attempt to transform subjective experiences into objective representations of those experiences. Human productions, be they tangible or intangible, physical or mental, are objective manifestations of subjective experience. The primary agents of externalization are language and typifications. When the psychotic patient says that his stomach is infested with snakes, and when Einstein expressed his theory of relativity, language was utilized to externalize a previously subjectively maintained experience or opinion. If, through social validation, these externalized productions are legitimated as "proper," "necessary," or "real," they are internalized as the true reality.

Objectivation is defined as the

> . . . transformation of man's products into a world that not only derives from man, but that comes to confront him as a facticity outside of himself. . . . The humanly produced world becomes something "out there." It consists of objects, both material and nonmaterial, that are capable of resisting the desires of their producer. . . . It stands outside the subjectivity of the individual as, indeed, a world. In other words, the humanly produced world attains the character of objective reality.[3]

Examples of objectivations are political ideologies, theoretical perspectives, roles, stereotypes, architectural barriers, and so forth.

Internalization is the resorption into an individual's consciousness of the externalized, objectivated and legitimated subjective experiences that constitute socially defined reality. Internalization is achieved through the socialization process in which the individual learns and identifies with the meanings in this social world.[3] Therefore, the occupational therapist's internalization of the social reality of occupational therapy is achieved through the socialization inherent in occupational therapy education. The internalization of the social reality of chronic disability is achieved through the socialization of clients into that reality as defined in hospitalization.

Einstein's theory of relativity is a good example of the dialectic. His expressions—verbal, written, and physical in terms of experiments and demonstrations—of his theory constituted externalization. Objectivation occurred as his theory was made available to various members of the scientific community; these people were confronted with a theory proposing an alternative view to the then dominant typification of Newtonian physics. Research and the scientific community's endorsement legitimated the theory of relativity. As internalization, scientists began to rely upon Einstein's work, to couch their research in the theory and to teach the theory to new and developing scientists.

Given the great variability in humans' subjective experiences, what is to prevent the objective or social reality from being rejected and replaced by multiple solipsistic realities resulting from the externalization of idiosyncratic experiences and meanings? The answer is legitimation, or social validation of the dialectical products. Legitimation is socially objectivated knowledge that explains and justifies the social reality. But, for these legitimations to be effective, they must be internalized or subjectively apprehended by the individual as real or valid. The primary vehicles for the maintenance and legitimation of social reality, both as the objective or social manifestation of that reality, and the subjective apprehension of that reality as valid, are language and interaction in the everyday world.[3,5]

"The plausibility and stability of the world, as socially defined is dependent upon the strength and continuity of significant relationships in which conversation about this world can be continually carried on."[4] In other words, the social reality is maintained via conversation with significant others. Also, the subjective apprehension of that reality as valid is maintained and legitimated through everyday, casual conversation. "Indeed, its [reality] massivity is achieved by the accumulation and consistency of casual conversation—conversation that can *afford to be casual* precisely because it refers to the routines of a taken-for-granted reality."[5]

METHODS OF SOCIAL CONSTRUCTION OF MEANING

Various ethnomethodologists have based their works on Schutz's and Berger's perspectives but have investigated the actual methods of the production of social reality employed by society's members. The outcome has been an identification of the concepts *"indexicals," "glossing,"* and the *"et cetera problem"* as major methods by which the socially real environment is understood and constructed. Ethnomethodologists further posit the existence of an underlying, unstated scheme of interpretive procedures that allows indexicals, glossing, and et cetera problems to provide meaningful accounts of objects, actions, and events in social reality. These interpretive procedures, referred to as *background expectancies,* also are utilized by humans to accord the status of "meaningful" or "real" to human objectivations.[6,7,12,13] Consequently, it appears that the ethnomethodological investigations provide a more definitive explanation of Berger's concepts of reality maintenance and legitimation, especially the communicative—verbal and nonverbal—means of maintenance and legitimation.

INDEXICALS, GLOSSING, AND THE ET CETERA PROBLEM

Indexicals are expressions, the meaning of which is the sum of the expression's typical meaning and its contextually determined meaning. Contextual determinants of meaning are biographical characteristics, that is, (a) who is making the expression, for example, a quadriplegic; (b) to whom the expression is directed, therapist or wife, for example; (c) where the expression is made, for example, home or clinic; (d) the social relationship between the teller and hearer; and (e) the purpose of the actor.[13,14] In short, indexicals refer to the practical, or use, context for the determination of meaning.[9]

Glossing is the occurrence of communicating more than what is said. It is the phenomenon ". . . whereby speakers in the situated particulars of speech mean something and are understood as meaning something different from what they can say in just so many words. . . ."[14]

The *et cetera problem* is accurately summed up by Sacks: "To any description of a concrete object (or event, or course of action, or etc.), however long, the researcher must add an et cetera clause to permit the description to be brought to a close."[22]

The latter two represent linguistic contexts for the determination of the meaning of an act, account, or object. It is through the use of these communicative characteristics—glossing, indexicality, and et cetera problem—that the socially accepted meaning of an account, event, or object can be communicated and understood (i.e., take on meaning) without a complete communicative expression of that account, event, or object.

BACKGROUND EXPECTANCIES

The background expectancies that enable these communicative characteristics to make meaningful and useful the accounts of everyday life are of three types: assumptions, emergence, and relativity. The assumptions are of (a) a taken-for-granted world shared by humans in a society, (b) a shared time perspective, (c) continuity and stability of events and objects, (d) trust that these assumptions hold true, and (e) reciprocity of perspectives on the part of members in a society.[7,12,13]

Paap provides an apt explanation of the background expectancies of emergence of meaning through time and relativity of meaning through space; therefore his words are presented verbatim:

> [According to McHugh (1968)] In time of orderly interaction, the "basic procedural rules" of "emergence" predominate. This means that "meaning" is a matter of joining events to an ongoing "theme," and anticipating the future and reconstructing the past in terms of this theme. However, when a "disruption" occurs, the emphasis shifts to basic procedural rules of "relativity." Here, meaning is found by focusing on the immediate arrangements in the environment (the "social present").[21]

That is to say that when a person is functioning in accordance with the common store of knowledge characterizing the everyday life of "abled" people, he or she obtains meaning for actions along a metachronological continuum indigenous to each person. Actions are executed, and their meaning understood in reference to a theme or trajectory expanding over past, present, and future. In other words, meaning emerges through time.[19] However, when the common store of knowledge of everyday life is no longer valid for a person due to disability, the person resorts to the procedure of relativity for understanding or meaning. That is to say that a disabled person may have to reject meaning as obtained in relation to long-term chronological plans if the disability eliminates capacities for those plans. Instead, the person has to obtain meaning in the here-and-now by executing and understanding actions in reference to objects in the immediate environments.[19]

Therefore, it appears that persons create meaning in their daily lives by relying upon these background expectancies. That meaning is, in essence, legitimation and maintenance of the socially defined reality, both objectively (externally) and subjectively (internally).

In summary, meaning is social reality, or the shared stock of knowledge found in the world of everyday life. The structures of this meaning are typifications and the we-relations; these structures represent (a) pragmatic methods for goal achievement and (b) socially confirmed and shared knowledge. Meaning in the form of typification allows for an individual's habituation; that is, typical procedures and understandings shared by members of a social group eliminate the need for conscious attention to and exploration of all objects or events in a person's life, thereby allowing a socially acceptable daily routine occurring on a habitual level. An individual's particular array of typifications, and the sequence in which these are acquired, are influenced by the person's interests, or pragmatic necessities relevant to that person's life.

The social reality or meaning is constructed through the dialectic process in which internal, individual experiences of humans are externalized, then objectivated or presented as a facticity, and if legitimated, internalized by humans as part of social reality. The legitimation and maintenance of this socially constructed meaning occurs through language and interaction in the everyday world.

Specific methods of the social constructions, legitimation and maintenance of meaning are indexicality, glossing, and the et cetera problem. These methods rely upon a constellation of background expectancies, specifically assumptions, emergence, and relativity.

DISRUPTION OF REALITY AND SOCIAL RECONSTRUCTION OF REALITY THROUGH OCCUPATIONAL THERAPY

DISRUPTION OF REALITY

As discussed earlier, Schutz recognizes the possibility of crisis, or disruption of the social reality, as a result of an imposed relevance in the form of disease or disability. But he only explores this phenomenon to the degree to say that, in such crises, "the traditional and habitual patterns of behavior or interpretation no longer are adequate methods by which to competently execute everyday activities."[24]

Berger pursues this issue further. He claims that in these crisis situations, where the taken-for-granted nature of everyday life is at least partially disintegrated, reality is redefined to a degree; but persons experiencing these crisis situations are often resocialized into the prevailing reality structure via explicit and intensive ritual techniques that confirm that structure.[3,5] Therapy is an example of such ritual. In therapy, the client is placed in an environment, or a plausibility structure, characterized by a specific social base and social processes endorsing the prevailing reality structure.[5] For example, a quadriplegic undergoing rehabilitation will be placed in a facility that has a social base constructed of cord-injured patients functioning within the context of the greater social structure— society. In this environment, significant others interact with the client to mediate the new or modified reality of quadriplegia in society to him or her. The therapeutic activities the patient will be required to engage in will function as ritual-like techniques resocializing the client.

Berger has provided an apt description of therapy from the existential sociological perspective. Ethnomethodologists, in their investigations of disruption of social reality, have identified conditions of such disruption in terms recognizable as the psychosocial consequences of emotional and physical disability. When a person experiences disability, his or her social reality is disrupted. The background expectancies the person had adequately relied upon to competently exist as a member of society prior to disability have been invalidated. As a result of that invalidation, certain psychosocial consequences occur. The consequences are easily recognizable in therapy:

> . . . Events should lose their perceivedly normal character. The member should be unable to recognize an event's status as typical. Judgments of likelihood should fail him. He should be unable to assign present occurrences to similar orders of events he has known in the past. He should be unable to order these events to means-ends relationships. . . . Stable and "realistic" matchings of intentions and objects should dissolve, by which I mean that the ways, otherwise familiar to him, in which the objective perceived environment serves as

both the motivating grounds of feelings and is motivated by feelings directed to it, should become obscure. In short, the members' real perceived environment on losing its known-in-common background should become "specifically senseless." Ideally speaking, behaviors directed to such a senseless environment should be those of bewilderment, uncertainty, internal conflict, psycho-social isolation, acute, and nameless anxiety along with various symptoms of acute depersonalization. Structures of interaction should be correspondingly disorganized.[13]

SOCIAL CONSTRUCTION OF REALITY THROUGH OCCUPATIONAL THERAPY

Thus, we have the central thesis of this chapter: By accepting the existential sociological perspective of the social construction of reality, and by viewing physical disability and mental illness as part and parcel of the disruption or disconfirmation of social reality, one can identify certain elements in the occupational therapy process that foster social reconstruction of reality in our clients. Physical disability and mental illness as disruptions of social reality represent an invalidation of previously valid typifications, as well as a disruption of the background expectancies which served to maintain and legitimate those typifications. Occupational therapy, as a plausibility structure or environment for the physically and emotionally disabled, and fostering the externalizations and subsequent objectivations and internalizations of the disabled, serves to generate the disabled's reconstruction of social reality. By fostering the acquisition of new typifications and the legitimation and maintenance of these through specific activities, based initially on the background expectancy of relativity of meaning through space, occupational therapy allows for the re-creation of meaning for the disabled within the prevailing reality structure. The disabled's new constellation of meanings is then compatible with the social reality; the disabled achieves a reintegration with the prevailing social structure.

In a study of the rehabilitation of spinal cord injured patients, Paap[21] concludes that rehabilitation involves a reconstruction of social reality and that the typifications giving shape to that reality arise primarily out of the patient's "here and now" bodily conditions (the immediate experience of body and mind disruption), interpersonal relations, and experiences of self during hospitalization. His work consists of an analysis of subjective experience as the foundation of the reconstruction of reality and an identification of the occurrences of externalization, objectivation, and reality maintenance in a rehabilitation setting. Even though Paap's work is delimited to a study of quadriplegics and paraplegics, he was investigating a phenomenon—the social reconstruction of reality—that characterizes the rehabilitation of both the physically and emotionally disabled. Consequently, I will generalize Paap's findings to an interpretation of the role of occupational therapy in the construction of social reality in our clients.

TYPIFICATIONS BASED ON BODILY CONDITIONS. Externalization and objectivation, as noted previously, are the "outpouring of human activity" and the attainment by those products of a socially validated, "objective," form that is no longer solely the subjective experience of the producer; in short, subjective experience is externalized as mental or physical activity and acquires an objective or socially shared status. However, products externalized initially in chronic disability and rehabilitation are often associated with confusion and depression and do not attain the status of objectivations; they are not socially validated as appropriate reconstructions of reality, for example, death wishes and hopelessness. The same applies to fantasy experiences of the initially disabled as well as denial experiences of the disability and its impact on the patient's occupational performance.[21]

Typifications as externalizations characterizing the "real" world for the chronically disabled in rehabilitation are initially and primarily based on the routines of patient care and treatment in the hospital; in other words, the disabled rely initially upon the background expectancy of the relativity of meaning through space as opposed to the emergence of meaning through time in an effort to understand and deal with their current condition. They focus on understanding the meaning of their disability in the here-and-now by learning what they are still capable of doing and what they are no longer able to do by attending to objects in the present; they no longer rely upon long-term plans to provide meaning inasmuch as they often are unable to achieve those plans due to disability.

Of concern to us are the "outpourings of human activity" in the form of occupational therapy that constitute externalization and objectivation. The initial externalizations by the patient largely pertain to the altered body and perceptions.[21] Schutz would claim that this initial focus is a result of the patients' practical interest fostering reflection upon their body and mind disruptions; this pragmatic-oriented reflection represents the chief principle by which disabled persons develop a perspective from which to reconstruct their reality, to give meaning to their altered beings.

The patient's common stock of knowledge, his everyday world, has lost much of its taken-for-granted quality; his previously effective course-of-action types and personal ideal types are now ineffective. The background expectancies of a shared, taken-for-granted world, trust, stability of objects and events, and reciprocity of perspectives have been disconfirmed. Consequently, the patient must develop new typifications, new personal ideal types and course-of-action types specific to his or her role as a disabled member of society. This is the fundamental problem in rehabilitation.

Occupational therapy fosters the development of new course-of-action types by addressing the issues of physical, emotional and interpersonal functions, activities of daily living (ADL), and vocational and prevocational exploration and training with clients. We help clients learn or acquire new typifications based on what they can do—physically, cognitively or psychologically, and socially—in light of their disability by engaging them in occupational therapy activities which are representative of the tasks of life they will be required to execute as members of society. When we help clients relearn or acquire modified versions of skills such as eating, dressing, and correctly computing the amount of change expected in a purchase, and when we allow clients to discuss their fears regarding difficulties in locomotion, sexual capabilities, and so forth, we are fostering their acquisition of new course-of-action types specific to the personal ideal types of their disability categories. These typifications, depending on their effectiveness and their social acceptability, will be validated by the therapy staff and other patients initially as socially appropriate.

Two objectivations that occupational therapists foster a redefinition of in clients and that directly impact the development of new course-of-action types and personal ideal types are time and space.[21] The client comes to accept a new meaning for space and its correlate, distance, by experiencing these phenomena anew as a disabled person. Such experiences could be attempting to fit a wheelchair through a door when there is not enough clearance, attempting to walk from the ward to the cafeteria when one's energy reserve is markedly impaired by psychotropic medications, or attempting to negotiate the use of a small bathroom when one is required to use a walker. A function of distance in the presentation of self is of particular concern to the physically disabled, especially those wheelchair-bound. At a distance of 10 to 12 feet, the entire body becomes the expressive unit; persons paralyzed have limited control over the impression given off by virtue of their physical status at that distance. However, if the disabled person is close enough to another so that the other can attend only to the face, arms, or hands, then the disabled person is better able to control the impression he or she gives.[21]

Time becomes a redefined objectivation due to the alteration in time requirements for the performance of practical activities.[21] Occupational therapists foster this redefinition by counseling the patient regarding changes in time requirements and energy conservation, by allowing the client to experience these changes first-hand, and by providing adaptive equipment and techniques for the quicker execution of time consuming tasks. An example of how occupational therapists impact this objectivation would be giving a client whose energy reserve is markedly impaired experience with utilizing time and motion saving techniques while washing, drying, and folding clothes. Other typical incidences that occupational therapists impact in regard to time are dressing, toileting, locomotion, and so forth.

Disability's disruption of the background expectancies of a shared, taken-for-granted world, and of a reciprocity of perspectives disconfirms personal ideal types and their imputed motives in the patient's interpersonal existence as well.[21] Not only are the personal ideal types and course-of-action types altered for the individual encountering disability, the typifications of other people with whom the disabled person has interpersonal relationships are also altered. The client, for example a quadriplegic, must develop new typifications that will allow him or her to function as a competent member of society while still remaining quadriplegic. He or she must learn new ways of dressing, eating, mobility, and so forth, that characterize quadriplegics and that are validated as acceptable by society. Additionally, the quadriplegic must redefine the personal ideal types and corresponding course-of-action types enacted by significant others in the quadriplegic's life. A classic example of this occurrence and the effort to impute new motives to a relationship is that of a cord-injured male's suspicions and perplexity regarding why his girlfriend still claims to remain devoted to him, thinking that she may be remaining in the relationship out of pity or sympathy, and not out of love for him as before his injury.

TYPIFICATIONS BASED ON INTERPERSONAL RELATIONS. Occupational therapy fosters the reconstruction of reality through interpersonal relations in two primary ways. First, therapists represent personal ideal types whose motives for interaction with patients can be taken for granted by staff and patients. These types provide some stability and continuity of events and objects for patients; they assume that the therapist is there for a specific purpose and will elicit their engagement in anticipated events and procedures.[21] Consequently, the occupational therapist is reconfirming certain background expectancies and helping the client reconstruct a set of personal ideal types with imputed motives.

The second way is by creating treatment settings that allow the client to engage in non-staff relationships of three major types. One type is the we-relations that Schutz acknowledges as the primary opportunity for a person to be experienced in his or her uniqueness, and not as a type. By creating groups in which patients can interact in ways not predicated by their disabilities and therapy, situations in which social activity, small talk, and friendly banter are the objectives, we allow patients to externalize elements of the self that go beyond being a disabled person.[21] These interactions provide for "a more generalized grounding for the everyday world"[21] than do the interactions with therapists; the latter, due to the restricted nature of the interaction, foster typifications characteristic only of the client's disability. Furthermore, the we-relation implies the existence of a self more diffuse than the disabled self that is taken for granted in such interactions; consequently, background expectancies are reconfirmed and the taken-for-granted nature of the everyday world is redeveloped.[21]

The remaining two types of non-staff relationships that occupational therapists foster as treatment for social reconstruction of reality are family therapy sessions in which both patient and family members examine, question, and negotiate new relationships and imputed motives, and outings into the community. The latter involves conscious typifications of motives for non-hospital personnel by the disabled,[21] a task the disabled will be undertaking post-discharge for as long as is required for them to fully reconstruct their social reality.

TYPIFICATIONS BASED ON EXPERIENCES OF SELF. Aspects of the client's self are also the products of externalization and objectivation in occupational therapy. By engaging in therapy, clients externalize aspects of self that they experience as real. This occurrence has been addressed earlier in terms of externalizing the self as disabled via experiencing the physical grounding and interpersonal grounding of the disabled self in the client's everyday world, specifically the physical and social activities predicated on disability and generated as occupational therapy. However, clients do not readily accept the definition of self solely as that implied in therapeutic activities; disability does not provide a positive and viable self-image in society.[5] Clients attempt to expand the definition of self by engaging in we-relationships, as discussed above. They also attempt to maintain a more valued sense of self by engaging in treatment routines and nontreatment activities in a manner that may be construed by staff as inappropriate.[21] Drug stashes, intoxication, bragging, and loudness regarding sexual exploits, as well as a cavalier approach to therapeutic activities and a denial laden belief in a return to normal function by the client can represent the patient's attempt to externalize a self that goes beyond the externalized self as disabled. How we, as therapists, and consequently as a major source of social validation of externalizations, respond to these efforts, and possibly even the timing of our responses, may have a significant impact on the eventually externalized self and self-image of the client.

Occupational therapy also fosters the externalization of self beyond the image of disabled by allowing clients to creatively express themselves in the arts and crafts activities that characterize much of our treatment modalities. Whether it is a grooming group in which patients learn to style their hair, or a leather group in which patients design and execute the engravings, these people are placing their benchmarks on products that represent the externalization and objectivation of a self broader than that defined by rehabilitation practices for the disabled.

ETHNOMETHODOLOGICAL FUNCTIONS OF OCCUPATIONAL THER-APY. Ethnomethodologically, occupational therapy contributes to the client's reconstruction of reality by providing background expectancies that function as broad limits defining what the patient will incorporate into reality and what externalizations by the patient will be validated as "real." Paap refers to these boundaries as "a priori 'givens' intrinsic to the context"[21] of the hospital and therapy settings. The first given is the previously addressed pragmatic orientation as the basis for the emergence of typifications; clients meet the requirements of their immediate physical and emotional situation as they engage in therapy. A second given intrinsic to occupational therapy environments is language. The nature of the clients' everyday world is influenced by the vocabulary they acquire during occupational therapy. The typifications of patients who are able to discuss their schizophrenia or quadriplegia are, in nature, recognizably different from the typifications of relatively naive patients. Clients knowledgeable of their disabilities are more likely to know their capabilities and limitations; this knowledge will be communicated directly and indirectly in their discussion. The sharing of this knowledge in actions and discussions during occupational therapy serves to legitimate the reality of the disabilities and to mediate the new reality to other members of the social structure of the clinic. Cultural givens endorsed and addressed in occupational therapy constitute a third major group of background expectancies controlling the emergence of typifications and the assignment of "real" to the client's externalizations. These givens deal with such issues as beauty, grace, and the value of work. A classic example of occupational therapy employing this given is the utilization of the task-oriented treatment group[11] to foster better reality testing.

We have already indirectly discussed occupational therapy as a given in and of itself by being a part of the routine of hospitalization. Patients experience occupational therapy as a source of background expectancies by engaging in the activities that constitute occupational therapy, by experiencing occupational therapy as a validator of externalization, and by experiencing occupational therapy as part of a routine of daily activities that dominate their everyday lives and are socially validated as a necessary part of that life.

Occupational therapy also plays a significant role in the client's maintenance and legitimation of the newly reconstructed everyday world of reality. The reality of the client's world, predicated on disability, is continually made manifest throughout the patient's daily activities.[21] As Berger would put it, the "massive facticity" of this aspect of the client's world is so overwhelming that it is self-maintaining. But other aspects of this reality built on the physical or emotional limitations characteristic of a client's manifestation of disability are not self-maintaining. These aspects are maintained by occupational therapy through the routines and trivia that can characterize therapy, through the utilization of the past, and through the opportunity for externalization and objectivation of aspects of self beyond disability.[21]

The routines in occupational therapy, and occupational therapy as a part of a greater daily routine called rehabilitation, convey to the patient a feeling of continuity of a world independent of the client. These routines eventually allow the development of taken-for-granted elements in the client's reconstructed reality; the client develops course-of-action types and personal ideal types which eventually allow the client to attend competently to daily activities without having to invest great quantities of conscious attention to the execution of these tasks.

The trivia that can occur in occupational therapy, such as idle discussions regarding football, weather, television programs, and the like, maintain the social reality by providing continuity with the patient's past, by reaffirming the existence of a reality beyond the hospital, and more importantly by allowing the re-emergence of the linguistic practices of glossing, indexicality, and the et cetera phenomenon. Through these characteristics of everyday speech with staff and similarly disabled persons, a client experiences reconfirmation of background expectancies and legitimation and maintenance of the new reality. The client experiences the new reality as intersubjective, or shared, and re-acquires a trust in the assumptions that constitute the background expectancies.

Occupational therapy utilizes the client's past for reality legitimation and maintenance in two major ways. First, we determine the client's assets. This step is essentially an identification of typifications that are still valid for the client. We incorporate these assets into therapy programs, thereby utilizing the past as a resource for some elements of reality reconstruction. For the client, this acknowledgment of the past is confirmation of the existence of a reality beyond the immediate experiences of rehabilitation and hospitalization. A second, but lesser, use of the past that occupational therapy endorses is reminiscence about one's history. Whether a life review with the elderly, or a discussion of a specific event in a client's history, we foster the acknowledgment of a past that also confirms the existence of a patient's reality as something larger in scope than the aspect identified in hospitalization.

The final way in which occupational therapy can foster reality legitimation and maintenance was discussed above. Not only through the provision for engagement in activities that reflect the client's physical and interpersonal grounding in his newly developing reality do we influence reality legitimation and maintenance. Also, through the provision of opportunities to externalize self beyond that of "disabled" via arts and crafts activities, occupational therapy fosters the legitimation and maintenance of a reality that is more satisfying to the client than a reality solely predicated on disability.

THERAPEUTIC PRINCIPLES

The information thus far presented supports the view that occupational therapy serves as a plausibility structure or environment for the disabled that creates situations which evoke externalizations specific to various disabilities. These externalizations, as physical, mental, and social typifications, are then disconfirmed or affirmed in the social order of the clinic, reflecting the greater social order of society. If affirmed, these externalizations are objectified as a facticity of the clinic and the disability; they acquire the status of real. These objectivations are then internalized and maintained by the clients via various therapeutic activities. This internalization represents the construction of a new reality, of new meaning for the disabled that is compatible with the reality of the greater social order in which the disabled will participate. Within this perspective, the ultimate goal of occupational therapy is to generate in the client a body of knowledge shared by abled and disabled members of society alike; this body of knowledge will be socially approved typifications that enable the disabled person to competently function as a participating member of society.

A systematic and conscious effort in occupational therapy to positively affect the client's creation of new meanings as a member of society can be achieved by adhering to several basic principles.

The most crucial principle is to *acknowledge and incorporate into therapy the fact that what the disabled person initially finds meaningful will be generated out of that person's practical interest alone.* The skills and interactions which will be of primary concern to the client will be those of pragmatic necessity; skills and functions, or typifications, which *the client* considers of major importance, not necessarily functions the therapist considers most important. In order to firmly establish the new and socially validated reality in the client, therapy must begin by identifying and subsequently addressing those skills the client finds most crucial. This means that in addition to evaluating for performance assets and liabilities, therapists should evaluate for those skills or performances the client finds the most meaningful. This evaluation and the therapy based upon it should be consciously recognized by the client as effort to re-establish the skills he or she finds most meaningful.

This identifcation of the most meaningful typifications for the client provides the foundation in therapy for an effective reconstruction of reality or meaning. The therapist will know specifically what skills the client is motivated to address; in other words, what redefined typifications the therapist will be most successful in facilitating for the client. With this knowledge the second principle of therapy can be utilized: *Typifications first facilitated in therapy should be based on the client's here-and-now bodily condition, and then based on interpersonal relationships.* The core of a client's new reality is based on his or her disability. No typifications regarding interpersonal relationships or self above and beyond disability can be validated until the client has acquired the necessary skills for adequate and feasible function within his or her nonhuman environment. The client must first know the range and limits of his functional capacity *before* he can adequately develop typifications regarding interpersonal behaviors inasmuch as the essence of those new typifications will be contingent upon what he is or is not capable of doing as understood by others.

Once the array of typifications based on the bodily condition is fairly established, typifications arising out of the interpersonal relationships should be facilitated. The third principle is that *typifications arising out of interpersonal relationships should be based on staff relations, we-relations, family relations, and community-based relations.* Interactions with staff, specifically with therapists, nurses, doctors, and so forth, provide an array of persons constant in their behaviors, performances, and expectations toward the client. As such, the staff represents personal ideal types with motives for interaction with the client that can be taken for granted by client and staff alike. The result is not only the development of typifications of human behavior and motives but also the reconfirmation of certain background expectancies, specifically the taken-for-granted nature of the world, and a reciprocity of perspectives.

The development of typifications based on staff relations occurs as a function of rehabilitation in general. However, typifications based on the other types of relations generally occur haphazardly. Conscious effort in therapy should be made to facilitate the development of typifications based on we-relations, family relations, and community-based relations in order for the client to have an adequate constellation of typifications necessary for reintegration into the social order. We-relations should be generated as a part of occupational therapy, accomplished by designing group activities parallel or participatory in nature that allow clients to interact in ways not defined by their disabilities or by traditional therapy. Clients should be allowed to interact with others in ways not restricted to the traditional aims of rehabilitation. They should have the opportunity to interact as unique individuals, not as quadriplegics, schizophrenics, and so forth, undergoing therapy. Such activities would be directed by the participants, not by the therapist.

The particular verbal or physical behaviors would occur spontaneously and would foster the externalization of elements of self unrelated to disability.

Therapeutic sessions should be generated in which the client interacts with family members so that all involved can redefine relationships and motives, if need be. Initially, the sessions should occur in the hospital environment, with the presence of a therapist who is abreast of the client's condition, progress, and prognosis. The therapist may intervene when discussions or interactions approach an invalidation of valid typifications held by the client. Then, as rehabilitation progresses, the client should be allowed home visits in which he or she will have to rely upon redefined typifications to function in a different physical and social environment. At any rate, the family members should be aware of what the client is capable of doing, so that their efforts to help will not result in the invalidation of the client's skills or typifications.

Community-based relations should also be generated as a conscious part of therapy. If a disabled person is to become a participatory member of society, he or she will have to be able to control interactions with others in society in such a way that his or her functional integrity is not compromised by the naive benevolence of others. The client must acquire the abilities to place limits on other people's efforts to help, and to withstand the prejudice and sympathy that may invalidate his or her role as a social member. Outings into the community where a client will encounter other people will provide direct experiences that can be examined and utilized for the development of such skills.

Inasmuch as disability does not provide a viable self-image in society, *therapy should foster the externalizations of self beyond those predicated on disability*. As a result, the client's self-image will be composed of perceptions not only of disability but of aspects unrelated to the disabling condition. Therapy can facilitate this broadened self-image in three ways. The first is to foster we-relations, as discussed above. The second is to recognize that the cavalier and sometimes obnoxious behavior of clients may be an attempt to externalize aspects of self beyond that of disability. The role of the therapist in this case is to tolerate such behaviors when those behaviors are perceived as an effort to claim an existence beyond that of disabled. Do not chastise or verbally ridicule the client in these instances. Allow the client the freedom to express oneself, even inappropriately, if the expressions are an attempt to identify an image beyond that of disability.

The third way by which occupational therapy can facilitate a broadened self-image is through creative activity. Through relatively unstructured activities, such as arts and crafts, and even some ADL, the client is able to create products that are neither a reflection of disability, nor a reflection of socially imposed standards. Whether sculpture, painting, sewing, woodwork, or whatever, the client is able to create a product that says "Look! I am not just a disabled person: I am also a person who can do this, or who sees the world this way, regardless of my disability."

To maintain continuity and stability of events and objects existing prior to and during disability, thereby maintaining some of the background expectancies, *typifications characteristic of the predisability existence but still viable should be incorporated into therapy*; this is the fifth principle. Evaluation should include an identification of those typifications still functional for the client; in other words, an identification of assets. These assets, in addition to providing a foundation for the newly emerging meaning for the client, confirm the existence of a reality and a self-image that transcends the immediate experiences of rehabilitation. As interests, valued goals, and career objectives, they also provide substance for the transition from the background expectancy of relativity of meaning through space to the background expectancy of emergence of meaning through time. Therapy up to this point will be characterized by a disruption of the acquisition of meaning as the appropriateness of actions within the context of a meta-chronological scheme; instead, meaning will be acquired by directly attending to human and non-human objects in the here-and-now. As therapy progresses and the client's ability to re-evaluate long-term plans, valued goals, and objectives that remain intact provide contexts in which the client can experience the meaning of his actions in a longitudinal or metachronological sense. By incorporating those goals and objectives into therapy, we reconstruct meaning for the client based on plans that are compatible with society at large, and that represent a reconfirmation of the background expectancy of emergence of meaning through time.

The final principle is to recognize that *occupational therapy functions as a provider of background expectancies, thereby fostering legitimation and maintenance of the newly constructed social reality* for the client. The therapy clinic, as a microcosm of society at large, serves as the immediate social order legitimating or invalidating the externalizations or new typifications of our clients. If legitimated, these typifications become part of the common stock of knowledge that all rehabilitants will be expected to acquire. The thoroughness of that store of knowledge, and subsequently the adequacy of that body of knowledge for allowing disabled persons to function in society, will largely be determined by the adequacy of therapy. Occupational therapy should expand beyond its traditional role in rehabilitation and reclaim its utilization of leisure and play activities with accompanying social dialogue as legitimate therapeutic endeavors. These activities and the characteristic social banter which generate typifications of self beyond that of disabled person provide a much needed complement to typifications predicated solely on disability in the traditional functions of occupational therapy. Only by acquiring a socially validated constellation of interpersonal and behavioral skills predicated on ability as well as disability, and based on the background expectancies common to all members of society, will the disabled person truly become once again a participatory member of society.

REFERENCES

1. ALTHEIDE, DL: *The sociology of Alfred Schutz.* In Douglas, JD, and Johnson, JM (EDS): *Existential sociology.* Cambridge University Press, Cambridge, 1977.

2. BARRETT, W: *The illusion of technique: A search of meaning in a technological civilization.* Doubleday and Sons, New York, 1978.

3. BERGER, PL: *The sacred canopy: Elements of a sociological theory of religion.* Anchor Books, New York, 1969.

4. BERGER, PL, and KELLNER, H: *Marriage and the construction of reality.* In DREITZEL, P (ED): *Recent sociology No. 2.* Macmillan, New York, 1970.

5. BERGER, PL, and LUCKMAN, T: *The social construction of reality.* Anchor Books, New York, 1967.

6. CICOUREL, AV: *Basic and normative rules in the negotiation of status and role.* In Dreitzel, HP (ED): *Recent sociology No. 2.* Macmillan, New York, 1970.

7. CICOUREL, AV: *The acquisition of social structure: Toward a developmental sociology of language and meaning.* In Doulgas, JD (ED): *Understanding everyday life: Toward the reconstruction of sociological knowledge.* Aldine Publishing, Chicago, 1970.

8. DENZIN, NK: *Symbolic interactionism and ethnomethodology.* In Douglas, JD (ED): *Understanding everyday life: Toward the reconstruction of sociological knowledge.* Aldine Publishing, Chicago, 1970.

9. DOUGLAS, JD: *Understanding everyday life.* In Douglas, JD (ED): *Understanding everyday life: Toward the reconstruction of sociological knowledge.* Aldine Publishing, Chicago, 1970.

10. DOUGLAS, JD: *Existential sociology.* In Douglas, JD and Johnson, JM, (EDS): *Existential sociology.* Cambridge University Press, Cambridge, 1977.

11. FIDLER, G: *The task-oriented group as a context for treatment.* American Journal of Occupational Therapy, 23: 43, 1969.

12. GARFINKEL, H: *A conception of and experiments with "trust" as a condition of stable concerted actions.* In Harvey, O (ED): *Motivation and social interaction.* Ronald Press, New York, 1963.

13. GARFINKEL, H: *Studies in ethnomethodology.* Prentice-Hall, Englewood Cliffs, NJ, 1967.

14. GARFINKEL, H, and SACKS, H: *On formal structures of practical actions.* In McKinney, J, and Tiryakian, E (EDS): *Theoretical sociology: Perspectives and developments.* Appleton Century Crofts, New York, 1970.

15. HEEREN, J: *Alfred Schutz and the sociology of common-sense knowledge.* In Douglas, JD (ED): *Understanding everyday life: Toward the reconstruction of sociological knowledge.* Aldine Publishing, Chicago, 1970.

16. KIELHOFNER, G: *Temporal dimension in the lives of retarded adults: A problem of interaction and intervention.* American Journal of Occupational Therapy, 33: 161, 1979.

17. KIELHOFNER, G, and BURKE, J: *Occupational therapy after sixty years: An account of changing identity and knowledge.* American Journal of Occupational Therapy, 31: 675, 1977.

18. KIELHOFNER, G, and TAKATA, N: *A study of mentally retarded persons: Applied research in occupational therapy.* American Journal of Occupational Therapy, 34: 252, 1980.

19. McHUGH, P: *Defining the situation: The organization of meaning in social interactions.* Bobbs-Merrill, New York, 1968.

20. NATANSON, M: *Introduction.* In Schutz, A: *Collected papers, Vol. I: The problem of social reality.* Martinus Mijhoff, The Hague, 1962.

21. PAAP, WR: *The social reconstruction of reality: The rehabilitation of paraplegics and quadriplegics.* Unpublished doctoral dissertation, University of Missouri, 1971.

22. SACKS, H: *Sociological description.* Berkeley Journal of Sociology, 8: 1, 1963.

23. SCHUTZ, A: *Collected papers, Vol. I: The problem of social reality.* Martinus Nijhoff, The Hague, 1962.

24. SCHUTZ, A: *Collected papers, Vol. II; Studies in social theory.* Martinus Nijhoff, The Hague, 1964.

25. SCHUTZ, A: *Collected papers, Vol. III; Studies in phenomenological philosophy.* Martinus Nijhoff, The Hague, 1966.

26. SHARROTT, GW: *Existential themes in occupational therapy literature from 1900 to 1978.* Unpublished masters thesis, University of Southern California, 1980.

27. TILLICH, P: *The courage to be*. Yale University Press, New Haven, 1952.

28. TILLICH, P: *Morality and beyond*. Harper and Row, New York, 1966.

29. YERXA, EJ: *Authentic occupational therapy*. American Journal of Occupational Therapy, 21: 1, 1967.

CHAPTER 11

WHO IS BOBBY? IDEOLOGY AND METHOD IN THE DISCOVERY OF A DOWN'S SYNDROME PERSON'S COMPETENCE *

David A. Goode

EDITOR'S INTRODUCTION

One of the more intriguing topics for any professional group is a discussion of how the group's activities appear from the perspective of an informed outsider. In this chapter the analytic skill of a sociologist is brought to bear on the most critical juncture of occupational therapy: the interface of therapist and client. The author is no stranger to clinical enterprise; he dissects the intricacies of professional ideology, clinical problem solving, micro interaction, and the construction of clients' clinical identity in a way that clinical personnel will appreciate.

Outsiders often call upon clinical personnel to accomplish some new task or standard, but offer few guidelines for remediation or operationalization. Some writers offer a strategy or give practical steps for accomplishing what they suggest. Only rarely does a writer construct an argument in such a way that the reader experiences what is recommended, as this writer does.

The sociological perspective in this chapter conceptualizes social life and reality as a situational process. According to the author's underlying thesis all reality we experience, including our identities, is fabricated in the social realm where people interact. From this basis the author examines the practical issue of how clinicians can discover the identities of their clients as part of a process of helping them. The concepts of etic and emic are used to differentiate how the clinician sees things from the way the client sees them. The emic perspective is the way that a person or persons experience reality. Etic refers to alternative definitions or perspectives constructed by outsiders. Simplisticly, the emic perspective is how one sees things; the etic perspective is how another erroneously thinks one sees things. The

---

* The research on the deaf-blind cited in the text may be found in Jacobs[7]. This chapter is dedicated to Bobby, who died in 1979.

chapter argues that clinicians are generally schooled in some paradigm or frame of reference which constitutes an etic perspective—one often at odds with the client's emic view. After detailing episodes demonstrating the consequences of this process, the author turns to a consideration of the paradigmatic basis of occupational therapy practice. Earlier discussions concerning the organization of knowledge in accordance with the need for clarity, scholarship, and broad perspectives are complemented by considerations of the immediate and practical implications of professional knowledge or ideology. This task is accomplished in an unusual way, which the author terms "sorcery." Before the reader's eyes an incompetent person is transformed into an informed and competent social actor. It is demonstrated, importantly, that competence changes only because the reader's perspective has changed. Thus, the author duplicates what the professional is called to do as a clinician.

This chapter shows the importance of operationalizing in clinical practice concepts from higher levels on the hierarchy of phenomena, as argued in Chapter 2. Here the hierarchical levels of human symbolization and social systems illuminate a problem which originates from the biologic structure of the client. The chapter also provides evidence for the failure of reductionism and the paradigm of inner mechanisms to serve all of the needs of chronically disabled persons. In concert with earlier chapters, the author does not call for discontinuing technologic approaches to caregiving. Instead, he documents the dangers of an application that is too one-sided, that ignores the higher level social and symbolic realities which are created when the structure of a chromosome is altered. Finally, the author concludes that occupational therapy's mandate, because of its moral treatment heritage, is to maintain the quality of life of disabled persons.

GK

. . . it is true both that some men are wiser than others and that no one thinks falsely. (Protagoras)

This chapter examines sociological and clinical issues that emerged in the course of two ethnographic studies with deaf-blind children diagnosed as having rubella syndrome. This research revealed the difficulties societal members have in understanding such children and how our most important response to them has been one of "fault finding."[*] Clinical personnel and lay persons, excepting parents, saw, experienced and exclusively explicated these children in terms of "faults" and remedial actions to correct their faults. My research challenged the deeply pejorative stance taken toward these children by demonstrating some of their true skills and competencies that were not apparent from the perspective of an average person. This was made possible through my attempts to experience the world from an alingual, deaf-blind perspective. I observed the details of these persons' daily lives, and simulated their organic deficits by means of artificial devices which limited my hearing and sight and thereby came to understand the sensibility and legitimacy of their subjective perspective and experience. While the prevailing clinical perspective on these children classified them among the lowest functioning human beings in our society, my work provided warrant for the idea that competence—

---

[*]The concept of fault finding is taken from the work of Harold Garfinkel (personal communication, 1975). The general approach taken in this work stems largely from his influence. The discussion of emic and etic knowledge owes to conversation with him and Melvin Pollner (personal communications, 1973-1978).

indeed the whole identity of a deaf-blind child—had to do with the *social context* in which the child was experienced as well as the *role and background* of the person describing or assessing him or her. Physicians and parents were in quite open disagreement about the capabilities and identities of particular children.

For example, the hospital file of one child, Chris, described her walking as "nonpurposive", "spastic", "atethoid" and having an "overly wide gait." This fault-finding version of the child's ambulation was the rationale for a remedial "walking program." Chris's mother, on the other hand, would point out what a good time Chris had doing her own version of walking from one place to another. When I accompanied her to school she would walk out of the ward door, take a few steps, spin around, stomp her feet, bend over and touch the ground, laugh, walk on a few more steps, sit down, roll, get up, run and so on. When clinicians applied an 'objective' behavioral framework of "normal" walking, only deviations or faults in Chris's actions were revealed. The mother used *Chris's* subjective perspective to arrive at a positive evaluation of her walking.

Objective, analytic, clinical, or research stances toward human behavior are called, in anthropology, 'etic' perspectives.[3] Etic perspectives are distinguished from the 'emic', native, subjective, or insider point of view. Etic frameworks are external to the situation under analysis, and very many etic or analytic models may be brought to bear on any situation. Ordinarily, the etic reality of the scientist is used as a superior criterion against which the native insider reality is judged. Emic or native viewpoints are discovered from *within* the situation under study. It is the perspective the person in the activities uses to produce the actions which the observer sees. As Evans-Pritchard[4] noted, it is no accident that etic perspectives lead to fault finding, while emic perspectives permit others to gain a better sense of the rationality, purpose, efficiency of native behaviors. Clinical frameworks tend to be exclusively etic and explicitly oriented to finding and eradicating flaws. Their descriptions of behavior inevitably find no value in deviation from accepted behavioral norms. The emic perspective necessarily emphasizes, in contradistinction, the value and creativity of deviant behaviors.

While it is not a question of which kind of description is ultimately right, my own observations revealed adaptive and rational features in Chris's faulted walking. She did indeed have an enjoyable time walking. Furthermore her form of walking made eminent sense within the context of the state institution in which she resided. Time is a highly available commodity in such places, and it was thus unnecessary for Chris to walk efficiently. In our normal walking, we are indifferent to our immediate circumstances; getting to the next place of business may make sense to us in institutions or elsewhere, but Chris had no such concern.

For a variety of reasons, hospitals and clinics are likely to produce faulty images and identities of deviant clients based on etic criteria applied to the person's behavior. This process is particularly insidious when we are dealing with chronically damaged persons who are likely to be career patients. I found that the clinical model of deaf-blind children's behavior completely dominated intervention strategies, programs, and placements. More positive evaluations of these children, found almost exclusively in parental testimony, were ruled (often on an *a priori* basis) invalid or even delusional. As a result, intervention reduced quality of life for many of these children as their own self-chosen behaviors, competencies, likes and dislikes were ignored in planning programs for them. Instead, their lives were guided by a list of professionally located faults and technical solutions.

Having unearthed and clarified some of these issues, I was asked to do research on a small group of occupational therapists who were providing services to developmentally disabled adults living in community placements.* This group consisted of therapists who were moving away from the purely neurologic, physiologic and psychoanalytic models of intervention associated with their profession towards an intervention paradigm that was humanistic and oriented to the everyday realities of their clients. Their intent was to focus their concern beyond etic descriptions of pathology, and to examine and aid persons with differing competencies in their struggle to master everyday life. They wanted to see how clients spent their time, what skills and deficits they exhibited in their daily routines, and how they experienced and felt about their lives.

This approach was resonant with the perspective I had developed while working with the deaf-blind. These therapists had already joined in collaborative work with an anthropologist and had begun to draw upon sociological principles in order to design effective intervention strategies with their clients. My role was to collect ethnographic observations and video tape their help-giving efforts. I set out to discover whether the arguments I had developed regarding deaf-blind children would also apply to adults who were biologically far less damaged. I focused on certain clients to whom the therapists were providing service. In case after case it became apparent that the fault finding procedures I found in the state hospital were precisely what these clients had experienced. Our collaboration of social scientists and occupational therapists enabled the latter to establish an emic perspective as a central part of their evaluation and service delivery. This did not happen overnight, but required a long period of self-examination and self-discovery in addition to close attention to the details of the retarded persons' lives. Partly because I had experienced success with the strategy twice before and partly because there is a growing tendency for social scientists and therapists to realize the competence of the devalued by taking their perspective, I chose to illustrate some of these processes through the case study of a single man named Bobby.

WHO IS BOBBY? THE CLINICAL IDENTITY

Robert, or Bobby as he preferred to be called, was a fifty-year-old man with Down's syndrome who had resided at the Sin San board and care facility for seven years before our contact with him. He had been separated from his parents at a young age, had lived with relatives for a short while, and was moved through varied living arrangements prior to his arrival at Sin San. While Sin San need not be described in detail here,† it should be noted that our ethnographic research led us to view such places as

---

*The Upward Mobility Project was conducted under the auspices of the Univesity Affiliated Facility at the University of California, Los Angeles Neuropsychiatric Institute. The project was a combined research and program development effort collaboratively directed by occupational therapists and social scientists. A description of the project may be found in Kielhofner, G. and Takata, N: *A study of mentally retarded persons: Applied research in occupational therapy.* American Journal of Occupational Therapy, 34: 252, 1980.

†For a description of this and similar board and care facilities see Bercovici, S: *Out of the hospital: an ethnographic account of institutional patterns in the community care of mentally retarded persons.* Unpublished doctoral dissertation, University of California, Los Angeles, 1980.

small scale institutions within the community. This understanding of his environment was crucial to our appreciation of the adaptive competence of much of Bobby's behavior.

I first came to know Bobby through his clinical records. He had a fairly substantial file that accompanied him wherever he moved, and that summarized his career in human service contexts.* His record was a kind of clinical biography that described his contacts with various helping professions, their assessments and descriptions of Bobby as well as any remedial procedures offered to correct his deficiencies. *These texts, what they did or did not contain, were testaments to the clinical identity Bobby had been given by clinicians.* Nowhere was Bobby discussed in terms of his having any sort of competence and human value; instead an exclusively fault-finding perspective was employed. The descriptions pointed to a series of encounters in which clinical standards of normality had been used as criteria to identify the constitutional faults of the client. This method afforded Bobby an essentially *devalued, incompetent* and *hopeless* identity. Consider the following excerpts from Bobby's file:

> *Medical assessment:* "Down's Syndrome . . . diabetes with peripheral vascular disease . . . edema of lower extremities."

> *Communication assessment:* ". . . speech or language therapy is not recommended as prognosis for improvement is poor . . . client can communicate basic needs but cannot express complex ideas and understands very little . . . difficult to communicate with. . . ."

> *Cognitive assessment:* A quick test of intelligence yielded a mental age of approximately 2.8 years. Clinician concludes that Bobby is "severely mentally retarded with severe brain damage."

> *Occupational therapy:* "Time and effort in this area are not suggested as prognosis for improvement is poor . . . maintain client in a protected environment as he can never function independently."

While these comments are out of context, *it is not* intended to exclude the "good" said about Bobby. There were none. The contents of clinical files typically display only lists of the faults of chronically damaged persons especially someone as "low functioning" as Bobby.

I had read many files like Bobby's before and had learned to regard them with some skepticism. Time and again I would read a file and then go and meet a child only to find that while the file did provide some valid technical data, it failed to provide anything which allowed me to understand the persons or work with, teach, or relate to them.† Thus we took Bobby's file as an etic account of his life. We wanted to allow these clients to develop a more positive identity for us. We read their files expecting to find discrepancies between them and our own video tapes and field notes. We even hoped for such differences.

---

*The concept of 'career' in mental health services was first presented by Erving Goffman.[6]

†The indifference of ward staff to clinical records is discussed in *A Rashomon of the Deaf-Blind.* Unpublished manuscript (available on request: David Goode, Wilkes College, Wilkes-Barre, Pa. 18766).

UNDERSTANDING BOBBY

As noted above, getting to know these individuals in emic terms was an unfolding process. In Bobby's case videotaping would have an important role. Occupational therapists on the project who had been working with Bobby for some time described him as a clinically low functioning individual with remarkable native skills. I went to Sin San, met Bob, and we began routinely to see each other regularly. At that time, the members of the project and I experienced Bob as a warm and friendly man whose presence (despite his sometimes poor self-care skills) was generally benign and positive. We all liked Bobby. He was bald and rotund with a simple perspective, which, even in the early part of our relationship, we had learned to appreciate as expressing competent self-awareness and knowledge of his immediate surround. I found Bobby intriguing and selected him as the client on whom I would concentrate my research efforts. It was clear that Bob was retarded and in many ways incompetent. We had considerable difficulty understanding Bobby when he spoke, and we spoke simply to him because he could not comprehend complicated matters. However, we had yet to appreciate his full competence and cognizance.

Only on reviewing video tapes of our interactions with Bobby were his competence and abilities fully revealed to us. About two months after our first meeting, a series of events occurred which radically changed our appreciation of Bobby's competence and our relationship with him.

Therapists and research staff had come to Sin San for the purpose of videotaping various clients, and we found ourselves in a room with three residents (including Bob) who waited while we set up our equipment. When we finished, one of the therapists asked Bobby to leave because we were going to videotape the other two residents— twin sisters—and we wished to ensure the privacy of their remarks. What followed was captured by accident on tape. Bobby insisted that he be allowed to remain during the taping. An altercation ensued increasing in vehemence until the situation was finally resolved.

An edited transcription of this incident follows:

Privacy Lost: An Interaction Between Emic and Etic Perspectives

Bobby — client
Gary — occupational therapist
Marty — research assistant with the project
Alice — another client whom we are going to videotape.

Audio Portion of the Videotape	Concurrent Action
Marty: Does it bother you to leave now?	Bob is sitting and looking down, dejected. He looks up at Marty while she talks.
Bobby: (unhearable utterance)	Bob turns his head away while talking.
Marty: When we film you, no one else is gonna be there except you and Bart (the facility cook) and all of us. I think it would make it alot	Bob looks at Marty while she speaks. During this explanation Bob turns his head down looking very unhappy. He moves his hands to his mouth.

Audio Portion of the Videotape	Concurrent Action

easier for Arlene and Alice to talk about what it is they want to talk about if they'd just be alone. O.K.? How do you feel about that?

Bobby: Bart Daniel! (The meaning of this utterance is not apparent)

Again Bob turns toward Marty using hand gestures voice and inflection in his answer to her.

Marty: Is it okay if you leave now and we'll get to you next, okay?

Looking at Marty he quickly turns away and clearly displays his displeasure.

Gary: Bob? did you wanna go first? Is that what you're mad about?

Bobby: Yeah.

Gary: Well uhh, the reason, the reason we're gonna do Arlene and Alice is because they have . . .

The names Arlene and Alice bring a raising of the eyebrows and shrugging gesture.

Bobby is adamant in tone.

Bobby: (interrupting) Bart say you talk to me!

Gary: *What?* We will, we will! We'll get time to talk to you.

Gary is startled, defensive tone and then reassures Bob.

Bobby: An, Bart Daniels.

Bob points to the kitchen and looks at Gary. He uses an assertive tone while shaking his head negatively.

Gary: We're gonna talk to Bart too. He said he was gonna be in the movie with you.

Bob watches Gary and Gary's tone is reassuring.

Bobby: Allre body in the room, Bart, too.

Again Bobby is assertive and shaking his head negatively. He is looking very bothered here. (At this point it appears Bob is trying to say everyone can stay in the room). As Gary apologizes Bob looks away & puts his hand on his chin, leaning.

Gary: Well I, aah, I am sorry Bobby. I didn't understand you. *What?*

Bobby: Bart Daniels is gonna to do another one?

Very distressed here Bob shakes head negatively.

Marty: Bart Daniels is gonna do another one? (Obviously not understanding, what this utterance means)

Bobby listens to Marty's repeat of his statement nodding agreement.

Bobby: An Alice too.

Still looking.

Arlene: Oh, he don't mean nothin! (referring to Bobby)

Gary: Okay, Bobby we'll set this up . . .

Bobby begins to look at Gary, but turns away.

(Continued)

Audio Portion of the Videotape	**Concurrent Action**
Marty: Since they (referring to Alice and Arlene) have to work in the morning we thought we'd get them filmed first. And then, right when we're finished, we'll come and film you and Bart in the kitchen.	Bobby with hand on chin, is looking at the floor with unchanging expression.
Gary: You know Bobby I'm sorry we hurt your feelings, but we didn't mean to. We didn't know it would make you feel bad if we did Arlene and Alice first.	
Bobby: (unintelligible utterance) . . . get somebody else.	Bob does an affrontive gesture—crossing the visual field with eyes turned down, indifferent to Gary's apology he stares off into space.
Gary: Are you gonna be mad at us all day?	Bob sneaks a look at Gary and turns away quickly. There is silence for 18 seconds as he stares out of the window.
Bobby: I'll sit, I'll take a chair over there.	Looks at Marty and gestures toward couch near window.
Gary: Oh, you said you'll sit back there?	Bobby looks at Gary and begins to grin when he hears Gary has understood him.
Bobby: Yeah.	
Marty: Oh you said you'll sit back there, oh I see Bobby.	Looks at Gary while Marty talks.
Gary: Bobby, I don't think that's fair, though, to Arlene and Alice in case they talk about things that are private.	Bobby looks at Gary, his face turns to a frown and he looks down and away. He pauses twelve seconds.
Marty: (starts another explanation) We'll probably do alot of films with everyone together, but this is a specific thing that is just for Alice and Arlene.	Bobby looks at Marty and turns away.
Bobby: I would turn my head and tell nobody else.	Bob's voice is very shaky and filled with emotion. He's more upset than before. [Here Bob clearly demonstrates he understands what privacy is all about]
Marty: You won't tell anybody else! Well, I don't know that they just might feel up-tight. Well I dunno. Why don't you ask them?	Bob still is looking out of window. The "vibes" are heavy here.
Gary: Yeah why don't you? Well what?	
Bobby: Well me and Jimmy . . . (unintelligible utterance)	Bob turns toward Arlene and Alice and camera follows to the sisters.

Audio Portion of the Videotape	Concurrent Action
Gary: Well, what about you Alice?	
Alice: That's alright for him to be in here.	Bobby smiles as Alice indicates his presence is fine with her.
Gary: You don't care?	
Alice: Don't care honey.	
Marty: Yeah.	
Gary: Well maybe it's o.k.	
Marty: Sure.	
Bobby: They don't care.	
Gary: (relieved) Okay, well then I guess it's all taken care of.	Bobby gets up.

Although this incident may seem unexceptional, it proved not to be so. At the time of the actual incident many of Bobby's utterances were not understood, but it was apparent that he had gotten his way. During the incident we were not cognizant of the mechanisms he employed, and we reasoned that if such mechanisms could be found, we could document competence inconsistent with Bob's clinical picture.

The videotape revealed expressions of competence immediately. Bobby's superior knowledge of his social environment and his relationship to the twin sisters was the actual issue. Specifically, Bob knew better than we the propriety of raising the issue of privacy with them. From his perspective, this issue was an imported (etic) concern of ours. It made no sense to insist on privacy, and his repeated, escalating protests reflected his frustration with our ignorance. Bobby had to rely upon the more competent client (one of the sisters) to formulate this in a way we could understand, but once expressed, the instructional value of Bobby's protests was clear. For these former inmates who had no locks on their doors or any other personal space, privacy was not a reasonable concern. Bobby had understood this and used this as a basis for his strategy. Partially because he was right, he was successful, and it was we who would have to adjust our ideas about such matters within the board-and-care context. It is for this reason that the transcription of the tape is titled "Privacy Lost."

As I watched the videotape repeatedly, an even more radical appreciation of Bobby's abilities to understand and communicate emerged. At the time of the incident and during our initial viewings of the tape, it appeared that many of Bobby's utterances were unintelligible (if not unintelligent). But after watching the tape a number of times, many 'unintelligible' utterances began to sound clear to us. While it was true that persons on the tape did not seem to understand Bob, the same persons watching the tape repeatedly could hear words where formerly they heard mumblings. We discovered that normal persons had a paradoxical reaction to Bobby's talk. They denied understanding him, but often took in more information than they were aware of. For example, on the tape the occupational therapist reacted to Bob's statement as if he did not understand it, then proceeded, to complete an answer to Bob's question. *We began to appreciate the degree to which Bobby's not making sense to us was as much our fault as it was his.*

Prior to this discovery, we had thought that there was a constant proportion of nonsensical utterances Bobby produced and we largely ignored them. When we mechanically altered Bobby's tonal qualities on the tape, many of these formerly senseless utterances became more audible. By means of mechanical readjustment they were reperceived as sensible (or sometimes potentially sensible) statements. Anyone who interacted with Bobby would perceive that his speech was apraxic. It was less obvious that his syntactically fractured talk had meaning, and especially that it was meaningfully related to the context of conversations. It had been our common assumption that Bobby did not understand much of what went on around him. But after watching the tape perhaps thirty times, a new definition of the situation emerged: Bobby's behavior seemed more like that of a foreign-speaking person than like a retarded one. Apart from his difficulties in making himself understood, *the transcript of that tape revealed that Bobby had followed the direction of the conversation, and had produced semantically meaningful (if ill-formed) utterances.* We began to appreciate that cognitively, Bobby was far more complex than we had supposed. He was clearly above the 2.8 year mentality assigned to him in his clinical record. His appreciation of abstractions such as privacy, as both a local and a larger cultural issue, and his fifty years of experience, distinguished Bobby's perception of the world from that of a three-year-old.

As we watched other tapes of Bobby, we heard how our participation with him determined, to a large degree, his competence. How *we* defined Bobby's participation, as in *our* abilities to understand his utterances, structured his potential competence with us. If this were true, we reasoned, perhaps a different communicational cohort—possibly his friends at the facility—could perceive more competence. We began to observe and tape Bob in peer group interaction and were astonished at the extent to which our supposition was true. Bobby's friends reported that as far as they were concerned he had no communication problems and "talked fine." His more intimate friends claimed that Bobby talked as well as you or I, but that "we just didn't understand him." It did not take long for us to understand that *familiarity* and *intimacy* were the key determinants in viewing Bobby as competent to communicate and think. As we shall see when we discuss Bobby's relationship to the facility cook, Bart, these claims were not merely fictions of Bobby's friends' imaginations. Peer interaction tapes showed that Bobby behaved more competently with his friends than with project staff. As one project member put it, Bobby's competence did not travel well because it was linked to a particular cohort of intimates within a closed residential system.

Once the videotape had alerted us to the possible semantic content of Bob's more problematic utterances, we began to understand his talk better. Furthermore, as we recognized the ecological specificity of his competence we could make use of the local context to increase his competence in interaction. For instance, one occupational therapist found that conducting a conversation with Bobby in his room practically eliminated communication problems.

BOBBY AND BART: EMIC AND ETIC PERSPECTIVES ON FRIENDSHIP

Our experience with the videotape discovery of Bobby's communicatory and interactional competence and his superior native knowledge naturally led us to a systematic search for a whole range of socially adaptive skills that we had ignored in our etic conception of him. These competencies were not obvious and involved taking off "clinical blinders." Our growing emic conception of Bobby meant that virtually every "pathological" behavior we and others had identified in Bobby was open for review.

For example, we recorded another videotape showing an "interview" of Bobby by his "normal" friend and benefactor, Bart, the facility cook.* The tape revealed a relationship in which Bobby was, in a clinical perspective, infantilized—treated as a child to the point where he called Bart, the younger of the two, his "daddy." Previously we saw Bobby as Bart's victim, since Bobby apparently lacked the communication and cognitive abilities to resist Bart's manipulations. Some of the scenes of infantilization on tape were horrific. At one point Bart recited his pet name for Bobby, "Bobby-Baby-Boo-Boo-Bow-Wow-Porky-Pig-Oink-Oink", and followed this with a request that Bobby 'bark' during the song "How Much Is That Doggy In the Window"? Paradoxically, Bart prided himself on being Bobby's best friend. Bobby called Bart his "daddy" and "best friend." Theirs was a contradictory relationship in which Bart clearly appeared to have the upper hand. For a while, everyone felt sorry for Bobby.

After our discovery of Bobby's competence in "Privacy Lost", we watched the scenes of infantilization with new interpretations of Bobby's behavior. It was not the case that Bobby was stupid and was manipulated by Bart. Instead we found ample evidence that Bobby was aware of and uncomfortable with his role, and at times resisted being cast in this devalued and patronizing position. Bobby had allowed this in order to reap certain material and psychological benefits which accrued by having a cook as friend and benefactor. Bart provided Bobby with special treats and evening snacks from the kitchen; he bought gifts and took him for rides in his car. Furthermore, Bart was sincerely affectionate, and employed his demeaning tactics in the belief that Bobby was not hurt by them. Bearing in mind the deprivations common to places like Sin San, the material and psychological advantages of having a normal friend who was also the cook become obvious. Moreover, competition for these scarce resources was fierce, and there were many at the facility with more skills than Bob could bring into play. Yet it was Bobby who secured a normal member of the staff as his special friend. This was a source of pride for him, apart fom the gifts, trips, and sandwiches. Given Bobby's situation at Sin San, he could have attained Bart's attentions in no other way than to act as his 'pet.' For Bobby, the role with all its costs was worth its benefits.

It is important to note that this emic account of Bobby's behavior was not simply a matter of wanting to find competence in his actions. Viewing the videotapes of him and Bart allowed us to switch frames of reference to a more adaptive theory of Bobby's relationship with Bart. This was not another etic version of Bobby's behavior but, rather, was an obvious (to Bobby at any rate) reality in his relationship to Bart. That is, Bobby was clearly aware of the costs and benefits of infantilization, although he had never been called upon to justify or explain his strategy to any of his friends.

The evidence that the adaptive version of Bobby's behavior was emic rests upon Bobby's own testimony. During the Bart-Bobby interview, I had become angry with Bobby because I felt he was not one who should tolerate such treatment. Failing to appreciate the rationality behind Bobby's strategy, I pulled him into a room and shouted, "How could you do that [the barking and so on]?" I was so displeased that I threatened

---

*For a detailed discussion of this tape see: Donald Sutherland, *Context and Competence,* unpublished doctoral dissertation, University of California, Los Angeles, 1980.

to leave because of his behavior. Bob kept telling me to "calm down" and that "it was OK." It was not until I viewed the tape and found the key to his strategy that I was able to appreciate his instruction. I visited him again and we had a talk. I formulated for him as simply as I could my new adaptive theory of his behavior with Bart. He clearly followed each point, indicating that he agreed with my description of why he "put up with Bart." He told me that he "did not like Bart that much." When I said something to the effect that it was not up to me to decide for him what was worth suffering for, he was vigorous in his agreement. As far as he was concerned, it was up to Bobby to decide what was all right and what was not. And he was right.

In Bobby's eyes, in his experienced world, he was effectively mastering his situation through his relationship with Bart. The genetic, psychological, and social resources through which this mastery was achieved were admittedly uncommon, but, as with most humans, there is generally little one can do about such givens. Bobby's control of his situation was in terms of his life limitations. Seeing him in this way put him on an equal footing with the rest of us—in a kind of existential parity.

Additional incidents on videotape, and further discussions with and observations of Bobby corroborated this improved image of his competence. We ceased using a high pitched, slow and patronizing clinical drawl with him. We had lost the clinical Bobby— the list of faults and hopelessness which constituted his on-record identity—and we began to talk to him as a person like ourselves.

THE ROLES OF PROFESSIONAL IDEOLOGY AND VIDEOTAPE IN ACHIEVING EMIC ASSESSMENTS

In our discovery of Bobby's identity two issues bear consideration: the clash of professional ideologies and the use of videotape. Certainly an important element of gestalt conceptual switches took place in our seeing Bobby. However, these changes in perceiving were much more efficiently accomplished with the technical aid of videotape. We had an opportunity to return to an event and construct another version of it from the one originally experienced.

There was a coordinated interaction between the conceptual processes which sought to achieve a competency, rather than a fault-finding stance and the perceiving processes which took place when viewing a tape. Classically the relationship of conceiving and active perceiving were juxtaposed. Neoplatonists and neohegelians emphasize the importance of the idea, the paradigm, while neomarxists consider the material forms which social action takes as paramount and determinative of thoughts. Having worked considerably with video, my experience revealed that any dichotomous formulations emphasizing either ideas or material form were absurd. In employing tapes there was always an obvious interaction between the two.

I often refer to this interaction as "sorcery" because in a real way something gets changed into something else: in goes the rabbit and out comes a pigeon. A substantial transformation of who Bobby was had taken place. This sorcery feature of videotape viewing impressed me in earlier work with deaf-blind children. One day while taping Chris, a blind-deaf child, I captured the following incident.

Chris had been playing with a record player, laughing hysterically; abruptly, and for no apparent reason, she began to cry hysterically. Such polar shifts in affect, seemingly not prompted by anything in the environment, were relatively rare, and it was not without some pride that I rushed a fellow researcher into the video room and played the tape. When I reached the point in the tape where Chris began to cry, I turned toward my colleague, expecting an acknowledgment of the unusualness of the behaviour, but got no reaction. When I asked him what he saw, he told me nothing unusual, just Chris playing and laughing. I played it again, even prompting him at the point where Chris switched affect, and still nothing. Frustrated, I called in another researcher to watch the tape, and she had the same reaction. When I watched the tape I saw the whole affect switch in detail while they did not see it at all!

I decided to tell them what it was I thought we had witnessed. Replaying the tape, I prompted them at the crucial point, and both reported that they saw what I was talking about. After a few more viewings, they were convinced that the tape was quite remarkable, and some weeks later at a group video viewing session, one of them was quick to point out the extreme shifts in Chris's affect (i.e., laughing to crying).

We had watched electronically coded magnetic tape played through a system designed to represent these codes as a motion picture version of reality. As these images impinged on our eyes and ears we translated them back into electrical energy, sent these to the brain and engaged in complex interhemispheric thought processes which resulted in our arriving at definitions of what we were seeing. These ideas were then externalized in conversation and debated. The ideas, in any descriptively adequate way I can conceive, grew out of the viewing situation and owe their existence to this situation. In this miraculous, almost alchemic, processing of electron codes on tape into images and images into interpretations, a "right" interpretation or "proper" way of seeing the tape was established by my being camerman and deaf-blind expert. It really was a kind of magical "now you see it, now you don't" type of thing.

Through this incident I became aware of the power of ideology and theory in framing what persons actually see on video tape and in everyday interaction. Of many possible interpretations of what is happening on the tape (or in the world), one is selected. There can be no doubt of the power of ideas in setting up perceptual expectations and categories of interpretation.

In selecting and emphasizing the emic, and therefore competent, interpretation of Bobby's behavior, one of many possible interpretations of his actions was advanced as the proper way of seeing the tape. Later on this interpretation extended to encounters with Bobby in everyday life. Certainly the basis for asserting that an emic description is clinically useful rests on matters of belief and value. We valued Bobby's experience and felt that he should be allowed to express a more positive social identity and to exercise his freedom of choice.

The videotape viewings of Bobby were definitely influenced by our readiness to accept this emic interpretation of his behavior. But the actual details of the tape, the material organization of the record of the interaction and of one discussion of the tape, were no less a part of the process of arriving at an understanding of Bobby. It is of course possible to embrace a competency model while recognizing the power of video tape in formulating and investigating it. The details of video use in Bobby's case are covered below.

Videotape played a dual role in our re-evaluation of Bobby's identity and our own attempts to help our clients at Sin San. As a method to generate alternative, more accurate and, in some senses, 'better' descriptions of behavior and interaction videotape was a *sine qua non*. It was especially powerful in allowing us to understand both problematic and successful helping efforts. During the "Privacy Lost" incident, it was through repeated reviews of the videotape that we came to realize how our own humanistic stance, though benign in intent (i.e., maintaining privacy), was insufficient since it was not yet emically informed. Video provided an opportunity and occasion to understand that which we had not perceived in the interaction by repeatedly standing 'outside' of our own interaction with Bobby. Eventually we saw ourselves importing an issue of privacy where it did not belong, to our client's detriment. Tapes were an avenue through which we could explore the nature of our own participation with the clients, and seemed never to fail to deliver news in that regard. There was always something, professional or personal, to be learned by watching our actions on tape.

Viewing tapes of what we had done put us in a paradoxical position regarding the "actual" state of affairs as we experienced it. On the other hand, the tape was used to recapture much of the detail of what was said or done by Bobby or by us. We consulted videotapes to get a deeper and more accurate perception of what had been a lived reality for us. On the other hand, in producing alternative and better accounts of what actually happened we took by definition a very unnatural stance towards that reality. During viewing sessions it was not uncommon to hear things like, "I didn't realize that Bobby was making so much sense" or "it was I who didn't understand him; that never occurred to me." These are interesting observations and accurate—with respect to our viewings of the tape—but they were absolutely unrelated to our thoughts during the actual situation. The observations were, instead, extrinsic to the lived situation and a product of repeated viewings of tape and our efforts to understand what had happened. Having achieved these situationally extrinsic definitions of who Bobby actually was or what we had really done, and reflecting on our stance during the interaction, we all felt that we had been ignorant of who Bob was as well as the organization of our activities. *Put as simply as possible, one can not avoid the impression that persons generally do not know, other than in practical ways, what they are doing while they are doing it.* Not that we do not have serious thoughts about what we were doing. Indeed, clinical rationales of action are often supported by voluminous articulations. But, these are, at best, partial understandings of our actions.

SOCIOGENIC IDENTITIES

In addition to relating the process by which we came to redefine Bobby's identity and our participation with him, I would like to offer a sociological explanation for these events. Such an exposition has to account for how it can be that the same person may have different identities and exhibit dissimilar behaviors depending on the interactional context (i.e., in the clinic or at home.) Thus we have to address the social bases for differential identity and competence in a single individual. A shorthand way of saying this would be that we have to understand how persons' identities are *sociogenic* (literally, socially-generated.) The explication of this idea will run counter to most clinical conceptions of competence as a stable trait.

The idea of context-dependent identities and skills, while discontinuous with a behaviorist or freudian-informed, atomistic and common-sense notion of personal identity and behavior, is not odd or unexpected for the sociologist. The conception of context-specific identities has been part of modern sociology for over fifty years. In addition, the current findings of social psychologists such as Asch,[1] Milgram,[10] and Zimbardo[11] establish the primacy of situational factors in determining behavior.

Videotapes of Bob in other contexts than those mentioned above reveal over and over again that Bobby's competence—indeed, the entire nature of his participation—seemed largely socially determined. Even with children such as the alingual, congenitally deaf-blind who have extremely limited behavioral repertoires, it is generally true that competence, participation, behavior and cognition, that is, basic constituents of who a person is in any situation, are largely matters having to do with the social organization surrounding them (for example, the clinic versus the home). An important part of the message of this chapter is that what has recently become known with respect to normal persons is also true of disabled persons. Such a correlation allows us to consider the implications of this for the logic and practices of the helping professions who serve disabled persons and to discuss the significance of a conception of human identities as context specific for our understanding of human behavior in general.

Sociology provides theories which explain sociogenic identities. One such explanation may be found in Mannheim's work, *Ideology and Utopia*. He argued that ideas and concepts (for our purposes we include identities) are relational. This is to say that ideas or ways of interpreting the world, which have as their product ideas (identities), *take on their meaning (and must be understood and appreciated) with respect to certain concrete social structures and processes that constitute the idea's (or method's) social situation*. Furthermore, to apprehend all thought as sociogenic is not necessarily to deny the validity of an idea, method, or identity. Instead, such an appreciation is a way to deepen our understanding of the partiality of any idea or identity. Any thought about the world is conceived as a partial, though socially and situationally adequate view of any phenomenon. According to Mannheim, knowing the sociohistorical conditions influencing the generation of a concept or paradigm (or for our present purposes, knowing the way a person's identity is part of its sociohistorical situation) allows us to see its incompleteness as a description of the person and to identify the vested interests, assumptions, and hidden motives of those persons who hold that idea about or identity of the person. In this way one can document the social conditions under which an idea, method, or identity is adequate and relevant. This entails understanding how meanings, facts, and methods are generated within social groups and how these form part of the collective life of that group. For Mannheim, truth was a practical and cooperative outcome of the affairs of men, and took on significance and value only with respect to these affairs. This history of truths in occupational therapy has been documented in an earlier chapter in this volume.

Harold Garfinkel's conception of persons as "organizationally incarnate"[5] is a more adequate and inclusive account of the social production of identities. Building upon the general approach suggested by Mannheim, Garfinkel argues that it is the social organization surrounding a person that gives him his identity and defines for him his participation, cognition, and so forth. Congruence or lack of congruence of identities in this approach is ultimately explained in terms of similarities or dissimilarities in social organization. Arguing in accordance with this position, physicians, occupational therapists, friends, and researchers tell different, partial, and organizationally sufficient truths about Bobby.

These truths are for all practical purposes adequate to the work of doctoring (as defined by the physician) at a particular clinic, being a friend, being in a research relationship, and so forth. There is absolutely no empirical requirement that what persons *say* about Bobby or *do* with him be consistent within each setting. Thus, minimally, the clinic or hospital-associated occupational therapist should be aware of the relative character of procedures and findings, and this awareness should affect practice with clients.

The implications of this theory for our conception of a person's competence are fairly clear. What most persons would call Bobby's competence (with emphasis on the possessive) is actually part of his socially produced, organizationally adequate identity. Any clinician's assessment of Bobby's competence reflects as much about the social organization of clinical work, the clinician's training, and a particular clinic's instruments and procedures, as it does about Bobby *per se*. Any researcher's belief about Bobby's competence reflects as much about the researcher, organization of the research, and so forth as it does about Bobby. As our history with Bobby demonstrates, radically different conceptions of his competence arose from different kinds of social relations with him. In this sense it should be no surprise that Bobby's friends felt he had no language difficulties and spoke with him freely while clinicians who were strangers to Bobby found him to have extremely marginal language skills.

Unfortunately, because of the medicalized, atomistic perspective of current clinical paradigms, this does surprise many clinicians. Partly because they have done their professional best with 'Bobby' (we'll use him in an exemplary way here), and partly because they believe in the validity of their tests and procedures, many clinicians find it difficult to accept that their clinically adequate procedures fail to detect Bobby's competence in other settings. Most often they are completely unaware of the problem, believing that their procedures capture Bobby's competence independent of any social situation. They perceive their test results as indicating attributes of Bobby, and thus they fail to grasp the social relativity of their own assessments and procedures. In so doing they also fail to understand the relationship between Bobby's clinically determined competence and his competence as experienced by his daily associates. For a profession with an 'everyday' orientation like occupational therapy, such a gap in knowledge brings into question the efficacy and validity of many intervention procedures.

IMPLICATIONS FOR CLINICAL PROCEDURE

It is essential for occupational therapists dealing with damaged persons to be aware of the sociogenic identity of their clients and of the possibility that there may be discontinuities between their assessments and experience of the client and those done by others in extraclinical settings. Since the paradigmatic concepts of professionals form much of their socially organized interpretations and actions vis-a-vis clients and patients, paradigms inevitably play a role in the sociogenesis of identities. An occupational therapist imbued with a neurologic, freudian, behaviorist, or other theoretical perspective, will formulate, in part if not totally, a neurologic, freudian, behaviorist or other clinical identity of the client or patient. This process of shaping clinical identities of persons by ideological preconceptions is a matter of no small import. More than any other group in society, those who are ill, disabled, or otherwise deviant receive ministrations from professionally trained persons. Their lives become, in so many ways, shaped and determined by those who administer service and therapy. The occupational therapist, more than he or she may be aware, shapes and determines the lives of human beings.

This being irremediably true, it would be unfair and unnecessary to leave the clinical reader with a feeling that all he or she knows is that he or she could be wrong about any particular client. Instead, there are clear procedural implications to be drawn from our work with Bobby. The paradigmatic grounding of any clinical discipline should allow for the construction of an emic description of the client's identity as an important part of the clinical profile. The earlier arguments in this volume that occupational therapists must construct, as part of their clinical knowledge about patients or clients, some representation of patients' and clients' image of the world, their symbolic self-representation of values and purposes, is a first step in this direction. This would help to assure that the sociogenic identity of patients and clients is not totally etic. Furthermore, it would inform the clinician's administrations in such a way that they might more successfully enable persons to enhance their competence in their lives and achieve a better quality of existence. The following observations may be useful in this process.

The natural availability of speech and behavior of chronically damaged persons in situations of clinical contact may be misleading regarding competence in other settings. Standard clinical procedures do not yield results that reflect skills in use in extra-clinical settings. Both observations reflect real differences in the social organization of clinical versus home turf life.

Because of this a number of procedural implications may be drawn. Communicative, cognitive, and behavioral competence should be assessed from within the client's life situation because recognition and production of competence is largely an interactional matter. The quality of communication and cognition is particularly influenced by the membership of the communicational cohort and their particular characteristics (especially their intimacy with the client). In addition to examining the client's individual abilities, the cohorts and families of clients need to be assessed as the natural unit they, in fact, are.

Cohorts may be assessed by means of videotapes of clients in their daily living situations. Video may be used to import records of the client's life into the clinic. By using videotape transcription one can begin to see, for example, how persons intimate with the client achieve competent communication with him or her.

Cohorts may also be useful on an in-house basis in aiding assessments which may prove more valid regarding the client's home situation. For example, simply asking a more competent member of the cohort to accompany Bobby and 'translate' for him would be useful in this regard. Cohorts may be useful in assessments done in extra-clinical settings. A video-social scientist-clinician team visiting the client's living situation would be the most ideal solution to the clinical problem our history with Bob raised. While from a resource point of view this may be impractical for every client, it would be highly beneficial if some information on certain clients could be collected by such teams. In this way we might begin to understand the relationship between in-house assessments and home behaviors. The clinician, especially those servicing deinstitutionalized clients, or those in special living situations (e.g., intermediate care facilities) needs to know more about the clients day-to-day situation. The logic of this argument applies to many populations with whom clinicians deal on an outpatient basis (for example, diseased, handicapped, mentally ill, retarded, and aged persons.) There is a conspicuous lack of information about the daily living circumstances of such persons and their relationship to supposedly objective clinical measures.

IMPORT AND RELEVANCE TO CONTEMPORARY OCCUPATIONAL THERAPY

Current occupational therapy is searching for coherence in theory and practice. As an outsider I see occupational therapists who embrace the disciplines of neurology, cognitive and developmental psychology, psychoanalytic theory and kinesiology, along with a medical style in applying these disciplines to enhance their client's welfare. I have also worked with occupational therapists who, while acknowledging the need for this knowledge, are more concerned with a holistic and humanistic form of help giving.

As noted in Chapter 1 moral treatment was the original ideology of occupational therapy. Resuming such a stance in contemporary America would involve, among other things, conceiving of occupation in its broadest sense, as that with which one is occupied on a daily basis. In all human activities persons seek to explore and master their world, to attain positive self-images and to perform activities in the company of others. Unfortunately, we are sometimes mastered by the world, fail in our exploration, feel poorly about ourselves and others, feel alone or abandoned. At such times it may be apropos to have specialized, technically trained help-givers to solve specific client problems, but it is even more necessary to have a help provider who is concerned with the welfare of the client as a whole in terms of the client's experience of his or her world. Occupational therapy is a profession with the historical mandate to fulfill this need.

It was possible and valid to see Bobby as merely a case of Down's syndrome or as a person, if judged by normal standards, with a host of related problems. But it was equally valid and far more beneficial for Bobby and us to see him as a man with an unusual countenance, different ways of thinking and evaluating, trying to explore and master his everyday world. The humanistic basis of such a description, too often absent from clinical evaluations, directed our attention away from a client's deficits—from the ways he was different from us—and towards one like ourselves who happened to have deficits in some areas and skills in others. Our experiences with Bobby showed that such a change was plausible and to the benefit of all concerned.

ACKNOWLEDGMENTS

Special thanks to Wolf Wolfensberger, Gary Kielhofner, Isidore Goode, Sylvia Bercovici, Herbert Grossman, Donald Sutherland and Robert Edgerton for comments on earlier drafts. Pamela Aregood provided excellent secretarial support.

REFERENCES

1. ASCH, SE: *Studies of independence and conformity: A minority of one against a unanimous majority.* Psychological Monographs, 70:9 (Whole No. 416) 1956.

2. BERCOVICI, S: *Educating Retarded Adults.* In Jacobs, J (ED): *Mental Retardation: A Phenomenological Approach.* Charles Thomas, Springfield, Ill, 1980.

3. EDGERTON, RB AND LANGNESS,LL: *Methods and Styles In the Study of Culture*. Chandler and Sharp, San Francisco, 1974.

4. EVANS-PRITCHARD, EE: *Witchcraft, Oracles and Magic Among the Azande*. Oxford University Press, London, 1937.

5. GARFINKEL, H: *Studies in Ethnomethodology*. Prentice-Hall, Englewood Cliffs, NJ, 1967.

6. GOFFMAN, E: *Asylums*. Anchor, New York, 1961.

7. JACOBS, J: *Mental Retardation: A Phenomenological Approach*. Charles C. Thomas, Springfield, Ill, 1980.

8. KIELHOFNER, G AND BURKE, J: *Occupational Therapy after 60 years: An account of changing identity and knowledge*. American Journal of Occupational Therapy, 31: 675, 1977.

9. MANNHEIM, K: *Ideology and Utopia*. International Library of Psychology, Philosophy and Scientific Method, New York, 1936.

10. MILGRAM, S: *Some conditions of obedience and disobedience to authority*. In Steiner, ID and Fishbein, M (EDS): *Current Studies in Social Psychology*. Holt Rinehart & Winson, New York, 1965.

11. ZIMBARDO, P: *A pirandellian prison*. New York Times Magazine. April 8, 1973.

CHAPTER 12

ROSE-COLORED LENSES
FOR CLINICAL PRACTICE: FROM A DEFICIT
TO A COMPETENCY MODEL
IN ASSESSMENT AND INTERVENTION

Gary Kielhofner
Shawn Miyake

EDITOR'S INTRODUCTION

Chapter 11 noted that therapists formulate clinical identities for patients or clients in terms of their own theoretical or paradigmatic frameworks. Heeding the instruction that this is a matter of great import for those who receive occupational therapy services, the authors of Chapter 12 propose a paradigmatic stance that recognizes inherent value in all clients—a kind of guaranteed-worth approach to clinical service.

The chapter also builds on the themes of earlier arguments. Chapter 1 proposed that the mechanistic thinking of reductionism is inadequate for the chronically ill. This chapter illustrates more clearly how this is so. The theme that humans are occupational creatures is implicit in the focus on each person's need to experience control and mastery and a positive sense of self as reflected in the verbalizations and actions of others.

The chapter can be viewed as complementary to Chapter 9, which explored the possibility for constructing a sociological model of service that enfranchises patients and that attempts to support their control despite their disability. The authors take these issues a step further, arguing that competence or control is largely a feature of the environment and that the severely disabled must have competence *in terms* of their disability. The authors propose that these issues can and must be addressed in clinical practice.

GK

GRANTED: I AM an inmate of a mental hospital; my keeper is watching me, he never lets me out of his sight; there's a peephole in the door, and my keeper's eye is the shade of brown that can never see through a blue-eyed type like me. (Gunter Grass, The Tin Drum)

Nothing is so puzzling, taxing, and seemingly insurmountable as the problems of chronically and severely disabled patients and clients. Occupational therapists know all too well the complexity of such persons' conditions since a substantial portion of their practice has traditionally focused on those with permanent, extensive disabilities. Reilly[11] suggests the true problem for occupational therapy appears when all efforts to reduce pathology have been exhausted and the patient's incompetence remains. The difference between removing deficits from clients and assisting them to gain competence is the theme of this chapter. By virtue of the patient and client populations of occupational therapy and its concern for the optimum functioning of persons, the concept of competence should be a guiding point of reference. However, as Goode illustrated in the Chapter 11, therapeutic endeavors often focus on deficits.

This chapter describes the process of moving from a deficit to a competency-oriented therapy. Our thesis is that the paradigm of inner mechanisms described in Chapter 1 resulted in a deficit perspective in clinical practice. Together with this we argue that the concept of competence should be an essential component of future thinking and practice in occupational therapy.

DEFICIT PERSPECTIVES: MEDICINE AND THE PARADIGM OF INNER MECHANISMS

Chapter 1 noted that occupational therapy's most recent paradigm imitated concepts borrowed from medicine. To understand how this paradigm resulted in a deficit perspective, one must first examine the medical model. The focus of this model is disease, conceived as disruption or disequilibrium of states of the organism.[13] In the medical model, disease is negatively evaluated on the basis of the "undersirability of bodily states leading to pain, disability, or death."[8] Consequently, the primary goal of the medical model is to prevent, eradicate, or minimize disease.[13] To do so, the physician must identify the disease that affects the patient. Thus, medicine involves a process of diagnosis that requires a decision as to the category of illness that fits each case.[3] Diagnosis is made possible by the classification of disease entities—usually on the basis of etiological factors and the disorders they precipitate. A disease is suspected through its manifestation in various symptoms. As part of the search for disease via symptoms, the physician looks for signs of the presence of a causative agent or trauma.

Judgments concerning the presence of disease processes in persons involve careful observation of the structures of the body and its functions. The criterion of assessment in medicine is classically the norm. Healthy physical and mental states are thought to be represented in statistical averages. Deviations from average are used to assess the undesirability of an individual's status.[9] With notable exceptions (e.g., a high intelligence quotient) persons who differ significantly from the average are candidates for attribution of an inherent disease process.

Classification of disease processes in medicine is necessary since diagnostic descriptions, including the etiology and nature of the disorder, suggest a course of therapy. Most treatment emanates from the logic of the germ theory of disease. This cause and effect approach involves location and removal of the factor causing the disease process. While germ theory is not the only mode of treatment in medicine, its influence on the cognitive structuring of the physician's orientation is substantial.[12] Most notable is the almost exclusive orientation of medicine to disease, its causes, its course of progression, and the most efficacious means of attacking the disease process. It might be said that the physician-healer seeks a neutral and objective stance toward the patient, but an antagonistic perspective vis-a-vis the disease process. Such an orientation is workable for many disease processes, since the patients share the physician's negative assessment of their condition and benefit from the physician's ability to remove or arrest the disease. Thus, judgments concerning the presence of disease are generally benign and helpful. However, this is not always the case.

When persons incur *permanent* conditions that deviate from the average, another set of problems emerges. A number of writers have argued that the identification of certain chronic diseases or dysfunctional states in persons lead to devaluation and worsening of their conditions.[2,5,9,15] Thus, the disease orientation that is successful and appropriate in acute remediable disorders is ill suited for intractable conditions.

In addition to its conceptual perspective, medicine's mode of interaction with patients also has significant implications for the chronically disabled. As noted in Chapter 8, Goffman's[5] conclusion is that, like many other occupations in the last two centuries, medicine has become a shop industry. He supports his argument by noting how the physician, like the car repairman, carries on his trade in a workshop suited to his own mode of "tinkering" that involves rearranging, repairing and replacing component parts. In order to receive service, clients surrender their property to the practitioner, placing their trust in the practitioner's tinkering and relinquishing control over the property. The usual personal jurisdiction over the mind and body and their functions is relinquished to the control of the physician who then alters their structure or function. The patient literally surrenders body and psyche to the examining room, the surgical table, or the analytic couch. The process of patient and physician social behavior is organized by this accepted definition of the physician's workplace.

The workshop model of medicine disenfranchises patients in order to permit necessary medical procedures. This feature of medical practice has been described as resulting in a special sick role. Parsons'[10] formulation of the sick role concept explains how patients and medical practitioners interact within the social model of medicine. The sick role obligates the patient to seek cure and to comply with the procedures of the professional. In return, the person in the sick role is temporarily excused from the requirements for productivity.

The conceptual orientation of medicine to disease, its tinkering model of practice, and the sick role invariably result in treatment of the human being as a mechanism. When disease interrupts the function of the human "machine," it can be identified and eradicated, limited, arrested, or compensated by rearranging the internal components, removing the disease or by some other intervention. This process is not without considerable success—especially in the case of acute remediable disease. It fails, however, as a modus operandi for chronic conditions. As noted in Chapter 8, the sick role readily becomes a disabling status for the chronically ill, or for those with permanent residual problems. In such cases the permanence of disease can be grounds for imputing an inferior or faulted status to persons.[2,9] The adaptation of medicine's disease orientation, tinkering model, and sick role to those with permanent, severe problems results in the kind of fault finding described in Chapter 11.

In occupational therapy the concern with function coupled with the diagnostic orientation of medicine resulted in a focus on *deficits which prevented function*. As pointed out in Chapter 1, deficits of motion, nervous system integration, ego maturation, and the like dominated clinical thinking. The deficit orientation emerged as an efficient way to translate the paradigmatic focus on disruption of inner mechanisms into a workable therapeutic schema. Together with medicine, occupational therapy focused on identifying and removing deficits.

TOWARD A COMPETENCY PERSPECTIVE

The recognition that a mechanistic and medically derived perspective is not suited for chronic disability and for the practice of occupational therapy requires a careful search among options for an alternative conceptual mode of organizing service. Chapter 11 showed that successful service to those with permanent disability requires a competency orientation. We agree with this conclusion and suggest that these issues are posed in the following questions: What constitutes competence? Can a highly disabled person ever be competent, and, if so, what is involved? How can occupational therapy turn its focus from pathology and toward competence without abandoning the knowledge needed for treatment? What mode of therapy should underlie practice and replace that derived from medicine?

THE NATURE OF COMPETENCE. The concept of competency typically connotes internal fitness for some environmental task or external set of requirements. Mechanistic conceptualizations of competency posit it as a characteristic of the internal state of the system. However, competence requires recognition of both internal and external factors, as White's definition suggests:

> The competence of a living organism means its fitness or ability to carry on those transactions with the environment which result in its maintaining itself, growing, and flourishing.[17]

Competence thus centers on the *interaction* between the person and the environment.

Because human beings survive by collective enterprise and cooperative efforts, the exercise of competent action by each member is a matter of concern to the entire group. An individual's competent contribution means that survival and quality of life for all are enhanced. Competence is also required by the makeup of the human psyche and its biologic roots. A feature of all higher life forms is that they seek to exercise their capacities and achieve some control over the world.[16] This propensity reflects the fact that the nervous system is programmed to seek opportunities for exercise of self-capacity. Competence can thus be viewed as an important requirement of both the group and the individual.

Competence always involves performance relative to the terms of one's life and situational perspective. Persons seek control over objects and processes that have meaning or purpose for them and that attract interest or serve some personal value. Individuals are able to experience themselves as competent when they can perform on their own terms, within the context of their immediate and historical experience. For the disabled, *a particular limitation becomes part of the perspective within which personal actions take on meaning.* The disabilities of individuals are part of their human condition and of the context wherein their competence must be achieved.

Individuals must adapt not only to an external world of demands and expectations, but also to an internal world of self-experience. Every human being is blessed and burdened by an awareness of his or her own existence. Awareness of self allows one to reflect on experience, plan for the future, develop personal potentials, and positive self-evaluation. Awareness of self also creates the need to positively experience self or, as Goldschmidt notes, human beings are "quintessentially concerned with the maintenance and furtherance of a positive self-image."[6] This positive self-image not only allows pleasurable experience of one's existence, but also serves as a springboard for deciding when and in what way to encounter the world in the future.[1,14] The degree to which a person views self as competent and worthy is an accurate barometer of future actions. Competent persons believe in their ability to accomplish things and to wisely choose activities or situations in which they can perform.[14,17] A person who has serious limitations of performance, but who retains a realistic belief in personal abilities in some area and who is able to accomplish a level of performance in that area may be said to possess a recognizable degree of competence. However, persons who have substantial abilities, but little belief in those abilities, appear incompetent since they are not disposed to exercise their capacity. Consequently, they limit the degree to which they will be able to meet internal and external demands.

Thus, our concept of competency must begin with individual experience and a personal view of the world, complemented by a set of beliefs about self. It must also recognize the right of individuals to choose and define their own areas of control and performance. In this way, subjective competence is important not only for its role in enhancing individual experience of self, but also for its ruling influence on individual courses of action.

Individuals' views of themselves are dependent in large part on the assessment of others. One comes to assess self positively or negatively in terms of others' definitions. As White notes, "it is nice to have other people love you, but even more pertinent to self-esteem is to have them respect your capacities."[18]

Most individuals who experience themselves as competent in some feature or aspect of their lives have access to environments, persons, and materials, that allow them to perform adequately, well, or superbly. Individuals who manage a positive existence do so both because they view themselves positively and because environmental supports allow them opportunities to perform well.

On close examination of competency we find that it is not as much the condition of an individual possessing this or that capacity (for even the most competent among us lack innumerable abilities) as it is having a positive self-assessment plus adequate environmental resources. This definition does not omit individual responsibility as a facet of competence. One must in some way perform to be competent. However, this view distributes the burden more equally among internal and external elements. The environment must not only demand, but allow and recognize competence. The individual's experience of self is as important as objective judgments by others.

In our view there are four essential elements of competence: (a) the abilities (and by implication the limitations of abilities) of the individual; (b) individual self-assessment;

(c) the objective or collective expectations of others for task performance in the person's environment; and (d) the range of opportunities and resources available to an individual in the environment.

COMPETENCE AND THE SEVERELY DISABLED. Occupational therapists daily witness a sector of the population that represents human failure and inability. When confronted with the profoundly retarded, those with head trauma, progressive paralytic or arthritic conditions, and others with devastating disabilities, the concept of competence may appear more idealistic than practical. However, we contend that this group, more than any other group, requires the careful application of a competency-based model. The great difficulty in discovering and nurturing competence in these individuals is cause for concentrated effort, not for pessimism.

As Smith[14] notes, the competency process can thrive in the most devastated body so long as the belief in control and self respect remain. Even in the face of serious brain injury an individual can continue the process of competency. Gardner relates the story of Zasetsky, a Russian soldier seriously brain injured from a gunshot wound:

> Zasetsky worked on his notebooks everyday for twenty-five years. Writing never came easily: some days he penned hardly a line, on many more he produced half a page, only on his very best days could he execute upwards of a page.[4]

Despite his limitations this man wrote an articulate and searching account of his own condition. He epitomized the potential for competence in disabled persons.

Our definition of competence suggests that ability (or the limitation of ability) is only one of four dimensions of competence. For most of us, these four components of competence are in some balance. We avoid circumstances where our limitations would hinder us. We seek resources to aid our performance in areas where we can be successful, and we find a reference group that respects our level of capacity.

The severely and chronically disabled person faces a situation in which limitation of ability threatens the balance among these factors. When ability is limited, other elements must shift to provide needed balance. As documented in Chapter 11, one of the most seriously limiting features of life for the severely disabled is the inability or unwillingness of others to recognize or grant competence to their efforts and performances because they differ from the average. The challenge raised is to discover how, when understood from the individual's perspective—albeit radically altered from our own—competence is both possible and necessary. The issues raised are more than idle philosophic questions. The question of whether the "faulty" walking of a blind-deaf child should be judged from her perspective or from that of a social world to which she has almost no access, points to a central problem in the care of the highly disabled. That they cannot accomodate the usual definitions of competent performance challenges those who serve the disabled to *construct* social versions of their competence as starting points for therapy. Such a *relativity theory of competence* would ask: What would be a good performance for the person with a radically altered brain or body? The answer to the question lies both in the perspective (however limited or deviant) of the individual and the ability of another to recognize and appreciate performance from the same perspective.

When discovery of competence is achieved by bridging the subjectivity with the patient or client, manipulation of the environment to maximize conditions for control

FEATURES OF OCCUPATIONAL THERAPY PRACTICE
AND THEIR IMPLICATIONS FOR CLINICS AND INTERVENTIONS

follows. The opportunity to express choice, even if only to select the texture of cloth he or she must rest upon day and night, or the color of a room's furnishings, are starting points. The ability to be competent in socially recognizable ways, even with respect to such simple behavior as cooperating with dressing procedures, or reduction of incontinence, can be personally meaningful. These kinds of performances should be elements of recognized competence in highly disabled persons. We can barely comprehend the importance such an insignificant amount of control may have for these persons; we can hardly afford to assume that it makes no difference in their lives.

FROM CLINICAL DIAGNOSIS TO CONTEXTUAL ASSESSMENT. In the medical model and in the inner mechanism paradigm of occupational therapy, diagnosis meant identification of inner states of disorder. While occupational therapy has always stressed commitment to discovering the strengths of an individual, the structure of mechanistic thinking leaves the therapist better prepared to deal with deficits than with strengths. This is because strengths have no place in a discovery mode derived from the dianostic fault-finding and eradication approach of medicine.

Part of the difficulty lies in the fact that mechanistic thinking assigns both weaknesses and strengths to qualities that inhere in an individual and that supposedly are the conditions that preclude or allow competence. One of the most important changes in the emerging paradigm will be an alternative conceptualization of patient circumstances via open system in place of solely mechanistic concepts. The function of any open system (and thus its competence) is determined by circumstances outside the system and the manner in which they interact with the system's internal state. Knowledge of the inner make-up of the system thus provides only part of the picture. An obvious question raised by such a conceptualization is how the therapist shall operationalize it. For example, the evaluation of inner mechanisms involves standardized testing to determine inner qualities. Contextual assessment, the open system mode of evaluation, seeks instead to determine environments in which the system functions well or poorly. In such a system of assessment one would, by definition, include information about competent performance. The therapist is required to continue altering environmental conditions until competent performance emerges. Alteration of environments may include a range of physical, symbolic, and social dimensions. For instance, relevant questions for a child with severe intellectual, motor, and perceptual impairment would be: With what objects can the child play and express some pleasure? What communications can the child interpret? By whose definition or by what social standards can this person perform a useful function? The answers, however meager, constitute the individual's competence.

Our experiences with severely retarded individuals confirmed the hypothesis that competence is, for the most part, a matter of the environment and the beholder. For instance, in first working with retarded individuals we found them engaging in what we perceived as patently incompetent behaviors. Clients fought over and gorged food; they stuffed their pockets, bras, and coats (the latter often worn in the heat of summer) with personal possessions. Their appearance and behavior violated socially appropriate norms. It was possible to offer a number of plausible mechanistic explanations for the behavior. These persons could be seen as psychodynamically immature, seeking need gratification in ways that violated social convention and reflecting their fixation at lower psychosexual stages of development. Alternatively, they could be seen as socially unlearned by virtue of improper reinforcement or inefficient learning capacity. These accounts judged the objective undesirability (or incompetent nature) of their acts and provided an explanatory framework for their faults.

Only later, as we became more knowledgeable about the circumstances of their lives, did we realize that the clients were not behaving in an incompetent manner *so far as their reality dictated*. These persons lived in social environments where competition for food and theft of personal belongings were everyday occurrences. Their behavior reflected practical attitudes toward managing these problems. Competing for food and hoarding personal possessions were optimal strategies. In similar fashion we began to discover additional evidence of personal competence. We were not persuaded to accept client's behaviors as desirable, but we understood the circumstance which made them reasonable and effective strategies to alter their environmental limitations and personal situations.

Thus, moving beyond a deficit perspective does not suggest that we ignore real limitations of our clients, or that we fail to secure accurate data on their inabilities. It simply requires that we understand them in terms of a larger context of competence in which the environment is a major element. Judging another's competence is not as much a matter of finding faults as it is to locate the current level of competent behavior in the individual relative to his or her capacities and environmental factors.

A FRAMEWORK FOR THERAPY. Our definition of competency compels a consideration of the patient's inner experience as he or she encounters the external world. This acknowledges that adaptive change must come from successful involvement in personally meaningful courses of action that serve to reinforce self-respect and confidence. The perspective requires that occupational therapy focus on the delicate process of structuring an external environment in which some measure of control may be found and which provides resources relevant to the perspectives, the values, and the interests of the client. Unlike the workshop of medicine with its foreign objects and procedures, the occupational therapy workshop must employ familiar and relevant resources and tasks that enfranchise patients. This is critical for the generation of competence in persons whose sense of control or abilities have been eroded by disease. It demands a structure of care fundamentally different from that of medicine. The patient should not function in a sick role with obligations for productivity eliminated. Occupational therapy must be organized to produce graded demands for productivity and performance in occupational roles, for this is the special form of caring which occupational therapy provides.

While it may be tempting for the authors and convenient for the reader to have specific guidelines for operationalizing a competency model in practice, it is not altogether proper for several reasons. First, the concept of competence offered here does not lend itself to neat, specifiable applications. Rather, it enjoins clinicians to ponder, query, and discover features of the clients' and patients' life experiences, capabilities, and circumstances. Second, each therapist is an important part of the social system which defines and attributes competence. Thus, each clinician must confront personal definitions, prejudices, and common sense that impact the competence of his or her patients and clients. Only after such a process of self-examination and after developing a set of personal principles and views can the therapist effectively elicit competence in others. Finally, the process of enhancing and supporting competence in others is not confined to the domain of technology. As Smith[14] notes, the metapsychology or philosophic assumptions of a field may be more important than its technology for effecting competence.

Chapter 1 pointed out that occupational therapy has its roots in moral treatment. We believe that three important facets of that era should be part of today's practice if we are to support the competence of those we treat: (1) A firm belief in the dignity of all human beings despite their immediate condition; (2) belief that many human problems, especially problems of daily living, result from persons' succumbing to the environmental circumstances about them; and (3) belief that all human beings, no matter how regressed or disorganized, possess some degree of self-control. These elements could constitute for occupational therapy what Smith terms the metapsychology of a field. Furthermore, they may serve as principles from which to develop theory and practice techniques. They sum up a very simple yet profound fact of life. Human value and competence are to be found where they are sought just as surely as faults are there for the finding. Ultimately, the practice of occupational therapy requires us to see competency where others do not because of the limitations of medical model and common sense orientations. Our *rose-colored clinical lenses* must permit us to see the positive elements of our patients and clients where others may see only faults. Unlike rose-colored lenses that ignore reality, ours must expose a very important reality which is all too often missed.

REFERENCES

1. DE CHARMS, R: *Personal Causation.* Academic Press, New York, 1968.

2. DEXTER, L: *On the politics and sociology of stupidity in our society.* In BECKER, H (ED): *The Other Side: Perspectives on Deviance.* The Free Press, New York, 1964.

3. FOUCAULT, M: *The Birth of the Clinic.* Pantheon Books, New York, 1973.

4. GARDNER, H: *The Shattered Mind: The Person After Brain Damage.* Alfred A. Knopf, New York, 1975.

5. GOFFMAN, E: *Asylums.* Anchor Books, New York, 1961.

6. GOLDSCHMIDT, W: *ethology, ecology and ethnological realities.* In COELHO, GV, HAMBURG, DA, AND ADAMS, JE (EDS): *Coping and Adaptation.* Basic Books, New York, 1974.

7. GRASS, G: *The Tin Drum.* Vintage Books, New York, 1961.

8. LEIFER, R: *In The Name of Mental Health.* Science House, New York, 1969.

9. MERCER, J: *Career patterns of persons labeled as mentally retarded.* In FRIEDSON, E, AND LORGER, J (EDS): *Medical Men And Their Work.* Aldine-Atherton, Chicago, 1972.

10. PARSONS, T: *Definitions of health and illness in the light of American values and social structure.* In Parsons, T (ED): *Social Structure and Personality.* NY: The Free Press of Blencoe, 1964.

11. REILLY, M: (ED). *Play as Exploratory Learning.* Sage Publications, Beverly Hills, Calif, 1974.

12. RILEY, J: *Western medicine's attempt to become more scientific: Examples from the United States and Thailand.* Social Science and Medicine, 11:549, 1977.

13. SEDGWICK, P: *Illness: Mental and Otherwise.* Hastings Center Studies, 1:19, 1973.

14. SMITH, M: *Competence and adaptation.* American Journal of Occupational Therapy, 28:11, 1974.

15. SZASZ, T: *The Myth of Mental Illness.* Dell Publishing, New York, 1961.

16. WHITE, R: *Motivation reconsidered: The concept of competence.* Psychological Review, 66:313, 1959.

17. WHITE, R: *Sense of interpersonal competence.* In White, R (ED): *The Study of Lives.* Atherton Press, New York, 1964.

18. WHITE, R: *The urge towards competence.* American Journal of Occupational Therapy, 25:271, 1971.

CHAPTER 13

DOING AND BECOMING: THE OCCUPATIONAL THERAPY EXPERIENCE*

Gail S. Fidler
Jay W. Fidler

EDITOR'S INTRODUCTION

This chapter presents the theme that human existence is bound up on one's acting in and upon the world. A pithy characterization of the chapter's thesis is that "one is what one does." The authors offer a glimpse of the vast literature that supports their underlying assertion, then show its applications in clinical practice.

The chapter echoes earlier arguments: the field's need to focus on occupation (here termed "doing") as its central business and major therapeutic strength, the importance of the patient's experience of meaning when engaging in occupations, and the recognition that humans are hierarchical phenomena in whom illness reverberates through several levels of structure and function. These themes are packaged in a coherent and persuasive prospectus.

It should be noted that the chapter exemplifies the kind of paradigmatic transformation this volume repeatedly calls for. Chapter 1 documents the contributions of these authors to a paradigm of inner mechanisms, while criticizing this perspective as inadequate for occupational therapy, and calling for an integration of its useful technology and knowledge into a new paradigm focused on occupation. The authors of this chapter admirably dispel the inertia which often comes with longstanding commitment to a point of view. They move forward in a most constructive way, retaining important ideas from a phase of occupational therapy's evolution (to which they significantly contributed) and incorporating them into a

---

*This chapter was adapted from a paper entitled: *Doing and becoming: purposeful action and self-actualization:* American Journal of Occupational Therapy, 1978, 32: 305.

new and timely framework. Behind their chapter is a metamorphosis of ideas, and thus its exemplary value supersedes what it has to say about occupational therapy.

GK

Now we realize our being in action (for we exist by living and acting) and the man who has made something may be said to exist in a manner through his activity. So he loves his handiwork because he loves existence. It is part of the nature of things. What is potential becomes actual in the work which gives it expression. (Aristotle)

During the centuries since Aristotle's proclamation, elaboration of the relationship between handiwork and individual development has been minimal. Although the critical relation of action to human existence and adaptation has been pursued by philosophers for many years, the characteristics and processes of action transformed into doing and human productivity have remained relatively unexplored in the behavioral sciences. While a balanced pursuit of work and leisure activity is recognized as characteristic of the life-style of an adaptive adult, and play is acknowledged as natural to the learning of childhood, the dimensions and characteristics of such activities have with few exceptions, received only superficial attention.

In the fields of medicine and mental health, bonafide purposeful activity continues to be viewed as peripheral to bonafide modes of treatment.

Consequently, the uses of activities in mental health, for example, are generalized and motivation for their use seems frequently to be avoidance of inactivity rather than providing help. In physical rehabilitation the limited focus upon constructive activities and their meanings is reflected in the dissociation of activities from the life context of the patient to an extent that implies that exercise is the sole virtue and purpose. As noted in Chapter 1, occupational therapy grew out of a conviction that activity is a potent agency of healing. More recently, the profession has to a considerable degree eschewed the association between handiwork and health care.

If health professionals are to assume major responsibility for designing environments and experiences for the prevention of illness and for the maintenance and restoration of health, they must achieve a more sophisticated understanding of *doing*. The word 'doing' is meant to convey the sense of performing, producing, or causing. It connotes purposeful action in contrast to random activity, in that the action is directed toward the intrapersonal (testing a skill), the interpersonal (clarifying a relationship), or the nonhuman environment (creating an end-product). *Doing* facilitates the development and integration of the sensory, motor, cognitive, and psychologic systems. It serves as a socializing agent and verifies one's efficacy as a competent, contributing member of society.

All organisms are born to act. Although lower animals come equipped with behavioral patterns enabling them to cope with the external world, humans are dependent upon their social and cultural environments for learning and developing the action patterns necessary for survival and satisfaction. Today, developments in social psychiatry, ethology, brain research, and developmental psychology reflect a growing sophistication in understanding the relationship of mental activity to motor behavior. There is an accumulation of significant data to support the thesis that the drive to action, transformed into the ability to "do," is fundamental to ego development and adaptation.

BECOMING "I"

The ability to adapt, to cope with the problems of everyday living, and to fulfill age-specific life roles requires a rich reservoir of experiences gathered from direct engagement with both human and nonhuman objects in one's environment. *Doing* is a process of investigating, trying out, and gaining evidence of one's capacities for experiencing, responding, managing, creating, and controlling. It is through such action with feedback from both nonhuman and human objects that an individual comes to know the potential and limitations of self and the environment and achieves a sense of competence and intrinsic worth.

The play of childhood is a striking manifestation of the natural drive to action in the service of exploration and discovery of the body, the self, and the external world. Bruner's studies of perception and learning emphasize the need for ongoing engagement with reality as the means by which behavioral patterns and strategies for dealing with the environment are learned. His recent explorations into the meaning and uses of play[4], provide impressive evidence of the critical value of all aspects of play in individual development and evolution. Piaget's observations[17] about play and other exploratory behaviors led him to define these as the processes by which the child assimilates experiences while accommodating to the world. His remarkable studies expanded the body of knowledge regarding adaptive human action in a world of objects. Reilly[18] views play as a "connectivity" phenomenon leading to competence and adult workmanship. She makes some valuable observations about the development of adaptive function and productivity. Erickson continues to emphasize the value of *doing* in achieving a sense of mastery, personal integrity, and in successfully participating in one's external world. His psychoanalytic background and ego psychology orientation are reflected in his focus on the expressive aspects of play,[8] and on *doing* in the process of self-actualization and acculturation.[7]

In his study of the nonhuman environment, Searles[19] convincingly argues that relatedness to nonhuman objects is a significant force in the development of the sense of self as human, as differentiated from the nonhuman. He describes how involvement with one's nonhuman environment is a means for learning about self and others, and for dealing symbolically and realistically with one's affective states, needs, and ideations.

In another work,[12] we hypothesized that when an activity relates realistically and symbolically to an individual's needs and personal characteristics, it is an agent for learning and growth. *Doing* within this context is seen as a means for communicating feelings and ideas, expressing and clarifying individuality, and achieving satisfaction. Our work and Edelson's[6] emphasize that *doing* in this sense can mediate between one's inner and outer world, nurture the capacity to invest, teach realistic responses to success and failure, provide concrete evidence of one's capacities and limitations, test the reality base of fantasy and perceptions, and validate the ability to achieve and influence one's environment.

The writings of John Dewey articulate the criticality of *doing* for developing a sense of "I" and in accumulating a store of action experiences essential for human functioning. Becker[1] explores how the sense of self is developed by and sustained in action. He adds a dimension to Dewey's earlier hypothesis by emphasizing the significance of the inherent feedback in the process in *doing*. He views such action as essential for coming to know the realities of self and the world, and for testing the truth of one's perceptions and mental images. Becker sees schizophrenia and other psychiatric disorders occurring when internal and external factors limit or preclude an individual's acting on—trying out—an idea or thought. In similiar fashion, the physically disabled must master changes in perception and their reactions to these new perceptions. They must also create new mental images for performance and self-knowledge to be achieved primarily through doing.

In defining "objective orientation," Black[2] states that the process of acting enables knowing or "taking account of" the presence of independent, material objects, emphasizing that it is such processes that make possible the distinction between reality and illusion. Doing is required for truly comprehending the new environment encountered by the developing individual, the distorted environment of the psychiatrically disabled or the changed interaction with the environment of the physically disabled. Each of us knows reality from our learned, predictable interaction with it.

Neurophysiologic theory seems to be converging on a similar description of behavior. In Karl Pribram's[16] intriguing use of the holographic paradigm, an organism will perceive a reality, conceive an intended reality or goal, and learn what motor activity is needed to achieve the goal through a constant series of "tests" to define each increment of change in perceived reality.

A counterpoint to *doing* as the means for defining reality is made by Don Juan as he explains *not-doing* to Castaneda.[5] The sorcerer discovers a separate or nonordinary reality by freeing himself from consensual reality. Don Juan explains, "that a rock is a rock because of all the things you know how to do to it . . . I call that '*doing*'. . . . A man of knowledge . . . knows the rock is a rock only because of '*doing*,' so if he doesn't want the rock to be a rock, all he has to do is . . . 'not-doing.' " As Sharrot shows in Chapter 10, reality and meaning are maintained in collective and individual cases by doing. Without such doing reality ceases to exist for humans.

BECOMING "COMPETENT"

In another context, each individual has personal evidence of the sense of well being, the excitement of challenge, the satisfaction of achievement that comes, for example, from a particular job success: mastering a calculator, planting a garden, repairing a carburetor, teeing off in good form, or painting a landscape. Whatever limitations there may be in the "artistry" of the end product from the viewpoint of the expert, there is keen satisfaction and a sense of competence in having accomplished it from one's own resources. Such gratification, the joy of being a cause, can be understood within the context of the human being's innate drive to master the environment.

Robert W. White[21] for a number of years has articulated the thesis that there is an innate human drive to explore and master the environment and that this drive can best be understood as motivation toward competence. White views a sense of competence and efficacy as emerging from direct encounters with and mastery of the environment. He further suggests that gratification from such mastery is intrinsic "in the sense that strictly speaking it requires no social reward or ratification from others. The child acts on the intention, for instance, to climb a stone wall; the outcome of the ensuing struggle between his muscles, hard surfaces, and the law of gravity is brilliantly clear to him even if no one is around to pronounce upon it."[22] White urges that the helping professionals become more knowledgeable about the phenomenon of competence and more alert to the patient's sense of competence. He suggests that to become "as sensitive to the client's feeling of competence as we are to anxiety, defensiveness, love and hate, would open a wide additional channel to being of help."[22]

When one's accomplishments, one's sense of competence are verified and valued by others, one's efficacy and value as a human being is confirmed. If, for example, climbing a stone wall has no relevance to the child's social group, the intrinsic gratification may be short lived or limited as an exploratory learning experience. The meaning and worth of one's doing or mastery is appreciably determined by the views and values of significant others. Humans are inextricably dependent upon others for learning, and thus for the feedback that verifies that something has been learned and that the new function has value to others. Self-esteem can therefore be understood as evolving from the intrinsic gratification of accomplishment and the feedback from others regarding the achievement.

The significance of doing and feedback from others in developing a realistic sense of competence and efficacy was illustrated in an experience with a patient group. The group was composed of patients who persistently rejected all aspects of occupational therapy programming. With few exceptions, members of the group acted provocatively and randomly in the community and in the hospital. It was decided to meet with them in a talking group and to move cautiously toward action with a purpose. It then became evident that action planned toward productivity and achievement generated tremendous anxiety. Their nonverbal behavior in this setting and their reflections on the experience, strongly suggested that to do was to risk verification of incompetence, lack of control over self and the environment, inability to master the environment, and "nonhuman-ness." Their expectation was that what they might produce, the fruit of their action, would replicate what they were. Their appallingly limited action-learning experiences and the negative or nonexistent feedback from the environment had left them with few action alternatives.

Many persons disabled by accidents show a reluctance to do in the presence of others. The physically impaired individual probably had adequate mastery of self-in-the-world, only to be robbed of competent action patterns. Although compensatory patterns of mastery develop from the process of new doing, the awareness of risk of failure frequently inhibits doing in the presence of others.

Action leading to achievement contrasts with random activity. Action is the product of a mental image that defines the objective. Action also is the creator of a mental image. The created mental image includes refinement of strategies for achieving the objective and an affective evaluation of the achievement. As noted by Kielhofner in Chapter 2, the created image is a prepotent factor in humanization. Without one's internal map of the world and the mechanisms for calculating and effecting one's actions upon it, the human would be an incompetent being. The actor builds a self-image as a competent actor, confronts the results of the action, finds the boundaries for reasonable objectives, and learns the social relevance of competent actions. When motivation or ability to act on mental images or ideation is blocked or inhibited by forces in the environment, by sensorimotor deficits, or psychologic distortions, coping behaviors and adaptive skills are not learned.

BECOMING A SOCIAL BEING

Humanization, becoming part of human society, may be defined as the process whereby the individual, beginning life as a biologic organism, becomes a person whose primitive actions are gradually transformed into behavior that satisfies individual needs and contributes to societal development. In this sense humanization can be viewed as the process of learning about self and one's world, of developing those perspectives and related performance skills essential to a functional society and a functional individual with satisfaction to both.

Mead[14] suggests that social roles are learned through the activity of play and games. Game playing teaches a perspective about significant others and begins the process of internalization of social roles and values. Let us return to the child climbing the wall. With the struggle to master the hard surface and the pull of gravity, the child is exploring, testing, and developing age-appropriate motor planning, physical skills, and agility. If peers share in the climbing experience, there is additional exploration and learning about "the significant other." If the activity becomes a game, it is reasonable to assume that the rules for playing the game will be defined according to the cognitive, psychologic, and social learning needs appropriate to the developmental level of those participating and congruent with their culture. If significant adults applaud the achievement, the efficacy of the action is acknowledged and verified as socially significant.

The task-oriented groups described by Fidler[11] are based on such hypotheses regarding *doing,* with the group providing consensual validation of the efficacy of action and interpreting social-cultural norms: the choices of tasks and the action process per se both reflecting and meeting the individual's developmental and learning needs.

Moore and Anderson[15] hypothesize that all societies have created "folk models" for dealing with the most critical features of their relationship with the environment. These models can be understood as games whose rules teach necessary perspectives and skills. The authors identify first the nonrandom aspects of nature; second, the random or chance elements: third, interactional relations with others; and fourth, the normative aspects of group living. These are correlated with four types of games: puzzles, which teach a sense of agency, the joy of being a cause; games of chance, which teach a relationship to events over which one has no control; games of strategy, which teach the individual to attend to the behavior and motivation of significant others; and aesthetic entities, or art forms, which teach people to make normative judgments and evaluations of their experiences. Learning experiences planned from this folk model are thus structured to include activities that incorporate varying aspects of these models, and are matched with the developmental level and personal characteristics of the learner.

As reviewed here, perspectives about *doing* bring into focus two critical dimensions for determining the value of any activity for a given individual. First, the activity or *doing* must match individuals' sensory, motor, cognitive, psychologic, and social maturation, as well as their developmental needs and skill readiness. Second, it must be recognized by the social cultural group as relevant to their values and needs.

Information available from the social sciences for research is impressive. However, what is not known about *doing* and human productivity and what is not being investigated is even more impressive.

CONSTRAINTS ON DOING

Middle class values place great stress on verbal skills. Professionals frequently reinforce the priority of this value in their educational and treatment orientations and practices regardless of what they know about learning and human functioning. Current scientific achievements encourage a search for technologic solutions to human problems. Drugs and surgical manipulations supplied by licensed agents diminish the personal desire to put effort into problem-solving and to extend coping skills. As a result, the role of action and feedback from action in self-realization becomes devalued. There is the familiar problem in mental health practice posed by those patients who, with impressive verbal skill, can describe the psychodynamics of their difficulties and articulate the psychotherapeutic process, but are much less able to act on such cognitive awareness. These are most frequently clients who disdain activity programs and view action and doing as irrelevant to their needs, problems, or lifestyle. Many physically disabled patients wait for technical interventions or external solutions to their complex problems. In those instances where personal struggle is combined with technical aids, the prognosis is more hopeful. Far too often patients eschew doing, tending to deny its relevance to their problems.

As community mental health health programs have broadened the base of psychiatric services, practice has come to include persons whose culture and learning place a priority on action. These persons frequently view talking as oblique to their needs, problems, and lifestyle. This does not always mean, however, that they see themselves and their actions as agents for change. Nevertheless, the therapist can capitalize on those cultural propensities to clarify the synergy between talk and action, acceptance of help, and initiation of self-help.

There is a need to pursue investigation into the neurologic, perceptual, and social components of action in relation to mental health. Simultaneously, conscious efforts to break down the stereotypes of introspective talk and technologic solutions are needed to enhance the awareness of *doing*. Both the quality and variety of *doing* are critical for ego development and adaptation. When treatment is viewed as a physical phenomenon only marginally related to the psychologic and social domains, the significant dimensions of mastery and sense of competence in relation to human performance are lost. In physical disabilities there is a critical need to examine the social, psychologic and adaptive potential of activities and to challenge the priority focus on therapeutic exercise. The nature and variety of doing are critical to the restoration, reaffirmation, or reconstruction of personal reality and ego integrity, to a sense of competence, and thus to coping and adaptation.

Social change and technologic development have altered the interaction of the person and the world. Direct life-supporting and life-threatening contacts with flora and fauna have been almost eliminated. Communication and information have been dramatically extended. People hear of events immediately but do not interact with them. The accuracy of reality testing is always dependent upon one's neurologic idiosyncrasies, perceptual distortions, the results of prior actions, and social responses. Contemporary psychopathology is fashioned by the current demands on all neurologic functions, on perceptual accuracy, on reduced opportunity for learning through action, and by the enlarged input of information and language.

One can, for instance, easily visualize the different possibilities in the world of John, who lives on a farm near a wooded hillside with his parents, grandparents, three siblings, and an uncle. He is responsible for a number of chores to maintain the household. He is free to explore nature with all manner of physical skills. He gets direct, consistent response from several generations while also observing them in their work roles. He receives indirect response from family members reacting to each other with value judgments. Finally, he has the direct and indirect responses available to all children at school.

Compare John to Peter, who lives in an apartment in the city with two working parents and a cat in a neighborhood that holds personal threat for much of the day and night. He may have some chores but they are unlikely to be viewed as critical to the maintenance of family life. He is given very limited freedom to explore. He receives some direct response from two people whose work he does not observe, except the housework which they complain about. He gets vestigial, indirect response from his parents and many hours of passively received and probably discordant, indirect response from television or radio. Finally, he has the direct and indirect responses available to all children at school. Once Peter has learned to manipulate his toys he is limited to exploring the behavior of his cat, which is limited in its own behavioral possibilities. A sense of mastery, especially for the new and unexpected, is difficult to achieve. A sense of value and social role identity is even more difficult. Feelings, actions, and meanings do not become integrated.

It has been hypothesized that the prevalence of senseless violence by children and adolescents who show no remorse may be generated by hours of viewing television violence that has no relation to their behavior and that is not accompanied by action on their part. When action does not follow thought, perception is distorted and the critical learning that comes from confronting the consequences of an act is precluded. Dissociation of thought, affect, and action so characteristic of schizophrenia follows the process of "learning without action." Schizophrenic dissociation may occur when neurologic and perceptual deficits preclude action, and when the environment inhibits doing, or does not support doing, in a variety of contexts. Limited learning of functional, adaptive skills that occurs when there is a paucity of opportunity for *doing* is emphasized by Winn.[20] She discusses faulty reality testing, loose distinction between illusion and reality, and the passivity of response evident in children whose daily hours are filled with TV viewing instead of psychomotor activity.

There is increasing evidence that limited action experiences are no less significant for the adult. Addressing the role of activity in maintaining normal human functioning and the consequences of sensory deprivation, Bruner points out that "an immobilized human being in a sensorially impoverished environment soon loses control of his mental functions."[4] Greenberg quotes Strainbrook commenting on thrill seeking as reflecting a search for individual mastery. "So much of our life has become sedentary, inhibitive action. There has been an over-emphasis on cerebration—thrill seeking behavior is expressing an almost desperate need for active, assertive mastery at something. We are programmed for action, but where there is so much less adaptive behavior which requires physical action, there is an insidious anxiety about the concept of mastery. We need to restore a sense of physical mastery and assertion; a sense of control, of self doing rather than merely thinking."[13]

PRESCRIBING INTERVENTION

The complexities of a rapidly expanding, industrialized society make it imperative for the health professions to attend to those factors that preclude or inhibit *doing*. A reduction in *doing* generates pathology. When pathology is identified, *doing* must be used in the service of personality integration. If treatment is heavily biased toward verbal communication or physical exercise, and if treatment responds to symptoms rather than to performance skill development and reinforcement, it will have a limited effect. Likewise, when activity programs fail to relate to the specific development of performance skills, their impact is more like random activity and much of their potential benefit is lost. The extent of carryover of learning and change from the treatment setting to the home environment is frequently determined by the degree to which treatment modalities are relevant to the adaptive and performance skill demands and expectation of the *home* setting.

Programming for the prevention of ill health or for the remedy of dysfunction must reflect an appreciation for and understanding of the interrelationship of internal and external systems in the generation and shaping of human behavior. Selective attention to one system, one skill area or component of coping, fragments the totality of the human being.

The question, then, is how to elaborate concepts about doing to create plans or prescriptions to enhance critical human functions. Different periods in the life cycle demand different configurations of skills, both those relating to the internal realities and those relating to the external realities. Performance can be understood as the ability, throughout the life cycle, to care for and maintain the self in a more independent manner, satisfy one's personal needs for intrinsic gratification, and contribute to the needs and welfare of others.

Planning and implementing intervention requires understanding the nature and complexity of such performance skills and their inherent interrelationships. Self-care and maintenance extend beyond dressing and feeding to maintaining one's self as independently as possible within a personal environment. It includes among other factors, individual value systems and the expections of significant others with regard to the dependent-independent continuum and role behaviors within the family or group. Personal need gratification relates to those doing skills that make it possible for the individual to pursue and experience personal satisfaction. This skill cluster represents a repetoire of activity skills that have as their primary motive the experience of fun, a sense of joy, and intrinsic gratification. Thus, these doing skills are focused more on personal needs and personal characteristics than on the values and expectations of others. The third skill cluster includes activity or doing skills directed toward making a discernible contribution to the needs and welfare of others. These skills are focused on making it possible to experience a sense of self as a productive, contributing, and necessary member of one's society. In delineating this cluster of skills for any individual, the priority is defined in terms of age-appropriate social roles, the individual's value system and the needs and expectations of others within the context of individual characteristics, interests, and abilities. The balance among these performance skill clusters, that is, the proportion of time, attention, and energy allocated to each is critical in achieving and maintaining a way of life that is satisfying to the self and to others and that is health sustaining.

The level and kind of skills and the balance among them at any one point are determined by age, developmental level, unique biology, and culture. For example, adequate levels of independent self-care and appropriate self-care activities will vary in accordance with age and cultural norms. Likewise, what is considered a healthy balance among caring for self, pursuing personal need gratification, and caring for others, changes with the different stages of life and varies according to one's culture. Intervention or treatment planning requires understanding these three aspects of performance as comprising an integrated, balanced system at any point in time, congruent with the unique needs and characteristics of the individual and his or her social and cultural orientations.[9] Planning for intervention therefore requires an initial assessment of the nature and level of the individual's intact skills, skill limitations, and balance among performance skill clusters. Once this profile has been made, it is necessary to identify those components or subsystems of performance that inhibit or prevent skill development. This description includes evaluations of the sensory, motor, psychologic, and social deficits as well as identification and assessment of human and nonhuman factors in the environment that impact being able to do.

When such data gathering and assessments comprise the first step in treatment, the priorities and focus of both immediate and long range goals can be more realistically addressed. Within this context, the use of a given modality and the design of a treatment plan are more apt to be perceived and influenced by the meaning of performance and adaptation to the patient and to the reality of his or her life-style performance needs. Thus, occupational therapy intervention is designed on the basis of four fundamental questions: (1) What performance skills are required at this time in order for this individual to be able to live with satisfaction to self and significant others? (2) Given such requirements, which performance skills are intact and what dysfunction or limitations exist? (3) What are the internal and external factors or forces that are impeding or impairing the ability to achieve an adequate level of skill performance? (4) What factors represent strengths and assets that can be used as resources to support and reinforce development and adaptation?

Concepts regarding the components of *doing* make it possible to analyze activities or doing experiences in relation to skill acquisition. Both the planning and implementation of treatment in occupational therapy requires that activities be understood and analyzed in terms of the level and kind of motor skill requirements, sensory integrative components, psychologic meaning, cognitive requisites, interpersonal and social elements. In addition, an analysis of an activity includes understanding both the real and symbolic meanings inherent in the activity. The dimensions of such meanings for anyone are defined by his or her real and symbolic, cultural, and idiocyncratic interpretations. For example, a baseball may be perceived for its realistic meaning, namely as a type of ball used in a definable, organized, competitive game. It may also be symbolic of success, failure, social structure and strategy, assertiveness, ineptness, competence, parental expectations and values or peer judgments. Following a pattern, cutting on a line, sanding a board or operating a jigsaw, may have meaning as these endeavors realistically relate to accomplishing a given task, producing an end product, or mastering a skill. Such activity may also symbolize or represent attitudes, feelings, and abilities with regard to doing what is expected: complying, controlling aggression, ordering one's world, defining boundaries, shaping one's environment, being an agent or a cause.

An additional dimension related to the meaning or significance of an activity for an individual concerns the end product of the activity. Whether it be in terms of an object created, a game completed or a skill mastered, the end product provides tangible evidence of the ability to do and to achieve. Mastery and competence are verified and become obvious in the reality of an end product. When the product resulting from an activity has social and cultural relevance to the individual and to his or her social groups, meaning is enhanced and social efficacy is affirmed. When only parts or segments of an activity are used, this important element of confirmation is sacrificed and Don Juan's "not doing" may characterize the experience.

Such knowledge is the basis for identifying and using activities or experiences that may be expected most effectively to elicit desired responses. The fit between the individual and an activity is crucial to the restoration or development of function in the sensory, motor, psychologic, cognitive, and social components of performance and to the integration of these systems. At another level, this match is essential if the choices of leisure, work, and self-maintenance activities are to result in a sense of intrinsic gratification, pleasure, and social efficacy for the individual.

In occupational therapy there is need to attend more seriously to the aspect of doing, of activity engagement that addresses the joy that is inherent in being a cause, and the fundamental human need to experience pleasure and fun. When these elements are viewed as tangential to the treatment process, essential integrative, motivational, and human factors are lost. When there is congruency between individual characteristics and the real and symbolic characteristics of an activity, there is greater likelihood that the doing experience will result in a feeling of pleasure and personal satisfaction, and that the essential learning will be integrated as an adaptive response.

On the basis of such data and constructs doing can be designed to provide the action-learning experiences necessary for the development of the critical components of performance and for skill acquisition. The following clinical examples may serve to illustrate some of the principles which have been presented.

Case I: Reconstructing Roles Through Doing

Mr. D. was 58 years old at the time he sustained a leg injury that made it impossible for him to return to his job. For 15 years Mr. D. had worked at the counter of an all-night diner, boasting about how he could manage the "tough characters" that frequented the diner during the night. One year after his accident he continued to refuse to consider other jobs, was sullen, depressed and became increasingly inattentive to his personal hygiene. He was finally admitted to a psychiatric hospital where he continued to refuse to participate in treatment or activity programs.

The treatment team finally suggested that he be assigned to the only paying job on the ward, which was responsibility for doing the laundry for the ward. The team viewed this assignment as "special" and thus helpful to his self-esteem and his values about work. The occupational therapist however, reasoned that considering Mr. D's "macho" values, and his need to confirm that he was a whole, strong male, the assignment would be nonproductive. The therapist pressed for placement in the hospital's compensated workshop, anticipating that the factory-like environment, the predominately male population and assignment to one of the more obviously male jobs, would be most therapeutic. This recommendation was reluctantly accepted by the team and Mr. D. was told of the plan and informed that he was expected to comply. He went sullenly and under protest. After two days in the workshop, his protests stopped and by the fourth day he was standing outside the ward, eagerly awaiting the bus. He became actively involved in the workshop, offering his help in a variety of situations and requested help in learning to become one of the machine operators. His general functioning improved rapidly and he began participating in group therapy, a vocational counseling group, and a male bowling group.

From an assessment of his previous lifestyle and interests of the patient it was possible to identify the features which had the greatest value in supporting his self-esteem and his conviction about his competence. If the staff had considered financial reward primary and ignored the undermining of male identity, the result would have been further symbolic castration to add to Mr. D's leg injury and increase his depression. By contrast, the task with the team of males allowed him to feel whole and competent again as compensation for the ego threat implicit in his bodily injury. This form of doing served also to reestablish a sense of contribution to others.

Case II: Achieving A Better Balance

Six men were in group psychotherapy as part of a research study of depression. All were successful businessmen, incapacitated by severe and recurring depressions. They were ambitious, upward striving individuals who shared lifestyles characterized by long working hours, little time with their families, and a sense that they would "never quite make it."

In their task-oriented occupational therapy group, they had reluctantly reached a consensus to make kites, as "the lesser of several evils." Their discomfort with a non-work task was reflected in their decision to make the kites for a boy scout troop. Plans for presenting the kites and the choice of the troop to receive them were engaged in as if they were business strategies. The group designed and constructed the kites, which were impressively complex. They became totally engaged in the construction, problem-solving, and theories of aerodynamics. When the projects were completed, the group decided on a test flight before giving the kites to the scouts. They flew the kites on a grassy hill, running, shouting, and laughing. Their pleasure in the fun and the horseplay was remarkable to see. When they returned to the group, they began to talk about how they had never really been children, never really played. They shared with one another their fright about being fathers, unable to play with their sons and the extent to which fun and pleasure had never been part of their lives.

The technical problem-solving required by this activity, the "political-volunteer" focus for the end product and the reassurance of the shared group experience allowed needs for self-gratification, intrinsic pleasure, and spontaneity to be expressed. Feeling more complete, the patients could face their self-doubts and shortcomings more honestly and openly.

Case III: Integrating Multiple Skills

Mary K. was an intelligent, 38-year-old woman with a graduate degree in engineering and a successful business career who had been badly injured in an automobile accident. Her physical rehabilitation was progressing well and it was expected that her residual disability would be minimal and would not impair mobility or interfere with her career.

However, Mary K. became depressed and although she had never been outgoing or socially spontaneous, she became even less responsive and her characteristic aloofness increased. She spent long hours reading alone and avoiding others. On interviewing Mary, an occupational therapist discovered that her structural, cognitive skills were coupled with a keen interest in art. Although she was not skillful in handling plastic media, her favorite leisure activity was visiting art museums, enjoying the visual appeal of composition, colors, and form. Matching this interest with her engineering skills, the therapist helped Mary K. to discover photography. Mary's delight in her new discovery and her skill in the activity opened new doors to creative expression and social relationships. A close friend commented, "Mary is a different person! There is a sparkle and sensitivity that we who have known her for a long time, never knew was there."

It is no discovery to note that many of us choose activities or vocations for misleading reasons. The result can be a disaster, or it may only be less than optimal. The occupational therapist helped this patient integrate functions that had previously been isolated. Such creative discoveries produce a healthy euphoria.

The planning for all patients must take into account the neurologic and psychologic functions underlying each human action. An act is performed within a particular social context and has its own specific values and meanings. Understanding the nature and relevance of *doing* to human adaptation makes it possible to plan intervention programs to facilitate learning and change, increase the chances of helping others maintain a state of health, contribute to a better understanding of the basis of pathology or dysfunction and, thus, develop more effective prevention strategies.

REFERENCES

1. BECKER, E: *The Revolution in Psychiatry.* The Free Press, New York, 1964.

2. BLACK, M: *The Objectivity of Science.* Bulletin of Atomic Scientists. 33:55, 1977.

3. BRUNER, JS: *On Knowing: Essays for the Left Hand.* The Belknap Press, Cambridge, Mass, 1962.

4. BRUNER, JS, JOLLY, A, AND SYLVA, K, (EDS): *Play: Its Role In Development and Evolution.* Basic Books, New York, 1976.

5. CASTANEDA, C: *Journey to Ixtlan*. New York: Simon and Schuster, 1972.

6. EDELSON, M: *Ego Psychology, Group Dynamics and the Therapeutic Community*. Grune and Stratton, New York, 1964.

7. ERICKSON, EH: *Childhood and Society*. WW Norton, New York, 1963.

8. ERICKSON, EH: *Play and actuality*. IN BRUNER, JS, JOLLY, A, AND SYLVA, K, (EDS): *Play, Its Role in Development and Evolution*. Basic Books, New York, 1976.

9. FIDLER, GS: *From crafts to competence*. American Journal of Occupational Therapy. 35:567, 1981.

10. FIDLER, GS: *The life style performance profile: An organizing frame for the evaluative process in occupational therapy*. In HEMPHILL, B, (ED): *The Evaluative Process In Psychiatric Occupational Therapy*. Charles B. Slack, Thorofare, NJ, 1982.

11. FIDLER, GS: *The task oriented group as a context for treatment*. American Journal of Occupational Therapy, 23:43, 1969.

12. FIDLER, GS AND FIDLER, JW: *Occupational Therapy: A Communication Process In Psychiatry*. Macmillan, New York, 1964.

13. GREENBERG, PF: *The thrill seekers*. Human Behavior, 6:17, 1977.

14. MEAD, GH: *Mind, Self and Society*. University of Chicago Press, Chicago, 1934.

15. MOORE, OK AND ANDERSON, AR: *Some principles for clarifying educational environments*. University of Pittsburgh, Research and Development Center, 1968.

16. PRIBRAM, KH: *Languages of the Brain*. Prentice Hall, Englewood Cliffs, NJ, 1971.

17. PIAGET, J: *Play, Dreams and Imitation In Childhood*. WW Norton, New York, 1962.

18. REILLY, M (ED): *Play As Exploratory Learning*. Sage Publications, Beverly Hills, Calif, 1974.

19. SEARLES, JF: *The Nonhuman Environment*. International University Press, New York, 1960.

20. WINN, M: *The Plug-in Drug*. Viking Press, New York, 1977.

21. WHITE, RW: *Motivation reconsidered: The concept of competence*. Psychological Review, 66:297, 1959.

22. WHITE, RW: *The urge toward competence*. American Journal of Occupational Therapy. 25:271, 1971.

CHAPTER 14

KNOWING WHAT TO DO: THE ORGANIZATION OF KNOWLEDGE FOR CLINICAL PRACTICE

Zoe Mailloux
Wendy Mack
Cynthia Cooper

EDITOR'S INTRODUCTION

Chapter 14 addresses the interface between theoretical issues and the practical concerns of clinical practice. Drawing upon their clinical experience, the authors explore important issues pertaining to what occupational therapists should know and be able to do with patients and clients. The chapter successfully integrates theoretical and clinical issues into a coherent discussion.

Two major themes from earlier chapters form part of the basic structure of this chapter. The first is the obligation of the field to focus on occupation as its central business. The authors use the term "theory" to refer to the clinician's use of concepts in practice. Readers may recall from earlier discussions that theories are part of the larger, inclusive paradigm of the field. Thus, in suggesting that occupation is a unique feature of occupational therapy theory and practice, the authors operationalize arguments about the paradigm in chapters 1, 2, and 3. In the same vein the second major theme of the chapter builds on the proposals of Chapter 2. The authors argue that systems concepts, especially concepts of open systems and hierarchy, are appropriate for organizing thoughts and action in clinical practice. This point is illustrated with examples and a discussion of clinical problems in theoretical terms.

The chapter serves as a reminder that many of the earlier themes of this volume are more than philosophical ruminations, demonstrating how they can be applied clinically. The chapter should leave most readers convinced that these themes must be applied to gain an effective and unique clinical service.

GK

If to do were as easy as to know what were good to do, chapels had been churches and poor men's cottages prince's palaces. (Shakespeare, The Merchant of Venice)

Clinical practice is the core of the profession of occupational therapy. Practical application provides the vehicle for enactment of the concepts, models, theories, and frameworks which comprise occupational therapy. West[29] describes practice as the "visible expression of our professional theories and goals and the methods we have devised to accomplish them," and as "the single greatest force determining our credibility." The majority of therapists—nearly 70 percent—are practicing clinicians,[1] and as in any service-related field, all theory, research, education, legislation, and professional development ultimately relates to practice.

Unlike most other health-related services, the scope of occupational therapy is staggering. Given its diversity and range, it is difficult to identify a common perspective for the field. The multi-dimensional aspects of human function that make occupational therapy interesting and indispensible also create a dilemma for the therapist attempting to organize knowledge for practice within a particular setting.

The extent to which occupational therapy practice relates to diverse areas of human function became apparent as we organized our thoughts for this chapter. Our own clinical practice provides an example of the dilemma. One author works in a large rehabilitation unit and sees problems ranging from decreased range of motion to occupational role dysfunction in a group of patients who vary widely in dysfunction, age, and cultural and social background. A second author deals with children who have been diagnosed as autistic, aphasic, learning disabled, or developmentally delayed. Treatment in this setting addresses neurologic dysfunction at a sensory motor level as well as disruption of social and emotional development. The third author deals in yet another arena of clinical practice, working with physically and emotionally disabled junior college students. In this setting problems range from motor and cognitive dysfunction to difficulty in coping with the demands of changing life roles. Our initial discussion of the diversity of practice in specialty areas led us to realize that our own practice exemplifies this diversity within a single setting and routinely in the treatment of only one patient. The problem of synthesizing apparently discrepant bodies of information is a dilemma that all practicing occupational therapists continually face. On one level, therapists must recognize their commonality in order to integrate specialty practice under a recognizable rubric. At another, more focal level, therapists must draw from many knowledge sources to produce strategies for addressing the problems of the individual patient. These strategies must acknowledge the multi-interactional effects of dysfunction within the context of the patient's occupational role. How can the therapist deal with this paradox of organizing disparate yet vital components of practice? And why should this exceedingly difficult task be attempted? Our purpose here is to demonstrate how various therapeutic approaches in clinical practice can be seen in relation to a unified framework for the benefit of the profession as a whole and for improving the treatment of the individual patient.

The importance of identifying and utilizing a cohesive occupational therapy framework has been highlighted by occupational therapists in recent years. Kielhofner and Burke[17] state that "the field of occupational therapy is currently without a universal conceptual foundation to shape its identity and guide its practice." Concern for a unified

FEATURES OF OCCUPATIONAL THERAPY PRACTICE AND THEIR IMPLICATIONS FOR CLINICS AND INTERVENTIONS

framework has arisen largely in response to the problem of identifying specialized areas of occupational therapy practice within the profession as a whole.

SPECIALIZATION: STIMULUS FOR A CONCEPTUAL CORE

Specialization can be considered a natural progression in the development of a profession. Given the proliferation of technical knowledge in occupational therapy and related fields, specialization may also be necessary to ensure competence within various practice settings. However, the dangers of premature specialization within a developing profession have been noted by several occupational therapists.[6,9,12,27] Specialized practice without identification of a common framework is likely to contribute to professional splintering, or as King states, "without a unifying theory to insure cohesiveness, specialization could easily become fragmentation."[19]

Another possible result of a poorly defined theoretical base is role confusion. The report of the Task Force on Target Populations[27] cautions that specialization trends in the absence of a unique and unified professional framework may ultimately bring occupational therapists into competition with other professions. Huss[15] cites the loss of the profession's original conceptual themes as contributing to the current overlap between physical therapy, occupational therapy, and other fields. Criticizing present trends of adopting other professions' modalities in the pursuit of specialization, she emphasizes the need for a common professional focus to develop modalities with a distinct perspective.

Identification of a unified conceptual framework is essential to the development of specialized professional practice, as specialization without such a framework may contribute to problems in professional role delineation.[15,12,27] The future of the profession may depend on its ability to integrate around common goals.[16] As continually increasing health care costs demand that professional service be identifiable and unique,[19] an inadequately delineated frame of reference may, in effect, threaten occupational therapy's viability. The need for a unified theoretical framework within the profession also directs attention to the role of such a theory base in clinical practice.

THEORY IN RELATION TO CLINICAL PRACTICE

The term theory is neither easily defined nor unequivocally employed across different areas of study. Rather, it is used to describe an elusive yet vital component of virtually all bodies of knowledge. According to Stevens,[26] some theories refer to principles which support or underlie specific actions or thoughts. Theories of this kind parallel Riehl and Roy's definition of a theory as "a scientifically acceptable general principle which governs practice or is proposed to explain observed facts."[25] At another level, theories may refer to an organized set of related constructs with extensive implications for guiding the development of the area to which they apply.[26] Regardless of the classification used to organize levels of theory, a central theme within the literature reflects the relevance of theory to practice.[7,23]

In terms of principles, most practicing occupational therapists use theory in every patient interaction. For example, a therapist working with a patient who has spastic paralysis may utilize an activity aimed at increasing range of motion. This practice is based on the theory that certain sets of motions performed regularly will prevent muscle and tendon tightness and formation of contractures.[28] A therapist using sensory integrative procedures may end a treatment session by encouraging an activity involving slow, rhythmical vestibular stimulation, based on the theory that this stimuli is calming to the nervous system.[2]

In a broader sense, occupational therapists work under a myriad of theoretical approaches or conceptual models. For example, sensory-motor, sensory integrative, neurodevelopmental, rehabilitative, biomechanical, psychodynamic and activity approaches are frameworks under which occupational therapists are aligned.[14,28] Martin[21] attributed the fact that professionals are "increasingly concerned with the nature of the kind of knowledge with which they identify themselves" in part to the rapidly expanding store of available information. With increasing sources of knowledge, occupational therapists face a greater dilemma in selecting theories appropriate for their practice. In addition to selecting approaches, therapists are forced to prioritize and integrate various principles of treatment.

Without a systematic means for addressing these demands, occupational therapists risk diffusing their profession even further into obliquity. In other words, if a profession cannot be differentiated by the theoretical approaches it utilizes in its practice, its utility as a unique service will be questioned. Perhaps even more significant is the likelihood that random selection, prioritizing, and integration of theories will not serve client needs.

Some aspects of theoretical approaches are incongruous and others are actually contradictory. For example, one of the concepts of the neurodevelopmental approach developed by Bobath and Bobath involves the use of therapist-imposed postures and movements.[4] This component of the theory is not compatible with the philosophy of a sensory integrative approach that emphasizes the importance of active involvement by the child.[3] This is not to say that these two theoretical approaches are discordant; on the contrary, much of each approach can be used in a complementary manner. Rather, this example illustrates the need for a systematic means to determine how diverse bodies of knowledge can be used appropriately.

GENERAL SYSTEMS THEORY AND PRACTICE

Disciplines such as psychology, nursing, sociology, anthropology, economics, and political science employ a systems approach to address the issue of integrating diverse bodies of knowledge.[5] The concepts of open systems, hierarchies, and adaptation as salient features of general systems theory for organization of occupational therapy knowledge and practice have been discussed here (see Chapter 2) and elsewhere.[18,24] This approach is a useful method of analysis and synthesis of the variety of phenomena, present in a single human "system," that must be addressed in order to appreciate an individual's abilities to function in daily life.

OPEN SYSTEMS

Within the treatment setting, the occupational therapist is involved with each aspect of the open system that characterizes human function. Individuals are provided with information through the processes of input and feedback.[17,18] An example of input in the therapy setting is the demands generated when an activity is presented. If a macrame project is used, the demand and information presented to the individual provide several types of input. Multisensory inputs are created by visual, tactile, and proprioceptive features of the task. In addition, there are cognitive, emotive, and perhaps social and cultural demands and meanings in such an activity. These characteristics of macrame provide input to the individual by making a demand at some level of the system. The therapist monitors the input by delimiting the demands of the particular activity.

Once presented with an input, the individual uses the process of throughput to organize and reorganize incoming information.[17] In a macrame project, the patient must organize all of the demands and information presented by the activity. Thus, each sensory input, cognitive demand, and emotional and cultural element must be perceived, assessed, and organized by throughput processes. The therapist may influence the process by providing structure, cues, or devices which will enhance the patient's ability to cope with the input.

The most salient feature of an open system for the therapist is the process of output, action, or "the mental, physical, and social aspects of occupation."[17] Action is the essence of an open system, providing the individual with purpose and meaning. Output not only allows the individual to have an effect or to produce, but also provides feedback, the second source of information to the system. Feedback is produced when an action occurs and is then integrated with input to begin the cycle again.[18] In the macrame example, the demands (input) are processed (throughput) and the individual makes a motor action (using his or her hands to form a knot), a cognitive action (using problem-solving skills to decide how to sequence the task), and an emotive action (responding in either a favorable or negative way to the activity). Each of these actions provides feedback that will modify performance on the next attempt. For example, if the patient cannot achieve sufficient shoulder flexion to complete a square knot, feedback (failure to perform the correct knot) provides information that the task is too difficult, and the position of the patient or the activity may be altered to allow for success. If the patient is able to complete the activity, a feeling of success serves as positive feedback to the system and enhances motivation to continue.

Output or action is dependent on all subsystems of the individual. Thus, the hands cannot make a knot without the muscles of the body, the problem-solving of the mind, and the spirit vitalized by the social and cultural significance of the activity. In order for the occupational therapist to decide how to work appropriately within the framework of an open human system in therapy, properties of hierarchies and subsystems must also be addressed.

HIERARCHICAL CONCEPTS FOR PRACTICE

Chapter 2 examined the possibility of hierarchy as a structure for the field's paradigm. Additionally, several occupational therapists have employed hierarchical models to conceptualize various aspects of occupational therapy theory and practice.[10,17,20] Kielhofner and Burke present a model of human occupation comprised of performance (skills), habituation (internalized roles and habits), and volition (personal causation, valued goals, and interests) subsystems. When properly operating, these subsystems function together to allow the individual to achieve mastery of the environment through successful and meaningful engagement in daily life activity. Lindquist, et al[20] describe a model of play development including sensory-motor, constructive, and social subsystems of play. Development of these subsystems is theorized to occur hierarchically, such that the proper development of higher levels of play (e.g., at the social level) are dependent on adequate development of lower levels.

Application of certain laws of hierarchy (see Chapter 2) to these models may further elucidate the nature of subsystems and relationships between subsystems.

(1) *The complexity of subsystems increases upward with higher levels incorporating lower levels.* The model of human occupation[17] identifies the volition subsystem, the highest and most complex of the levels, as incorporating lower levels of performance and habituation. Volition chooses and enacts behavior, habituation maintains it, and the performance subsystem produces the necessary skills. That is, the volition subsystem draws upon available skills, habits, and roles from lower subsystems in the formation of specific interests and goals. Similarly, the model of play development outlines various aspects of play, the highest level of social play with peers being the most complex manifestation of play. Social play incorporates sensory-motor and constructive play, as evidenced, for example, in children playing "hide and go seek" (social play incorporating sensory-motor play), or children cooperating to build an "airport" of blocks (social play incorporating constructive play).

(2) *The highest subsystem directs all lower subsystems.* The model of occupation conceptualizes the volition subsystem, driven by the urge to explore and master the environment as the controlling influence over lower subsystems. Thus, the volition subsystem, through developed personal causation, interests, and goals, governs the choice of specific actions as system output. For example, a stroke patient may have developed an interest in weaving prior to the CVA which can be utilized to guide the performance subsystem in therapy to maintain range of motion and increase functional use of the affected side of the body.

The model of play development similarly utilizes social play to influence the output of lower subsystems of play. Once social play has developed to become the major focus of play, a child will enact various types of constructive and sensory motor play in social play.

(3) *A disturbance in one subsystem will affect all others.* An example of this within the model of human occupation may be a person suffering a chronic psychiatric disorder who has experienced recurrent failure in daily life. This person's sense of personal causation (volition subsystem) may be that of one who is not in control of his environment, and who perceives himself as controlled by external forces. This person's volition subsystem may choose to avoid future failures and not enact output at all, thereby deteriorating through disuse previously developed skills and habits, while also failing to develop critical skills and habits that might help to develop new roles for daily activity. Thus, a disturbance in a higher subsystem disorganizes lower subsystems.

A disturbance in a lower subsystem, however, may act to constrain the function of higher subsystems. This may be evidenced within the model of play development in a child with a sensory integrative disorder. The child's deficits interfere with effective use of the body in space and subsequently affect the development of sensory-motor play. If the child is unable successfully to engage in sensory-motor play, development of constructive play will most likely also be affected, as adequate mastery of body movements fail to develop to control, combine, and creatively use objects in the environment. In addition, social play with peers will be constrained as the child avoids activities which make these deficits more apparent to others.

These illustrations are intended to familiarize the reader with systems concepts for application to clinical practice. Understanding a systems approach lays the foundation for conceptualizing these attributes in relation to a client's daily life function. The laws of hierarchy in relation to the clinical setting are covered in a subsequent section.

ADAPTATION THROUGH OCCUPATION

The properties inherent in open systems and hierarchical processes enable the human system to respond adaptively to environmental demands. Occupational therapists enter into the adaptation process through occupation.

Consideration of the process of adaptation has long been a critical component of occupational therapy. As early as 1922, Meyer discussed the "value of work as a sovereign help in the problems of adaptation."[22] Since then adaptation has continued to develop as a central concept within the profession. Impressed with the significance of adaptation within occupational therapy, King proposed in her Eleanor Clarke Slagle Lecture that the adaptive process can be seen as a unifying theoretical framework. She cites Ayres' use of the phrase, "eliciting an adaptive response" as a "succinct and accurate description of what an occupational therapist does."[19] In their model of human occupation, Kielhofner and Burke organize aspects of occupational behavior central to human existence and adaptation. They state that "occupational therapy clinics tap the deepest and most powerful adaptive response—the ability to find challenge and meaning in one's daily undertaking, one's occupation."[17]

Occupation is thus the cornerstone of occupational therapy practice. Wolfe defines an occupation as a "culturally defined and organized activity which, when performed by a person, engages the person's mind and body in purposeful, meaningful, organized and self-initiated action."[30] Its commitment to occupation as an organizing framework enables the occupational therapist to influence individual adaptation. Emphasis on purposeful activity to facilitate adaptation, that is, "the process of reacting favorably to environmental influences to preserve function and maintain a state of equilibrium"[14] is the recurrent theme that unites and distinguishes occupational therapy practice.[29] As Englehardt states, it is "*activity,* or more importantly, interest in human activity that most clearly identifies occupational therapy."[8]

Within the context of viewing the individual as an open system, the use of active, purposeful participation through occupation allows a meaningful output to occur. In Chapter 10, Sharrott elucidated the occupational therapist's role in the patient's experience of meaning. Yerxa states, "Through the use of media the client is involved intellectually and emotionally in discovering what is purposeful to him. He is also involved in relation to objects, actions and persons. Through these relationships he is helped to come to grips with his particular reality including his disability, his emotional reactions, his will and his potential."[31] Meaningful outputs are emphasized for the organizing effect they have on the individual. For example, a seven-year-old severely gravitationally insecure girl became suddenly motivated to learn to do a sommersault. Although the prospect of engaging in what was perceived as an intensely threatening activity was somewhat overwhelming, she was driven to succeed. She seemed to know that if she did it once, she would have the ability to repeat it. The first sommersault was traumatic, with false starts, squeals, and perspiration. Once completed, however, she was able to do one after another, each one with more freedom than the last. The action provided feedback that was organizing to the system, allowing an adaptive response to occur.

Within a systems view, the use of occupation to facilitate adaptation is also inherently a hierarchical process. That is, activity that has meaning to the individual cannot affect a subsystem in isolation. If we see the sommersault example within the context of the Kielhofner and Burke model,[17] we can see how this action or output has a multi-level effect on the system. Sensory (proprioceptive, tactile, vestibular, visual), as well as cognitive, psychologic and emotional processes were involved in providing input and feedback to produce a skill from the performance subsystem. The rules of skilled action were further clarified by the initiation and experience of this motion. Internalized roles of a seven-year-old girl include that of peer and player. In light of the importance that skills such as sommersaults hold for a seven-year-old, the effect on the perception of each of those roles can be imagined. New friends, new games, and new social activities may be associated not only with the gain of a skill, but even more importantly with the appreciation of expanded possibilities which accompanies such growth. With the realization of new possibilities, the implications for the volition subsystem governed by an urge towards exploration and mastery can be seen. The subsystem, functioning to enact, helped the child initiate the action through her motivation to achieve. The subsystem will also be subsequently influenced by the positive experience, contributing to feelings of success and mastery. A "person's sense of personal causation, or belief in their proven efficacy in some sphere of action is necessary for the output of competent occupational behavior."[17]

The application of open systems, hierarchical processes, and adaptation is fundamental to the use of occupation in practice. Utilization of these concepts provides the foundation for organizing theoretical knowledge in the clinical setting.

KNOWING WHAT TO LOOK FOR

Initiation of occupational therapy practice lies in the evaluation process. According to Gillette, "the evaluation process determines the baseline, provides a springboard from which the objectives are formed and thus serves as the foundation for the program of treatment or readjustment. It permits the identification of those problems which can and those which can not be mediated through the occupational therapy process."[11] However, in order to determine the problems that may or may not be addressed by occupational therapy, the evaluation process must be structured around an organized framework. A systems approach to evaluation provides the occupational therapist with such a foundation, and evaluation based on this method allows for recognition of the interrelationships between human subsystems. Without a structural base for the evaluation process, there is the danger of gathering varied information which is beyond the scope of occupational therapy, outside the realm of purpose to the client, or unrelated to the total treatment process. For example, a therapist utilizing what he or she might consider an eclectic approach may use the same set of evaluations for every client to assess function in several domains. The numerous ways in which disability differentially affects individuals limit such an approach in dealing with interrelationships. Why do some people with significant clinical limitations have better occupational role performance than others with fewer clinical problems? What is the relationship, if any, between self-image and the changing of hand dominance after a cerebral vascular accident? How might slurred speech compound these problems? If the information gathered is not organized, processed, and interpreted in relation to other information and to the overall functional level of the individual, therapists relinquish their professional judgment to perform mere technical skills.

Consideration of the interrelationship of subsystems and hierarchical characteristics of assets and limitations provides the context in which the therapist may express the unique goals of occupational therapy. Approaching a problem in this manner allows for the use of a wide variety of evaluation techniques, rather than limiting the scope of the tools utilized. A group of occupational therapists continually faced with the necessity of relating evaluative findings to each other and to the overall functional state of the client are those who treat children with sensory integrative dysfunction. Among several reasons for the presence of the issue in this area of practice is the fact that ramifications of sensory integrative dysfunction are not as clearly consequential as with other disorders. For example, that hallucinations associated with schizophrenia may interfere with an individual's ability to develop social relationships is generally understood. However, that inability to process tactile input may be related to hyperactivity or that poor vestibular processing may be associated with difficulty in reading[2] is less easily recognized. Therapists are thus continually forced to draw associations between the problem and the interference of function that occurs. In addition, the interrelationship between sensory processing and adaptive development, and the inherent hierarchical nature of sensory integrative functions make the use of an organized systems approach a requisite tool for interpreting evaluation findings in a meaningful way. A systems approach in this area of practice may allow therapists to use a wide variety of evaluation instruments and methods in assessing clients' sensory integrative status as it is associated with age-related occupational roles of student and player. In this manner, somatosensory function is not evaluated in isolation, but rather in relation to academic, social, and emotional parameters which also contribute to the child's development. Employing such a method within any area of practice will promote appropriate diversity rather than artificial constraints.

The evaluation process utilized may identify a professional to the same degree as the treatment process employed. As such, it is vital for the occupational therapist to take stock of the uses of evaluative findings. Without the organizing framework of occupation it is difficult to distinquish that which fits in the realm of occupational therapy from that which belongs to physical therapy, recreation therapy, social work, or nursing. In evaluation and treatment, occupational therapy must approach patient or client as an open system that experiences adaptation through occupation. In knowing what to look for the following questions must be asked before, during, and after the evaluation process:

(1) What was the patient's pre-onset occupational role?
(2) What is the patient's current occupational role?
(3) What is the patient's clinical status?
(4) What is the relationship between the patient's occupational role and clinical status (i.e., how do the findings affect other subsystems)?
(5) What are the patient's values (including socio-cultural factors) and expectations regarding recovery of pre-onset occupational role?

Once the findings of an assessment are interpreted within the context of these questions, the therapist is prepared to explore the prospect of knowing what to do.

KNOWING WHAT TO DO

Occupation is the organizing framework within which a systems approach can be utilized in the treatment setting. The therapist addresses the spectrum of subsystems that must function together to permit the individual to experience adaptation within the environment. For example, an adult male suffering a traumatic hand injury experiences disruption at several levels of function. The physical disability concurrently affects aspects of occupational role performance such as self-care, work skills, leisure activities, and social relationships. Treatment must address not only physical rehabilitation, as in muscle strengthening, range of motion and so forth, but must also address related areas as well. If the person was a carpenter prior to injury, a woodworking project may be a more appropriate therapeutic modality than weight-lifting. The fact that the activity is related to previous and perhaps future role performance engenders greater meaning and purpose, and occupation in such activity enhances organization of subsystems for future adaptation.

In this context, the therapist's role is to design environments to aid the client in organizing his actions (or output). By eliciting adaptive or successful outputs within purposeful activities, ability to interact competently within the environment is enhanced. Most importantly, successful occupation in *meaningful* activity will influence the client to function better in daily life.

To design such environments is certainly no easy task, and requires attention to all inputs which might have positive or negative effects on elicited outputs.

The following clinical guidelines, extracted from systems concepts, address the occupational therapy process as it relates to human occupation in environmental interaction and adaptation.

(1) In designing specific activities to remediate deficits in lower subsystems, the therapist must also address higher subsystems and the possibility of these impeding or facilitating the treatment process. For example, a therapist may attempt to develop independent function in two blind patients with similar clinical pictures. In designing an activity to encourage independent community mobility, it becomes evident that one patient is highly motivated to achieve these skills, while the other seems disinterested. The unmotivated client may have a past history of perceived failures with risk-taking experiences, and thus perceives herself as unable to exert internal control to successfully impact the environment. This client may avoid all situations in which failure may occur, or may prefer to remain dependent on others to avoid unsuccessful interactions. In this case, it is not enough to address only mobility skills within the treatment process. Rather, higher level motivational processes that influence the patient's ability to take risks must also be considered.

(2) The therapist should avoid focusing on just one subsystem in a therapeutic activity. It must be remembered that human occupation involves all components of human function, and that the failure or success of an activity may depend on a subsystem factor other than the one addressed. For example, a gravitationally insecure child interacts with another child in a sociodramatic play situation involving a trip on a "spaceship to the moon" on a large swing. When the child plays alone, he may not be able to overcome his fearful associations with vestibular activities in order to ride the swing. However, in a play situation, the child is involved not only in a

vestibular-based activity, but one that also has inherent emotional and social components. In this situation, it is the social component that provides the meaning and motivation to engage successfully in this otherwise fearful activity. On the other hand, a therapist working with emotionally disturbed children to encourage social interactions in play must keep in mind the sensory motor demands of the activity. For some children, these demands may make the task so threatening that organizing appropriate social interaction becomes impossible.

(3) When faced with chronic, irremediable deficits in a subsystem, another (usually higher level) subsystem may be utilized to compensate. For example, a therapist may help a patient to use cognitive strategies of energy conservation and work simplification and counseling on the use of time to overcome physical deficits of a systemic disease such as rheumatoid arthritis.

(4) The therapist utilizes and adapts the environment to help the individual organize successful outputs to activity demands. This involves careful activity analysis to address all aspects of the activity and environment which impinge on the client and influence output patterns. For example, a schizophrenic woman may have difficulty utilizing public transportation to reach a work training center. Analysis of the activity may reveal that the individual has no difficulty coping with the demands of the task except that she becomes disorganized when required to present the correct fare to the bus driver. By simplifying the task (i.e., by selecting the correct amount of change in advance) this individual will be more likely to succeed.

(5) Therapeutic activities should be designed to be meaningful for the individual for whom they are intended. Depending on results of an assessment of each subsystem of human function, a unique constellation of needs is revealed. It is therefore inappropriate for every stroke patient to engage in the same therapeutic exercise or self care task. While a craft activity may provide a purposeful means for one individual to achieve selective finger motion, a specific work-related activity such as typing may be more meaningful to another. Consideration of individual differences along the entire spectrum of human function is essential.

However technical, complex, simple, or common a modality may be, the occupational therapist must consider its implications for the entire human system. Relating the variety of treatment approaches to the common rubric of occupation provides the basis for "knowing what to do" in the treatment setting.

KNOWING WHY

The concerns of the practicing occupational therapist are indeed multifaceted. In addition to client-oriented problems, there are administrative, interdisciplinary, and intraprofessional issues which arise daily. Organizing theory and technique within a framework which binds clinical practice to the conceptual core of occupational therapy is not often considered within the daily regimen of clinical problems. Energy directed toward this process, however, ultimately could provide a medium for more efficient and purposeful management of clinical concerns.

Understanding, or knowing why, is one of the most crucial elements sustaining identity in clinical practice, and is greatly facilitated by organization of knowledge within a frame of reference. Although it may be easier to explain an activity in isolation, an association with overall purpose and process can be much more fruitful. For example, a therapist working on grooming with a mentally retarded adolescent probably could justify that activity with no difficulty. Consideration of the task alone should not lead to controversy because good hygiene is generally valued. In view of the gestalt, however, many questions could arise. Why is this a problem the occupational therapist should address, not the nurse? How does this activity relate to goals of occupational therapy? Why encourage independence in this activity when others may perform the task more quickly? A well-developed theoretical structure allows the therapist to meet questions from administrators, other professionals, families, clients, and, perhaps most importantly, questions that may arise from within oneself as a therapist. As Chapter 7 showed, theoretically articulate models of practice may be prerequisite to the future marketability of practice. Organizing practice within an overall occupational therapy context allows the therapist to recognize and explain how grooming is related to overall occupational role performance and adaptation to the environment as steps toward independence. All treatment programs, whether acute remedial intervention or long-term rehabilitation should be geared toward such functional goals.

An emphasis on meaningful occupation and an appreciation for the impact such activity (or lack thereof) has on an individual's life provides the occupational therapist with distinctive principles upon which to base practice. Recognition of those theoretical frameworks consistent with these principles of meaningful activity allows the therapist to realize the *feasibility* of utilizing diverse bodies of knowledge in practice. Understanding the scope of occupational therapy and its relation to one of the most fundamental of human processes, that is, occupation, compels the occupational therapist to recognize the *necessity* of doing so.

REFERENCES

1. American Occupational Therapy Association, Division of Operations and Research, 1981.

2. AYRES, AJ: *Sensory Integration and Learning Disorders.* Western Psychological Services, Los Angeles, 1972.

3. AYRES, AJ: *Sensory Integration and the Child.* Western Psychological Services, Los Angeles, 1979.

4. BOBATH, K AND BOBATH, B: *The neurodevelopmental approach to treatment.* In PEARSON, P AND WILLIAM C (EDS): *Physical Therapy Services in Developmental Disabilities.* Charles C. Thomas, 1972.

5. CHIN, R: *The utility of system models and developmental models for practitioners.* In BENNIS, WG, BENNE, DK AND CHIN, R, (EDS): *The Planning of Change: Readings in the Applied Behavioral Sciences.* Holt, Rinehart, & Winston, New York, 1961.

6. CROMWELL, F: *Sociological perspectives on specialization.* American Journal of Occupational Therapy, 33:29, 1979.

7. DICKOFF, J, JAMES, P AND WIEDENBACH, E: *Theory in a practice discipline, Part 1: Practice oriented theory.* Nursing Research, 17:415, 1968.

8. ENGLEHARDT, H: *Defining occupational therapy: The meaning of therapy and virtues of occupation.* American Journal of Occupational Therapy, 31:666, 1977.

9. FIDLER, GS: *Specialization: Implications for education.* American Journal of Occupational Therapy, 33:34, 1979.

10. FIDLER, G, AND FIDLER, J: *Doing and becoming: Purposeful action and self-actualization.* American Journal of Occupational Therapy, 32:305, 1978.

11. GILLETTE, N: *Occupational therapy and mental health.* In WILLARD, HS AND SPACKMAN, CS (EDS): *Occupational Therapy,* Ed 4. JB Lippincott, Philadelphia, 1971.

12. GILLETTE, N, AND KIELHOFNER, G: *The impact of specialization on the professionalization and survival of occupational therapy.* American Journal of Occupational Therapy, 33:20, 1979.

13. HALL, AD, AND FAGEN, RE: *Definition of a system.* In BUCKLEY, W: *Modern Systems Research for the Behavioral Scientist.* Aldine Publishing, Chicago, 1968.

14. HOPKINS, H AND SMITH, H: *Willard and Spackman's Occupational Therapy,* Ed 5 JB Lippincott, Philadelphia, 1978.

15. HUSS, AJ: *From kinesiology to adaptation.* American Journal of Occupational Therapy, 35:574, 1981.

16. JOHNSON, JA: *Occupational therapy: A model for the future.* American Journal of Occupational Therapy, 27:1, 1973.

17. KIELHOFNER, G, AND BURKE, J: *A model of human occupation, Part 1. — Conceptual framework.* American Journal of Occupational Therapy, 34:572, 1980.

18. KIELHOFNER, G: *General systems theory: Implications for theory and action in occupational therapy.* American Journal of Occupational Therapy, 32:637, 1978.

19. KING, LJ: *Toward a science of adaptive responses.* American Journal of Occupational Therapy, 32:429, 1978.

20. LINDQUIST, JE, MACK, W AND PARHAM, D: *A synthesis of occupational behavior and sensory integration concepts in theory and practice, Part 1. Theoretical foundations.* American Journal of Occupational Therapy, 36:365, 1982.

21. MARTIN, W: *The Order and Integration of Knowledge.* University of Michigan Press, Ann Arbor, 1957.

22. MEYER, A: *The philosophy of occupational therapy.* Archives of Occupational Therapy, 1:1, 1922.

23. POPPER, K: *Conjectures and Refutation: The Growth of Scientific Knowledge.* Harper & Row, New York, 1968.

24. REILLY, M: *Play as Exploratory Learning.* Sage Publications, Beverly Hills, Calif, 1974.

25. RIEHL, J AND ROY, C: *Conceptual Models for Nursing Practice.* Appleton Century Crafts, New York, 1974.

26. STEVENS, B: *Nursing Theory: Analysis Application and Evaluation.* Little Brown and Co., Boston, 1979.

27. *Task force on target populations.* American Journal of Occupational Therapy, 28:158, 1974.

28. TROMBLY, CA, AND SCOTT, AD: *Occupational Therapy for Physical Dysfunction.* Williams & Wilkins, Baltimore, 1977.

29. WEST W: *Historical perspectives.* In *Occupational Therapy: 2001 A.D.* American Occupational Therapy Association, Rockville, 1979.

30. WOLFE, R: *Defining occupation.* Unpublished manuscript, University of Southern California, 1981.

31. YERXA, EJ: *Authentic occupational therapy.* American Journal of Occupational Therapy, 21:1, 1967.

CHAPTER 15

THE ART OF OCCUPATIONAL THERAPY

Gary Kielhofner

EDITOR'S INTRODUCTION

Preceding chapters have addressed in various ways the process involved in the delivery of occupational therapy service. The authors offered prescriptions, caveats, and structures to serve as guidelines for clinicians. These chapters were girded by logical theses which were operationalized in some way relevant to practice.

Chapter 15 builds on the recurring theme of examining clinical practice from the point of view of the patient or client. Its format is more descriptive because it attempts to demonstrate the art of practice. The descriptions are drawn from the experience of the author over a period of several years of practice with a variety of patients and clients. A common thread throughout the chapter is that, in Marshall McLuhan's terms, the media is the message. What is offered as therapy and how it is offered, and, most importantly, the context in which it is offered, are proposed as determining the meaning of the therapy to the patient and the effect therapy will have.

The chapter concludes by focusing on the powerful theme of occupational therapy identified in Chapter 1. The same theme echoed throughout the remainder of the book: Occupational therapy works for a multitude of reasons. Some are physiologic, others psychologic, but the central, determinative factor in the practicality of occupation as a health-giving force is that, in the course of engaging in occupations, human beings—and specifically patients and clients—discover meaning. Meaning, in turn, infuses and energizes the culture, personality, and physiology of the individual. It is the core of the efficacy of occupation as therapy. Finally, this chapter proposes that it is transmitted when therapy is practiced as an art.

GK

I have to tell you that what (occupational therapists) operate is, in a simpler and more old-fashioned language, a mystery. What the theologians would call a sacrament. You are the administrants of an outward and visible activity, and your hope is that the patient will receive, through your administrations, an inward and spiritual grace. . . . The modality is somehow to be the carrier for a message to the patient. A message about himself, his relationship to the human universe and the relationship between himself and you. . . . But, I warn you, the business is not so simple. Unless the priest—and I mean you—feels that the modality matters more than any other thing in the world, the deeper message is rather liable to fall by the wayside (Gregory Bateson, 1956)

The idea of writing a chapter on the art of occupational therapy occurred to me when this volume was in the planning stage. It seemed appropriate that a text devoted to scientific, theoretical and otherwise rigorous topics should end with a discussion that would temper previous considerations. Thus, the idea of an "art" of practice seemed an appropriate finale.

I have come to believe that there is an element of healing which supersedes the technical and—if you will—scientific elements of practice. As Riley[25] notes, a large portion of medicine's successes may be attributed to a placebo effect which is rooted in the cultural rather than technical aspects of medicine. In their defense of the medical model, Seigler and Osmond[26] argue that the physician's aesculapian authority and the patient's confidence in the healing role of the physician are indispensible parts of the success of medical care. Smith notes that:

> There is still much more artistry than science to both educational and therapeutic endeavors and the broad strategies that guide us in the working with people still depend more on the underlying assumptions about the nature of man than upon firmly established findings.[28]

The art of a field, he points out, depends on its metapsychology or philosophical preconceptions. In occupational therapy the broad assumption that energizes its art is the belief that human beings require and experience meaning in their daily activities.

The elements that the therapist manipulates as part of the field's art are, not surprisingly, those that have eluded scientific description and analysis. They include values, aesthetics, morale, ritual, and other modes of being and doing that seem to defy the neat structures of science. One way of characterizing the difference between art and science—a way that sets the stage for our considerations of the art of therapy—is that science may be described as textual while art is contextual. When we speak of the facts of science and when we employ them in therapy, we are engaged in a literal translation of ideas; when we follow the dictums of science we operationalize a text of knowledge. Thus, science can be prescriptive in a most exact sense.

In saying that art is contextual, I refer to the fact that while the production or product of art may have a literal aspect (the play script or the color combinations of a painting) its meaning is always nonliteral. Context, or the relationship of the art object or performance to some larger dimension of life, is always involved. That is precisely why we *understand* scientific facts, but we *appreciate* art.

The science of a field yields its technology; however, its art is embedded in the way technology is choreographed in the therapeutic event. The clinical judgment that a patient will need an assistive device or a splint is a matter of science, and can be specified by recourse to exact knowledge. The art of orchestrating the event of a patient's trying out the new splint or device to achieve a desired experience involves a deep and important contextual dimension. It is this concept of context and its relationship to the human experience of meaning that are our concerns here.

THE ORGANIZING FUNCTION OF ART AND MEANING

I would like to propose that the dimension of art in therapy has the special property of ordering and giving meaning to human emotion, thought, and morale. This derives from the generic character of all art forms.

The meaning in art and in therapy is an intermingling of intellectual and emotional elements that yield pleasure by evoking some higher value. The pleasure of appreciating art uplifts, enhancing the morale of the audience and bringing forth deep appreciation of some aspect of humanity or nature. Thus art has an important role in synthesizing human emotion and intellect, evoking value, and enhancing morale—processes not unlike our vision of occupational therapy. In his discussion of art, Kepes notes that:

> As common perception gathers a number of sense impressions into a *gestalt,* a pattern-vision, this heightened perception of artistic vision collates sense impressions into vision of the high patterning of works of art, with their harmony, balance, melodic sequence and rhythm.[17]

The process of ordering is perhaps the central key to how properly orchestrated therapy (i.e., therapy artfully executed) influences the healing process. The dynamic of this process is the transference of some meaningful order in the external world to the internal world of the patient or client. We are well aware of how external disorder is transformed to internal dysfunction; schizophrenia provides an example of such a process.

The original insight of occupational therapy was that establishing a meaningful external order with harmony, balance, and explicit values has the effect of positively transforming disordered internal affairs. The art of occupational therapy lies in creating such an order for patients and clients in which their participation imprints itself on the internal disarray, restoring or bringing order via the meaning the participants experience.

MEANINGFUL ACTIVITY. As Sharrot and Engelhardt showed in earlier chapters, occupational therapy involves the creation of meaning through the use of occupation. Yet, nothing is more elusive in occupational therapy than meaningful activity. While few therapists would deny that they rely on meaningful activities as an important part of their service, most would be hard pressed to offer a systematic, if not theoretical, explanation of how they manage to make activities meaningful. Indeed, while the field has maintained a verbal and practical commitment to the importance of meaningful activity, no serious attempt has been made to ferret out the nature of meaning or the process by which meaning is created in human action. One of the most important challenges to occupational therapy is to understand how to orchestrate what we have so blithely called "meaningful activities." In Chapter 10, Sharrot offers the first important examination of the nature of meaning in human action. My intention here is not to present such a sweeping thesis, but to illustrate a few features of human meaning which bear on the art of clinical practice.

The meaning of anything is the impact or change it warrants in the perceiver's framework of knowing about the world.[4] Thus, the meaning of an activity is in part determined by a person's accumulated experience and the way in which it predisposes the person to attribute significance.

Simultaneously, external context is a powerful determinant of meaning. For the present discussion my characterization of context is derived from the work of Bateson[2] and Goffman,[11] especially the latter's concept of dramaturgical context. Goffman proposes that individuals interact and produce public behavior in terms of various socially defined situations within which they find themselves behaving. Thus, behavior is never simply behavior per se, but part of an action sequence belonging to some type of event, whether a friendly greeting, business encounter, social occasion, or a religious ceremony. Each of these dramaturgical contexts has its proper stage or setting, identifiable props (behavioral or material), roles, and a script which the social actors follow with remarkable predictability. Goffman's conceptualization of dramaturgical context points out the important truth in Shakespeare's famous line "all the world's a stage." Bateson[2] refers to this aspect of context as "metacommunicative." Context tells about its contents, how they are to be understood, what their meaning will be. In short, persons derive their 'instructions' for how to experience and behave from a cultural set of contexts.

These dramaturgical contexts are largely matters of social convention. That is, the social sphere provides the possibility for a given context by virtue of having such contexts in the cultural tradition, and it provides for the possibility of persons recognizing and participating in contexts of action by virtue of their shared nature. Cultural members come to agree upon, or more properly, take for granted the existence of certain contexts of action and they recognize and produce them through agreed upon conventions. When we speak of a cultural tradition providing for the possibility of contexts, we are referring to the fact that contexts are the products of culture—their existence is in the collective tradition. A culture which does not contain, as part of its tradition, the context of healing through the ministrations of a witch doctor, does not give its members a framework within which it becomes reasonable or natural to engage in behaviors which are recognizably required for and understandable as witchdoctoring. Thus, acts that derive their meaning from such a context appear ridiculous to us. On the other hand, the contexts of modern medicine provide cultural members with a definitional framework within which another range of acts becomes sensible. The patient does not faithfully take the physician's prescription because he understands the physiologic rationale for the efficacy of a drug. Rather, the context of "being cared for by the doctor" provides sufficient definitional background. Taking the pill is an act made sensible by the context.

We also note that cultural members recognize that contexts pertain to situations by virtue of conventional signs. The physician's garb, his black bag and stethoscope are just as important as signs that a context pertains as they are as functional implements of the trade. These accoutrements speak for the context; they announce its pertinence. As Goffman[11] notes, times, places, artifacts, attire, and a plethora of other material and nonmaterial elements serve as indicators of a dramaturgical context, that it is now—so to speak—the frame within which actors will carry out and experience their action.

Bateson[2] also stresses the importance of context as a determinant of meaning and experience. He notes the importance of individual recognition that a particular context

FEATURES OF OCCUPATIONAL THERAPY PRACTICE
AND THEIR IMPLICATIONS FOR CLINICS AND INTERVENTIONS

or frame pertains to their behavior and their employment of that frame as a means of interpreting and participating in ongoing events. Without context, Bateson shows us, there is no meaning. He proposes that all learning, and thus all competent behavior, involves the acquisition and use of metacommunicative contexts that define the nature of what is learned or undertaken. For instance, he notes that play is not a particular act or action; rather, it is a context for action. Play serves as a context for actors to acknowledge that they are acting in a "make believe" fashion—as when their aggressive acts signify not aggression, but a parody of aggression. Actions that might be considered offensive, harmful, or idiotic take on totally different meaning within the context of play, the practical joke, and so forth. Thus, part of the nature of context is its role as a mutually agreed upon definer that sets ground rules for all interpretations and actions within it.

Let us examine what this signifies. The meaning of an activity can be shown to change as it is examined in various contexts. An occupational therapist doing needlework will serve to illustrate the point. Imagine the therapist in the following contexts drawn from my observations: at home after work, in the clinic while teaching a patient a craft, and in a group of therapists being addressed by a United States senator. The meaning of the activity shifts as we imagine it within these contexts. In other words, as we reframe any activity, we can manipulate its meaning.

This consideration of the nature of meaning and contexts returns us to the role of art in occupational therapy. The thesis of this chapter is that occupational therapy as an art can influence the internal order of a human system by virtue of its control over the meaning that activities have for patients or clients. Such a perspective presumes the importance of context in determining meaning, the manipulability of context, and the importance of meaning in organizing behavior. In Chapter 2, it was proposed that the organization of the human organism is a hierarchical phenomenon in which higher levels ruled the lower. At the apex of human system is the capacity for the system to experience meaning—a symbolic capacity that involves acquiring and adhering to values. Meaning thus has the ability to organize behavior by virtue of its position in the hierarchy of phenomena which comprise human life. Meaning lies at the core of both art and the organization of human action. As Kepes[17] notes, human order is always in terms of value; it is the highest, ruling dimension of human experience. The ordering of experience and behavior to some higher value or values gives meaning to life.[10]

CONTEXTS FOR THE ART OF HEALING THROUGH OCCUPATION

We come now to the special problem of identifying the kinds of dramaturgical contexts that may be used in occupational therapy. Our problem is to define metacommunicative frames we can construct around our activities to influence the meaning that these occupations will have for patients.

A great deal of interest has been generated in recent literature concerning the play frame and its derivations. Play has always been an important part of occupational therapy; as noted in Chapter 1, some early therapists saw occupational therapy consisting entirely of occupations that belonged in some sense to the domain of play.

The contexts derived from play which will be discussed in the following sections are exploration, festivity and ritual, sport, and craft. Although most readers may have been accustomed to thinking of these as activities (i.e., performances consisting of throwing balls, moulding clay, toasting a friend, etc.) we will examine how each of these serves as a frame to define the behavior and experience that goes on within them.

EXPLORATION. One of the most basic frames of human experience, and one that occurs early in the developmental process, is exploration. Within the context of exploration curiosity is the reigning spirit.[23] Actions have one important meaning in this context: they are oriented to the task of finding out. Exploration is perhaps one of the few situations that has no possibility of failure, since what is found out is not at issue; rather, finding out serves as an end in itself. As Bateson notes:

> Exploration is self-validating, whether the outcome is pleasant or unpleasant for the explorer. If you try to teach a rat to not explore by having him poke his nose into boxes containing electric shock, he will . . . go on doing this, presumably needing to know which boxes are safe and which unsafe.[2]

The most important dimension of the exploratory context is this absolution from failure. Participants in exploration find that they are free to discover aspects of the material, human, and symbolic world with impunity. The context asks of us only that we seek to find. This context gives license to individuals to vary their actions in finding their consequences and limits. Behaviors that would otherwise appear senseless or nonpurposeful take on meaning in the exploratory context. Whether it be a child investigating a new toy, or an adult testing the limits of a newly purchased sports car, exploration represents the context of ultimate freedom in human experience. The context of exploration also provides a vehicle for some of life's most fundamental learning. As humans approach and experience their material and symbolic world they are exposed to characteristics, consequences, values, and a whole range of information that otherwise would be unavailable or hidden to them.

A number of elements may facilitate or block contexts of exploration. Physical and social variables make exploration a pertinent context or mitigate against it. We all recall as children those situations, places, times, and persons presented as contexts for exploration. An empty lot, an attic, or a grandparent's lap presented ready exploratory contexts. However, church, adult meetings, and the school principal more or less forbade an exploratory attitude. The exploratory context requires a degree of familiarity and safeness juxtaposed with novelty or complexity to provide opportunities for discovery. Social definition always provides an exploratory context. The announcement that a particular event will begin with "getting to know one another" or "getting the feel of" some procedure allows freedom of exploration. By the same token, social demands which are too consequential destroy the possibility of exploration.

Many individuals lack ability to enter the context of exploration. This is found among the young who cannot play and who, as a consequence, learn little about their environments. It may be found among the disabled and elderly who find it too painful to entertain novel modes of existence, to search for new sets of values and interests. Yet, for all these individuals the context of exploration is an important avenue from a state of disorganization and unhappiness to a more satisfying and organized existence.

FEATURES OF OCCUPATIONAL THERAPY PRACTICE
AND THEIR IMPLICATIONS FOR CLINICS AND INTERVENTIONS

Thus, human beings who encounter the world in the context of exploration have an opportunity to learn about the objects, people, and events about them, to acquire a better sense of themselves (especially if the self is a drastically changed one, as in physical trauma), and to discover new interests and values. Exploration is the prime context in which individuals can incorporate new information about their world and their existence.

Our clinics were once organized to be contexts of exploration. Slagle spoke of the kindergarten model of therapy for the emotionally disturbed. She offered the stimulants of color, sound, simple materials, and activities as arenas for discovery. Tracy[30] proposed that therapists could elicit the exploratory context by serving as models of the pleasure to be gained in exploration. They realized that the context of exploration required a degree of laissez faire, an attitude of frivolity, and freedom from the pressures of survival. To the degree that our modern clinics are devoid of such playfulness and attend to the "serious business" of therapy, we revoke the possibility of the exploratory context for patients.

The following story, which I have related elsewhere, serves to illustrate something about the necessity of creating a context of exploration for our patients:

> John was an intellectually normal 13-year-old with a diagnosis of adolescent adjustment reaction. He exhibited a paucity of skills, disorganized behavior, and extreme anxiety and rigidity in the face of novel situations or tasks. In the first occupational therapy session when offered clay, John, having only touched it, promptly enclosed himself in the storage closet, refusing to emerge. The occupational therapist (one of the authors) suggested that John simply sit and watch the therapist as *he* made something of the clay, hoping to decrease John's anxiety over encountering the craft. As if nothing could go right, the therapist proceeded to spill a bowl of clay slip over his pants. In a good natured exchange of joking about the accident, the therapist and a student managed to clean up the mess and the pants, while John watched on.
>
> Thinking the episode must have eliminated even the slightest urge on John's part to make something with clay, an alternative was offered. John, however, remarked that the clay looked like it might be fun and offered to give it a try which he did with some success. Over the course of therapy John learned to try out many new crafts with an increasing sense of control, investment, and satisfaction.
>
> Only later by reflecting on the original incident did it become apparent that the accident with the clay and its subsequent "nonserious" treatment was just what John needed. It revealed to him that the occupational therapy clinic was a place where even the worst could happen without ill consequences. It was safe to play.[32]

Often, such human intervention or demonstration is required to convey to the patient the message that it is safe, that the context of exploration pertains.

In summary, exploration as a context for human behavior and experience is an important determinant of a person's ability to learn about and achieve some degree of comfort with the material and symbolic world. Through the designs of our clinics and through the attitudes we engender within them we can either facilitate or mitigate against this context.

SPORT. Sutton-Smith[29] proposed that sport involves four dramatic roles: player, co-player, coach and spectator. In sport, player and co-player are responsible for initiating and responding to each other under a set of ground rules that determines the nature of their endeavor. Thus, player and co-player take action with reference to each other in terms of a rule-bound structure. The coach monitors the playing process to make sure that players adhere to rules. The role of coach may be assumed by one player or more; thus, it is not always represented in a single individual. Finally, there is an audience to witness the outcome. The sportive metaphor, or frame may serve as a context for both group and individual action. As Sutton-Smith[29] notes, even children in solitary play assume roles of player, co-player, coach, and audience as they engage, respond, set the ground rules, and witness their own actions and their results. An adult version is the game of solitaire, in which the element of competition is preserved. Sport is a kind of dialectic in which outcome is a function of the effort, skills, and cunning of player and co-player.

While sport is ordinarily thought of in terms of competition, it may also involve cooperation as two players work together to achieve an effect. Some of the games in which children or adults attempt to prolong a sequence of events (i.e., jumping rope, volleying a ping-pong ball). The New Games movement is another example of cooperative sport. In such events the competitive element of the game is supplanted with the dialectic between players' efforts to maintain processes of high improbability and the odds of its failure.

The organizing dimension of a game or sport is found in the juxtaposition of skills and strategy against a situation of risk.[33] Most importantly, behavior is organized so that the dimension of "how much risk is feasible" becomes apparent. While sport involves risk, it also tempers it. The risk is not burdened by harsh consequences; thus, the sporting frame serves as an important context to minimize or control consequences of risk. Bruner offers an excellent example of this in the following story about a child with a learning block:

> Take the eleven-year-old boy who at one of his first sessions said to the tutor that he was afraid to make an error in reading because his teacher yelled at him. The tutor asked whether his teacher yelled very loud, and upon being assured that she did, volunteered that he could yell louder than the teacher, and urged his patient to make a mistake and see. The boy did, and his tutor in mock voice yelled as loud as he could. The boy jumped. Tutor to patient: "Can she yell louder than that?" Patient: "Yes, lots." Tutor: "Make another error and I'll try to get louder still." The game went on three or four rounds, and the tutor then suggested that the patient try yelling when he, the tutor make an error . . . After a few sessions, a playful relation had been built up about the mistakes in reading . . . Soon the child was able to take satisfaction in the skills in which he was achieving mastery.[5]

The sporting metaphor served to redefine the entire act of sentence construction by changing the ground rules. The activity no longer meant failure but mastery to the child.

In a program using sports with mentally retarded adults, we became aware of the importance of introducing and maintaining the game context. Many retarded men simply did not grasp the idea of a sport context and could not contribute to its maintenance. Therapists not only had to participate as co-players, coaches, and audience in the game process, but also had to maintain a game attitude:

> Part of the game context was an attitude of playfulness. When an atmosphere of playfulness or fun replaced a more serious mood, it elicited participation, thus resolving many of the motivational problems acknowledged by others who were working with these men.[18]

The game context is one of the most basic modes of human interaction. Thus, it is particularly suited as a context for therapeutic interaction with the disabled. For instance, Goode, in a sociological study of deaf-blind retarded children, relates the following incident:

> Chris maneuvered me in such a way that she was lying on my lap face up and had me place my hand over her face. By holding my hand she eventually maneuvered it in such a way that my palm was on her mouth and my index finger was on her right ("good") eye. She then indicated to me that she wanted me to tap on her eyelid by picking my finger up and letting it fall on her eye repeatedly, smiling and laughing when I voluntarily took over this work as my own (She has also "shown me," by moving my body, that she wanted me to speak in her ear and flick my fingers across her good eye.) While I tapped Chris's eye, she licked and sniffed my palm occasionally and softly hummed seemingly melodic sounds. *We did this* for about 10 or 15 minutes.[12]

Games with persons who have vastly altered neurologic and sensory apparatus may serve as important contexts for establishing communication and giving these individuals some access to the external meanings of our world. In addition, as Goode argues, we are enriched with a vision of such persons' inner worlds.

One of the most important functions of the sport context is its ability to equalize or level relationships between players. Through the process of "handicapping" and through team composition games seek to give equal advantage and opportunity to players or teams. The game process often provides an opportunity for individuals to experience themselves as valid and competent social members. We found this to be the case in our use of games with mentally retarded adults. Persons who otherwise related to us as therapists with authority and control over them, experienced us as equals in a process. The game context, by virtue of this equalizing process, often elicited competent, organized performances from persons who were otherwise behaviorally disorganized. Mead[19] notes that sports offer individuals miniature models of society within which they can organize their behavior. This contextual property of games is an important one for the occupational therapy process of ordering human experience and behavior.

FESTIVITY AND RITUAL. One of the most ordering experiences of human life is the participation in feasts and rituals. According to Cox, "Festivity, by breaking routine and opening men to the past, enlarges his experience and reduces his provincialism."[6] Festivity and ritual are marker events. Not surprisingly, feast and ritual often signal the end of, or mastery over suffering, struggle, personal sacrifice or loss. "At such times we affirm life and gaiety despite the facts of failure and death."[6] Commenting on the origins of ritual, Duthie notes:

> Thus Man, as a conscious-living or 'minded' organism, facing the certainty of death and the likelihood of illness, accident and natural catastrophy, discovered in ritual a means of making the inchoate less awful and thus more understandable and bearable.[9]

By commemorating the struggle, accomplishment, and suffering of the past, by celebrating the moment and attaching our hope to the future, festivity and ritual fuse past, present, and future. The ordering process of festivity and ritual is the collation of the three dimensions of time under the rubric of hope that is made possible when we transcend suffering, see the fruits of our efforts or struggle, find present joy and hope for that which is to come. Duthie notes that ritual is

> a method whereby individuals are able to project the important happenings in their own lives against the background of man's collective experience: events and happenings in our own lives are, through ritual, given significance on being related to a wider human experience.[9]

Duthie's view of ritual approximates that of Durkheim,[8] who distinguished the sacred from the profane in everyday life, relegating ritual to the domain of the sacred. We generally think of the ritual dimension of life as pertaining only to hallowed or exalted times, places, and persons. However, recent writers such as Blanchard[3] and Handleman[15] suggest that ritual also has a mundane form. Thus, we recognize the ritual aspects of much daily discourse.

Affirmation of membership in a group is a major function of ritual. Whether it be donning clothes of a certain type, sitting down to a common meal, or participating in some "inside process," such contexts provide the frame within which an individual's behavior or identity is affirmed, as sharing common features with a larger collective.

In the same way that an individual may be brought into a group by participation in its rituals, one may achieve a connection to others and the larger values they represent by performing personal rituals in which others participate. When the boss, minister, or president comes to dinner, it is not he or she who has joined us, but rather that we have been made part of the collectivity which they represent.

Participation in ritual reminds the individual that his or her personal experience is simply a variant of a much greater human condition. Through ritual individual experience is connected to and interpreted in terms of the group collectivity and its values which impart meaning to behavior. The bar mitzvah and the confirmation affirm adulthood and membership in a group with its reigning values and interpretation of behavior. Less widespread rituals such as the initiation rites of high school and college groups, or even the highly stylized greeting of certain cultural subgroups, are ritual means of enlisting individuals within a larger group.

Miracle[21] proposes that it is both possible and desirable to create and implant rituals in institutions. He sees institutional ritual as a means of influencing the spirit or morale of members. The implication for occupational therapy is that local rituals should be in place for participation by patients. Nursing homes, long-term board and care facilities, and halfway houses—all are institutions that would benefit from the incorporation of festive and ritual contexts. In one psychiatric facility where I worked, annual events during holidays were organized by therapists. One adolescent unit prepared a Thanksgiving feast for parents and families; all units participated in a grand Christmas production. The normalizing effect of these festive and ritual occasions was apparent in the sudden decrease of disorganized activity, acting out, and similar maladaptive behavior by patients. If the proposals offered by those who favor festivity and ritual are correct, we can assume that these events also served the lasting purpose of realigning otherwise alienated individuals to the larger group and its values. We need only recall how many psychiatric patients find themselves alienated from the holidays, celebrations, and rituals of their culture. It is not so much that they recall painful experiences associated with these times, but that they must face their inability to celebrate and their alienation from the larger group.

A further implication for occupational therapy is that we must learn to recognize and cultivate the natural rituals of patients and clients and their subgroups or families. Patients bring with them a personal history of celebrative and ritual styles that could have important functions in organizing their behavior and experience. Allowing patients to create their own celebration and ritual is an important consideration in allowing patients to find meaning. The following story illustrates this point.

I once worked with an elderly patient who had suffered a cerebrovascular accident that had rendered her wheelchair-bound and robbed her of effective use of one upper extremity. When I interviewed this woman about her life I ascertained that she had worked, raised children, and had a successful marriage that culminated in years of caring for an ailing husband. With her newly acquired disability and advanced years, she had determined that it was her lot to be a helpless cripple until she died. Her younger sister, a woman with deep religious feelings, also had accepted that it was God's will that she should care for her sister in her remaining life. Her well intentioned but deadly plan was to wait on her sister and require nothing of her in return.

As an individual and as a therapist, I found this an intolerable prospect and I told her that I saw a large reservoir of remaining capacity which she not only could but should exercise. Furthermore, our mutual exploration of her past revealed an activity that had meant more to her in everyday life than anything else: baking cookies, breads, and so forth. The ritual context in which this activity had meaning involved her loving relationship with her husband and the nurturing of her children. Each afternoon she carefully planned and baked goods which would be fresh and waiting as her children and husband returned from school and work. The sequence of her careful preparation and execution of the activity, her growing excitement and hurried preparation as the time of arrival of husband and children neared and the warm and satisfying episodes that ensued were the epitome of Frankl's[10] notion of finding meaning in the immediacy of life. That she should lose every remnant of this activity seemed an intolerable condition for her remaining years. Her sister's household to which she would return was populated with children and adults who could enjoy and value her baking.

When I shared this idea with her, she protested, noting that her ravaged body and failing health prevented her from engaging in such activities. After some exhortation, she agreed to try a cooking session (in which she adamantly predicted failure) only because I was "such a nice young man."

In preparation for the event, I examined the clinic kitchen, fabricated needed adaptive equipment, borrowed a recipe of her favorite baking project (chocolate chip cookies), and rehearsed the sequence and steps of the needed performance.

On the appointed day, amid mild protests, she began the activity. With the aid of adaptive devices, some ad hoc instruction, and a bit of help, she completed the task, noting (inaccurately) that I had "done it for her." Finally, she crumpled the recipe and tossed it in the wastebasket.

As planned earlier, ward and therapeutic staff appeared at the door and set to greedily eating the cookies, showering compliments and gratitude. During this sequence her affect slowly changed as she proudly announced that she had "done it all alone." When everyone left, we washed the dishes and put the kitchen in order. As we were about to leave the room she stopped to ask if she could retreive the recipe from the wastebasket.

Celebration and ritual in their varied forms are important contexts for restoring morale and renewing commitment to values while providing continuity of experience with the past and with the world outside. They are too often absent from or ignored in occupational therapy today.

CRAFT. The experience of craft stands against some of the other contexts we have examined. In a sense it is the most tangible of contexts, one which brings individuals closest to everyday reality. Richards characterizes craft as follows:

> Part of the training we enjoy as craftsmen is to bring into our bodies the imagination and the will we enact. The handcrafts stand to perpetuate the living experience of contact with natural elements—something primal, immediate, personal, material, a dialogue between our dreams and the forces of nature.[24]

Further, craftsmanship provides a context for experiencing control, independence, and self worth. In the craft context there is no ulterior motive; work is done for the products and the process of creation.[20] Thinking and action are fused in craft, which provides the most immediate context for Reilly's[22] vision of occupational therapy as a process binding hands and will to common purpose.

Craft involves a tradition of "know-how".[16] The craftsman learns attitudes and skills from a mentor through imitation. Thus, the context of craft is infused with the notion of accumulated wisdom and technical know-how that defines what is worth accomplishing and how it can be accomplished. Craft also embodies a set of values, as identified by Mills:

> As ideal, craftsmanship stands for the creative nature of work, and for the central place of such work in human development as a whole. As practice, craftsman stands for the classic role of the independent artisan who does his work in close interplay with the public, which in turn participates in it.[20]

Trupp offers the following as a set of craft values that characterizes American craftsmen:

> *Pride* in able workmanship, *performance* to the highest standards of his craft, *protection* of his honor and his reputation through quality control, *pleasure* in the completion of a job well done, and the rewards of personal satisfaction and gain.[31]

In the craft context the participant is brought into the presence of these values and can attach his performance to these standards while incorporating them as part of his own ethic of performance. Craft is one of the most organizing of contexts. It requires attention, patience, persistence of effort, and rigorous following of rules, all tempered with personal creativity. Craft provides a coherent metaphor for life and its organizing processes. The context of craft requires an orderly environment with proper tools and materials, and with models who emulate the craft experience. I like to think of myself as an accomplished craftsman in carpentry. When working with patients, it seemed to me that one of my most important assets was an ability to create a context which encouraged the adaptive struggle of patients by providing examples of how careful effort is rewarded. For instance, for several months a cotherapist and I ran a woodworking shop for a small group of cerebral palsied men. One of the rules of the shop was that therapists had to be working on projects that the clients observed as they began their own. What a tremendous difference there is between the individual brought into a clinic and offered a choice of some activity and one who is brought into the presence of a craftsman whose performance invites participation! In our shop these cerebral palsied men turned out products of remarkable quality despite their motor impairment. Their struggle against the limitations of their bodies was maintained and organized by the craft context, and I am convinced that nowhere else could they have accomplished as much. Further, the men gained a significant degree of self-worth and confidence through their identification with the process and their identification with us.

Craft is one of the powerful traditions in occupational therapy, but its use as a context of therapy has unfortunately declined. Hall,[14] Haas,[13] and Dunton[7] were early occupational therapy proponents who advocated craft as one of the most uplifting and organizing human experiences, since it combined order, precision, creativity, planning and concrete reality. They perceived a need for occupational therapists to be thorough craftspersons. The ideal of the occupational therapist as craftsperson seems to be dying, and this is a tremendous loss to the art of the field.

CONCLUSION

This chapter has proposed that the generation, alteration, manipulation and maintenance of contexts constitute what may properly be called the art of occupational therapy. Further, by virtue of its ability to create, modify, and maintain meaning this art constitutes a fundamental aspect of the healing process in occupational therapy. When contexts are artfully used in the process of therapy a special organizing influence comes to bear on the behavior of patients. Realization of this requires that we understand how meaning is the governing process in the organization of human behavior. Without meaning, everything slowly decompensates; with meaning, even the most disorganized mental and physical processes can be reorganized.

In physical disabilities our patients share the condition of being disenfranchised. At the level of bodily insult we recognize those who have lost the ability to sense and to move. However, a deeper and more debilitating disenfranchisement takes place: the loss of the ability of these persons to make sense of their lives and to be moved by the values of their world. Life takes on meaning in the minute-by-minute reality in which we experience ourselves achieving the ordinary things that sustain a sense of the commonplace, a security in the very ordinary nature of most of our experience. We are anchored in the familiar reality of our daily lives. Mundane though it may be, it is the stuff of our sanity. Beyond this unreflective involvement in moment-by-moment life, we are attached to a larger world—one bounded by an extension of time to past and future, of self to relationships with others, and of personal purpose to the grander scheme about us. This I have referred to as our attachment to value.

In similar fashion psychiatric clinics are populated with persons whose major source of debilitation is disengagement from everyday life and from the values of the social group. The adverse effects of this alienation and meaninglessness are substantial, as we know.

In these cases we hope to restore some sense of meaning, some attachment to value, some morale for daily life. Occupational therapy is a negotiative process in which we seek to arbitrate between the disorganized inner contexts of our patients and the outer contexts we manipulate to give meaning. The situations we create, and the tasks, opportunities, challenges, and celebrations we provide are the dimensions of our art. It is our belief that the organizing features of the contexts we create will transfer to patients' internal context—that they will acquire abilities to explore, celebrate and ritualize, engage in sport and craft as ways of being, and that they will become more competent, more ready for the tasks, disappointments, and joys of life.

REFERENCES

1. BATESON, G: *Communication in occupational therapy.* American Journal of Occupational Therapy, 10:188, 1956.

2. BATESON, G: *Mind and Nature: A Necessary Unity.* Bantam Books, New York, 1979.

3. BLANCHARD, K: *Sport and ritual in Choctaw society: Structure and perspective.* IN SCHWARTZMAN, H (ED): *Play and Culture.* Leisure Press, West Point, NY, 1980.

4. BOULDING, K: *The Image,* University of Michigan Press, Ann Arbor, 1973.

5. BRUNER, J: *On coping and defending.* IN COLEMAN, J (ED): *Psychology and Effective Behavior,* Scott, Foresman and Company, Glenview, Ill, 1969.

6. COX, H: *The feast of fools.* Harper and Row, New York, 1969.

7. DUNTON, WR: *Reconstruction therapy.* WB Saunders, Philadelphia, 1979.

8. DURKHEIM, E: *The Elementary Forms of the Religious Life.* Free Press, New York, 1969.

9. DUTHIE, JH: *Athletics: The ritual of a technological society.* IN SCHWARTZMAN, HD (ED): *Play and Culture.* Leisure Press, West Point, NY, 1980.

10. FRANKL, V: *Man's Search for Meaning: An Introduction to Logotherapy.* Washington Square Press, New York, 1962.

11. GOFFMAN, E: *The Presentation of Self In Everyday Life.* Doubleday Anchor Books, New York, 1959.

12. GOODE, D: *The world of the congenitally deaf-blind: Toward the grounds for achieving human understanding.* IN JACOBS, J (ED): *Mental Retardation: A Phenomenological Approach.* Charleles C. Thomas, Springfield, Ill, 1980.

13. HAAS, L: *Practical Occupational Therapy.* Bruce Publishing, Milwaukee, 1945.

14. HALL, H: *O.T.: A New Profession.* The Rumford Press, Concord, 1923.

15. HANDLEMAN, D: *Re-thinking naven: play and identity.* IN SCHARTZMAN, H (ED): *Play and Culture.* Leisure Press, West Point, NY 1980.

16. JANSON, HW: *History of Art.* Narry N Abrams, New York, 1970.

17. KEPES, G: *Comments on art.* In MASLOW, MA (ED): *New Knowledge In Human Values.* Henry Regnery, Chicago, 1959.

18. KIELHOFNER, G AND MIYAKE, S: *The therapeutic use of games with mentally retarded adults.* American Journal of Occupational Therapy, 35:375, 1981.

19. MEAD, GH: *Mind, Self, and Society.* University of Chicago Press, Chicago, 1962.

20. MILLS, CW: *Power, Politics and People.* Ballantine Books, New York, 1963.

21. MIRACLE, A: *School spirit as a ritual by-product: Views from applied anthropology.* IN SCHWARTZMAN, HB, (ED): *Play and Culture.* Leisure Press, West Point, NY, 1980.

22. REILLY, M: *Occupational therapy can be one of the great ideas of 20th century medicine.* American Journal of Occupational Therapy 16:1, 1962.

23. REILLY, M: *Play as Exploratory Learning.* Sage Publications, Beverly Hills, Calif, 1974.

24. RICHARDS, M: *Centering.* Wesleyan University Press, Middletown, Conn. 1964.

25. RILEY, JN: *Western medicine's attempt to become more scientific: Examples from the United States and Thailand.* Social Science and Medicine, 11:549, 1977.

26. SIEGLER, M AND OSMOND, H: *Models of Madness, Models of Medicine.* Harper and Row, New York, 1974.

27. SLAGLE, EC: *Training aides for mental patients.* Archives of Occupational Therapy, 1:11, 1922.

28. SMITH, MB: *Competence and adaptation.* American Journal of Occupational Therapy 28:11, 1974.

29. SUTTON-SMITH, B: *A "sportive" theory of play.* IN SCHWARTZMAN, H (ED), *Play and Culture.* Leisure Press, West Point, NY, 1980.

30. TRACY, S: *Studies in Invalid Occupation.* Witcomb & Burrows, Boston, 1912.

31. TRUPP P: *The Art of Craftsmanship.* Acropolis Books, Washington, DC, 1976.

32. VANDENBERG, B AND KIELHOFNER, G: *Play in evolution, culture, and individual adaptation: Implications for therapy.* American Journal of Occupational Therapy, 36:20, 1982.

33. VONGLASCOE, C: *The work of playing "redlight".* IN SCHWARTZMAN, H (ED), Play and culture Leisure Press, West Point, NY, 1980.

INDEX

An *italic* number indicates a figure.
A "t" indicates a table.

DEFICIT perspective(s), medical model and, 258-259
Depersonalization, elimination of, 207
Developmental activities, 113
Dialectic. *See also* Meaning.
  defined, 220
  legitimation and, 221
Differentiated systems, 62
Disability, chronic
  competence and, 262-264
  self-image and, 232
  sick role and, 204
Disease, hypokinetic, 98
Disease, chronic, medical model and, 259
Disease process, deficit perspective and, 258-259
Disuse syndrome, 98-99
Dubos, Rene, 155, 181, 183, 187, 200, 201
Dysfunction. *See also* Occupational dysfunction.
  mental illness and, 81, *82, f*
  occupational, 191
  spinal cord injury and, *81, f*

EDUCATION, professional, 96, t
Emic perspective
  defined, 239
  videotape and, 247
Environment(s)
  competence and, 263-264, 270-271
  culture and, 106
  designing of, 290-291
  as determinant of occupation, 105-106, 107, t
  expansion of, 106
  as factor in intervention, 109, 113
  group behavior and, 106
Enculturation, 77
Ethnomethodology, occupational therapy and, 228-230
Etic perspective, defined, 239
Evolution, human, work and, 104-105
Exploration, importance of, 300-301

FREUD, Sigmund, 128-129
Freudian principles, 36-37
Functional activity, 34

GAMES. *See* Play.
Gradualism, in treatment, 19-20

HABIT dysfunction, 15-16
Health, defined, 183
Health care
  consumer and, 168-169, 171
  future trends in, 186-188, 193
  iatrogenesis and, 198-199, 201
  impact of changes in, 169-170
  marketing and, 171-174
    description of service, 172
    research procedure, 173
  overlap of services, 175
  service sectors of, 183-185
    curative, 184
    health promotion, 185
    preventive, 185
    restorative, 184
Health care industry, U.S. Government and, 165
Health insurance, 166
Health professions, conflict within, 167
Hierarchy
  clockworks and, 60
  concept of, defined, 56, 59
  cybernetics and, 60
  differentiated systems and, 62
  frameworks and, 60
  iconic systems and, 62-63
  laws of, 66-68, *69, f*
  occupational therapy knowledge and, 58-59
  open systems and, 61
  paradigmatic view and, 68-73
    biologic phenomena and, 69-70
    psychologic phenomena and, 70-71
    social phenomena and, 72-73
  rules for therapy, 85
  schema of levels, 59-60
  social systems and, 66
  symbolic systems and, 63-65
Hippocrates, 181
Historical method, 5-12
Homeostasis
  defined, 27
  reductionism and, 27
Hospital(s)
  change in services offered, 165-166
  expansion of, 165-166
Hygeia, 181

IATROGENESIS, social, 199, 201

Iconic systems, 62-63
Identity, sociogenic, 250-252
    importance of, 252-253
Idleness, effects of, 14-15
Illich, Ivan, 199-200
Illness, social-psychologic model of, 107
Image
    as network of information, 63
    psychologic phenomena and, 71
Inner mechanisms
    deficit perspective and, 260
    paradigm of, 30-42
        criticism of, 31
    treatment approaches and, 38, f
Intervention
    emic perspective and, 240
    performance skills and, 275-276
    planning for, 276

KUHN, Thomas, 5-9, 32, 57

LIFESTYLE, as factor in disease, disability, 191

MANNHEIM, Karl, 251
Marketing, health care and, 171-176
Mead, George Herbert, 131, 272
Meaning. See also Dialectic.
    background expectancies and, 223
    concept of, 216
    external context of, 298-299
    shared knowledge and, 217-218
    social construction of, 220-223
        dialectic and, 220-221
            externalization, 221
            internalization, 221
            objectivation, 221
        methods and, 222
            et cetera problem, 222
            indexicals, 222
            glossing, 222
    in symbolic systems, 65
Medical diagnosis
    role in therapy, 16, 258
Medical marketplace. See Health Care.
Medical model, criticism of, 40-41
Medicine, Western
    historical roots of, 180-182
    traditional values of, 155, t
Mental attitude, importance in treatment, 18

Mental health
    activity and, 268, 273
    pathologic approach and, 11-12
    in the professional, 3
Mental illness, dysfunction and, 81, 82, f
Mentally ill, the, moral treatment and, 11, 97
Mind-brain unity, 74-76
Moral treatment movement, 9-11, 97, 143
    demise of, 11
    humanistic approach in, 11
Mortality, sick role and, 203-204
Motivation
    behaviorism and, 129
    dynamics of occupation and, 70-71
    effectance and, 129
    Freud and, 128
    need states and, 129
    occupational behavior and, 101
    personal causation and, 130
    tension reduction and, 130
    tension-seeking and, 130
    in treatment, 19-21
Mystification. See also Sick role.
    failure of, 203-204
    process of, 201-203

NEUROPHYSIOLOGY
    mental phenomena and, 74-75
    occupation and, 30
    sensory input and, 74
    symbolic processes and, 75

OCCUPATION. See also Occupational behavior.
    adaptation and, 287-288
    complexity of, 127-136
    defined, 136
    developmental opportunities and, 109, 113
    as a goal of therapy, 23
    as a health determinant, 98-99, 100, t
    interdisciplinary knowledge and, 125-136
    as intervention, 109-113, 114, t
        process of, 108-109
    paradigm of, 12
        clinical puzzles in, 14-16
            balance, failure of, 15
            habit breakdown, 15
            idleness, 14-16
            medical diagnosis and, 16

Play
  adult occupations and, 103
  competence and, 269
  development of, 96
  enculturation and, 77
  games and, 131, 302-303
  importance of, 13
  loss of, 15
  motivation for, 127-128
  social roles and, 272
  symbolic processes and, 75
  worker role and, 101
Practice model(s)
  medical marketplace and, 171-176
    consumer demand and, 171
  need for, 170-171
    occupation theory and, 171-174
Principles, therapeutic, 230-233
Profession(s), goals of, 140
Programming, evolutionary
  humans and, 64-65
  mammals and, 64
Puzzle solving
  paradigm and, 8-9, 14
  therapeutic occupation and, 82-85
Puzzles, clinical, redefined, 79. *See also* Occupational dysfunction.

REALITY, social
  disruption of, 224
  social reconstruction of, 225
Reductionism
  criticism of, 30, 182
  defined, 27, 156
  homeostasis and, 27
  inadequacies of, 39-40
  inner mechanisms and, 31
  medical model and, 27
Regression, principle of, in treatment, 19
Rehabilitation, 184, 188
  chronic disability and, 204
  failure of, 214
  reconstruction of social reality and, 225
Remediation, in therapy, 85
Research
  at advanced level, 118
Research
  marketing health care and, 172-173
  methodologies, quantitative, 116

Ritual(s) 144
  importance of, 304-305
Role dysfunction, occupational, 107-108, 109, t
Role theory, 107-108, 131-132
  behaviorist perspective and, 132
  gestaltist perspective and, 132, 133
Roles, professional, 140-141

SCHIZOPHRENIA, 274
Service delivery. *See also* Practice model.
  health apprentice role and, 206-207
  planning for, 172-174
  professionalism and, 174
    research and, 173
Sick role
  concept of, 202-203
  failure of, 203-204
  medical model and, 259
  mystification and, 201-203
  physician and, 153-154
Social Darwinism, 11-12
Social groups, occupational role and, 72
Socialization
  defined, 135
  premise of occupation and, 136
  process of, 135-136
Socialization
  in treatment, 21
Social organization, 66
Social roles. *See also* Social groups.
  development of, 77-78
  function of, 78
Social science, selection of concepts from, 128
Social systems, 66
  human behavior and, 77
  individuals and, 76-77
Sociology, existential, 215-216
Specialization, dangers of, 283
Spinal cord injury, 80, *81, f*
Sport, importance of, 301-303
Symbolic interaction
  defined, 131
  role theory and, 131-132
Symbolic processes, as link to action, 75-76
Symbolic systems, 63-65
  meaning and, 65
  values and, 65
Symbolization, 65